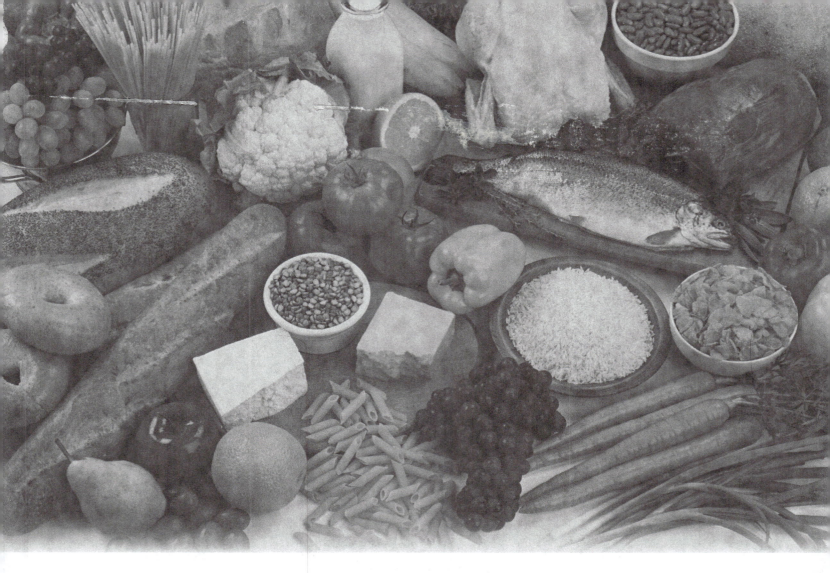

FOOD COMPOSITION TABLE

 **Higher Education**

Boston   Burr Ridge, IL   Dubuque, IA   New York   San Francisco   St. Louis
Bangkok   Bogotá   Caracas   Kuala Lumpur   Lisbon   London   Madrid   Mexico City
Milan   Montreal   New Delhi   Santiago   Seoul   Singapore   Sydney

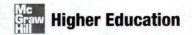

Higher Education

FOOD COMPOSITION TABLE

Published by McGraw-Hill, a business unit of The McGraw-Hill Companies, Inc., 1221 Avenue of the Americas, New York, NY 10020. Copyright © 2009 by The McGraw-Hill Companies, Inc. All rights reserved. No part of this publication may be reproduced or distributed in any form or by any means, or stored in a database or retrieval system, without the prior written consent of The McGraw-Hill Companies, Inc., including, but not limited to, in any network or other electronic storage or transmission, or broadcast for distance learning.

Some ancillaries, including electronic and print components, may not be available to customers outside the United States.

This book is printed on acid-free paper.

2 3 4 5 6 7 8 9 0 QSR/QSR 0 9 8

ISBN 978–0–07–340256–7
MHID 0–07–340256–7

Publisher: *Michelle Watnick*
Executive Editor: *Colin H. Wheatley*
Senior Developmental Editor: *Lynne M. Meyers*
Senior Marketing Manager: *Tami Petsche*
Project Coordinator: *Mary Jane Lampe*
Senior Production Supervisor: *Kara Kudronowicz*
Senior Media Project Manager: *Tammy Juran*
Manager, Creative Services: *Michelle D. Whitaker*
(USE) Cover Image: *© Mitch Hrdlicka/Getty Images*
Senior Photo Research Coordinator: *John C. Leland*
Compositor: *S4Carlisle Publishing Services*
Typeface: *10/12 Giovanni Book*
Printer: *Quebecor World Dubuque, IA*

Library of Congress Cataloging-in-Publication Data

Food composition table / the McGraw-Hill Companies, Inc.—1st ed.
    p. cm.
  ISBN 978–0–07–340256–7 — ISBN 0–07–340256–7 (hard copy : alk. paper)
1. Food–Composition–Tables. 2. Nutrition–Tables. 3. Brand name products–Composition–Tables.
I. McGraw-Hill Companies.

TX551.F6858   2009
613.2—dc22   2008016240

Contents

Food Composition Table

The following table of nutrient values of foods represents a small portion of the database found in the NutritionCalc Plus diet analysis program available from McGraw-Hill. The nutrient data in the software and in this appendix comes from the ESHA Research database. Some nutrient or food component values for some foods are not included in the database because no *accurate* data values exist. The nutrient or component may in fact be present in the food, but insufficient laboratory analyses have been performed to establish an accurate value. These missing values are indicated by a – (dash) in the appropriate nutrient columns.

Name-brand foods often have missing values because manufacturers are only required to analyze for nutrients that must appear on Nutrition Facts labels and only to the level of accuracy required by the nutrition labeling regulations. All missing nutrient or food component values are clearly marked in the table.

Abbreviation Key

Unit/Amt = Unit Amount
Wt (g) = Weight in grams
Energy (kcal) = kilocalories
Prot (g) = Protein
Carb (g) = Carbohydrate
Fiber (g) = Dietary fiber
Fat (g) = Total fat
Sat (g) = Saturated fat
Mono (g) = Monounsaturated fat
Poly (g) = Polyunsaturated fat
Chol (mg) = Cholesterol
Vit A (RE) = Vitamin A
Thia (mg) = Thiamin
Ribo (mg) = Riboflavin
Niac (mg NE) = Niacin
Vit B-6 (mg) = Vitamin B-6
Vit B-12 (μg) = Vitamin B-12
Fol (μg) = Folate
Vit C (mg) = Vitamin C
Vit D (IU) = Vitamin D
Vit E (mg AT) = Vitamin E
Cal (mg) = Calcium

Iron (mg) = Iron
Magn (mg) = Magnesium
Phos (mg) = Phosphorus
Pota (mg) = Potassium
Sodi (mg) = Sodium
Zinc (mg) = Zinc
Wat (%) = Water
Alco (g) = Alcohol
Caff (mg) = Caffeine

g = gram
mg = milligram
μg = microgram
mg AT = milligrams of alpha
   tocopheral
mg NE = milligrams of Niacin
   Equivalents
oz = ounce
lb = pound
Tbs = tablespoon
tsp = teaspoon

PAGE KEY: 2 Beverage and Beverage Mixes   4 Other Beverages   4 Beverages, Alcoholic   6 Candies and Confections, Gum   10 Cereals, Breakfast Type
14 Cheese and Cheese Substitutes   16 Dairy Products and Substitutes   18 Desserts   24 Dessert Toppings   24 Eggs, Substitutes, and Egg Dishes   26 Ethnic Foods
30 Fast Foods/Restaurants   44 Fats, Oils, Margarines, Shortenings, and Substitutes   44 Fish, Seafood, and Shellfish   46 Food Additives
46 Fruit, Vegetable, or Blended Juices   48 Grains, Flours, and Fractions   48 Grain Products, Prepared and Baked Goods

Code	Food Name	Unit/ Amt	Wt (g)	Energy (kcal)	Prot (g)	Carb (g)	Fiber (g)	Fat (g)	Sat (g)	Mono (g)	Poly (g)	Chol (mg)	Vit A (RE)
BEVERAGE AND BEVERAGE MIXES													
Carbonated Drinks													
4794	Lemonade, cnd, Country Time	1 cup	247	90	0	23	0	0	0.0	0.0	0.0	—	0
20055	Soda, 7 Up	1 cup	240	100	0	26	0	0	0.0	0.0	0.0	0	0
20207	Soda, 7 Up, diet	1 cup	240	0	0	0	0	0	0.0	0.0	0.0	0	0
20006	Soda, club	1 cup	237	0	0	0	0	0	0.0	0.0	0.0	0	0
20147	Soda, Coca Cola/Coke	1 cup	246	103	0	27	0	0	0.0	0.0	0.0	0	0
443	Soda, cola, caff free	12 fl-oz	372	156	0	40	0	0	0.0	0.0	0.0	0	0
4796	Soda, Dr Pepper	1 cup	246	100	0	27	0	0	0.0	0.0	0.0	—	0
4797	Soda, Dr Pepper, diet	1 cup	246	0	0	0	0	0	0.0	0.0	0.0	—	0
20530	Soda, fruit punch	1 cup	251	117	0	32	0	0	0.0	0.0	0.0	—	0
20031	Soda, grape	1 cup	248	107	0	28	0	0	0.0	0.0	0.0	0	0
20032	Soda, lemon lime	1 cup	246	98	0	26	0	0	0.0	0.0	0.0	0	0
20271	Soda, Mountain Dew	1 cup	240	113	0	31	0	0	0.0	0.0	0.0	0	0
20272	Soda, Mountain Dew, diet	1 cup	240	0	0	0	0	0	0.0	0.0	0.0	0	0
20161	Soda, Mr Pibb	1 cup	249	97	0	26	0	0	0.0	0.0	0.0	0	0
20029	Soda, orange	1 cup	248	119	0	31	0	0	0.0	0.0	0.0	0	0
20166	Soda, Pepsi	1 cup	240	100	0	27	0	0	0.0	0.0	0.0	0	0
20167	Soda, Pepsi, diet	1 cup	240	0	0	0	0	0	0.0	0.0	0.0	0	0
20009	Soda, root beer	1 cup	246	101	0	26	0	0	0.0	0.0	0.0	0	0
20454	Soda, root beer, diet, w/nutrasweet	1 cup	240	0	0	0	0	0	0.0	0.0	0.0	0	—
20163	Soda, Sprite	1 cup	249	96	0	26	0	0	0.0	0.0	0.0	0	0
4815	Soda, Squirt	1 cup	246	100	0	27	0	0	0.0	0.0	0.0	—	0
Coffee and Substitutes													
20312	Coffee Substitute, inst, dry	1 tsp	3	10	0	3	—	0	0.0	0.0	0.0	0	0
20592	Coffee, cappuccino, w/lowfat milk, tall	1.5 cup	244	110	8	11	0	4	2.5	—	—	15	80
20639	Coffee, cappuccino, w/whole milk, tall	1.5 cup	244	140	7	11	0	7	4.5	—	—	30	60
20439	Coffee, espresso, prep at restaurant	1 cup	237	5	0	0	0	0	0.2	0.0	0.2	0	0
20659	Coffee, latte, iced, w/lowfat milk, tall	1.5 cup	392	90	7	10	0	3	2.0	—	—	15	60
20023	Coffee, reg, inst, prep w/water	1 cup	238	5	0	1	0	0	0.0	0.0	0.0	0	0
Dairy Mixed Drinks and Mixes													
44	Drink, carob, prep f/dry mix w/milk	1 cup	256	192	8	22	1	8	4.6	2.0	0.5	26	69
14	Drink, chocolate, dry mix	2.5 tsp	22	75	1	20	1	.1	0.4	0.2	0.0	0	0
40	Drink, strawberry, dry mix	2.5 tsp	22	85	0	22	0	0	0.0	0.0	0.0	0	0
12	Hot Cocoa, dry mix	3 tsp	28	113	2	24	1	1	0.7	0.4	0.0	2	0
48	Hot Cocoa, prep f/dry mix w/water	1 cup	275	151	2	32	1	2	0.9	0.5	0.0	3	1
62057	Instant Breakfast, French vanilla, dry mix, pkt	1 ea	36	130	4	27	0	0	0.0	0.0	0.0	3	350
101	Instant Breakfast, prep w/1% milk	1 cup	281	233	15	36	0	3	1.8	—	—	14	469
25	Instant Breakfast, prep w/2% milk, pwd	1 cup	281	253	15	36	0	5	3.1	—	—	24	469
26	Instant Breakfast, prep w/whole milk	1 cup	281	280	15	36	0	9	5.3	—	—	38	630
30	Malted Milk, chocolate, dry mix	3 tsp	21	79	1	18	1	1	0.5	0.2	0.1	0	1

Thia (mg)	Ribo (mg)	Niac (mg NE)	Vit B6 (mg)	Vit B12 (μg)	Fol (μg)	Vit C (mg)	Vit D (IU)	Vit E (mg AT)	Cal (mg)	Iron (mg)	Magn (mg)	Phos (mg)	Pota (mg)	Sodi (mg)	Zinc (mg)	Wat (%)	Alco (g)	Caff (mg)
—	—	—	—	—	—	0.0	—	—	—	—	—	—	—	90	—	91	0.00	0.00
—	—	—	—	0.00	—	0.0	—	—	—	—	—	45	—	50	—	89	0.00	0.00
0.00	0.00	—	0.00	0.00	—	0.0	—	—	—	—	—	—	—	35	—	100	0.00	0.00
0.00	0.00	0.00	0.00	0.00	0.0	0.0	—	0.0	12	0.01	2.4	0	5	50	0.2	100	0.00	0.00
0.00	0.00	0.00	0.00	0.00	0.0	0.0	0.0	0.0	7	0.07	2.5	36	2	5	0.0	89	0.00	30.67
0.00	0.00	0.00	0.00	0.00	0.0	0.0	—	0.0	11	0.07	3.7	48	4	15	0.0	89	0.00	0.00
—	—	—	—	—	—	0.0	—	—	—	—	—	—	—	35	—	89	0.00	27.20
—	—	—	—	—	—	0.0	—	—	—	—	—	—	—	35	—	—	0.00	27.20
—	—	—	—	—	—	0.0	—	—	0	0.00	—	0	13	10	—	—	0.00	0.00
0.00	0.00	0.00	0.00	0.00	0.0	0.0	—	0.0	7	0.20	2.5	0	2	37	0.2	89	0.00	0.00
0.00	0.00	0.03	0.00	0.00	0.0	0.0	—	0.0	5	0.17	2.5	0	2	27	0.1	90	0.00	0.00
—	—	—	—	0.00	—	0.0	—	—	0	0.00	—	0	—	47	—	87	0.00	36.66
—	—	—	—	0.00	—	0.0	—	—	0	0.00	—	0	—	23	—	100	0.00	36.66
0.00	0.00	0.00	0.00	0.00	0.0	0.0	0.0	0.0	—	—	—	29	14	7	—	90	0.00	27.00
0.00	0.00	0.00	0.00	0.00	0.0	0.0	—	0.0	12	0.15	2.5	2	5	30	0.2	88	0.00	0.00
—	—	—	—	0.00	—	0.0	—	—	0	0.00	—	35	—	23	—	88	0.00	24.67
—	—	—	—	0.00	—	0.0	—	—	0	0.00	—	27	5	23	—	—	0.00	24.00
0.00	0.00	0.00	0.00	0.00	0.0	0.0	—	0.0	12	0.11	2.5	0	2	32	0.2	89	0.00	0.00
—	—	—	—	0.00	—	—	—	—	—	—	—	—	—	30	—	100	0.00	0.00
—	—	—	—	—	—	0.0	—	—	—	—	—	0	0	23	—	89	0.00	0.00
—	—	—	—	—	—	0.0	—	—	—	—	—	—	—	15	—	89	0.00	0.00
—	—	—	—	—	—	0.0	—	—	0	0.00	—	—	—	0	—	0	0.00	0.00
—	—	—	—	—	—	2.4	—	—	250	0.00	—	—	—	110	—	—	0.00	90.00
—	—	—	—	—	—	2.4	—	—	250	0.00	—	—	—	105	—	—	0.00	90.00
0.00	0.41	12.34	0.00	0.00	2.4	0.5	—	0.0	5	0.31	189.6	17	273	33	0.1	98	0.00	502.44
—	—	—	—	—	—	1.2	—	—	250	0.00	—	—	—	100	—	—	0.00	90.00
0.00	0.00	0.56	0.00	0.00	0.0	0.0	—	0.0	10	0.10	7.2	7	72	5	0.0	99	0.00	61.97
0.10	0.44	0.34	0.10	1.08	12.8	0.0	—	0.1	251	0.63	25.6	205	335	118	0.9	84	0.00	0.00
0.00	0.02	0.10	0.00	0.00	1.5	0.2	—	0.0	8	0.68	21.2	28	128	45	0.3	1	0.00	7.78
0.00	0.01	0.01	0.00	0.00	0.0	0.1	0.0	0.0	1	0.10	0.2	1	1	8	0.0	0	0.00	0.00
0.02	0.15	0.17	0.02	0.37	0.0	0.5	—	0.2	40	0.34	23.5	89	202	143	0.4	2	0.00	5.09
0.03	0.20	0.21	0.03	0.49	0.0	0.5	—	0.2	60	0.46	33.0	118	269	195	0.6	86	0.00	5.48
0.30	0.14	5.00	0.40	0.60	99.7	27.0	0.0	6.8	250	4.50	79.7	100	249	95	3.0	—	0.00	0.00
0.40	0.47	5.48	0.52	1.53	117.7	30.9	100.0	5.4	406	4.86	118.5	392	731	267	4.1	79	0.00	0.00
0.40	0.47	5.48	0.52	1.50	117.7	30.9	100.0	5.5	403	4.86	118.5	390	726	264	4.1	78	0.00	0.00
0.40	0.46	5.46	0.51	1.50	117.7	30.7	100.0	5.5	396	4.86	117.1	386	721	262	4.1	77	0.00	0.00
0.03	0.03	0.41	0.02	0.03	10.7	0.3	1.0	0.0	13	0.47	14.7	37	130	53	0.2	1	0.00	7.76

4

PAGE KEY: 2 Beverage and Beverage Mixes 4 Other Beverages 4 Beverages, Alcoholic 6 Candies and Confections, Gum 10 Cereals, Breakfast Type 14 Cheese and Cheese Substitutes 16 Dairy Products and Substitutes 18 Desserts 24 Dessert Toppings 24 Eggs, Substitutes, and Egg Dishes 26 Ethnic Foods 30 Fast Foods/Restaurants 44 Fats, Oils, Margarines, Shortenings, and Substitutes 44 Fish, Seafood, and Shellfish 46 Food Additives 46 Fruit, Vegetable, or Blended Juices 48 Grains, Flours, and Fractions 48 Grain Products, Prepared and Baked Goods

Code	Food Name	Unit/ Amt	Wt (g)	Energy (kcal)	Prot (g)	Carb (g)	Fiber (g)	Fat (g)	Sat (g)	Mono (g)	Poly (g)	Chol (mg)	Vit A (RE)
Fruit Flavored Drinks													
20004	Drink, breakfast, orange, prep f/pwd	1 cup	248	122	0	31	0	0	0.0	0.0	0.0	0	191
20385	Drink, cherry, swtnd, prep	8 fl-oz	254	60	0	16	0	0	0.0	0.0	0.0	0	0
20737	Drink, fruit punch	8 fl-oz	252	110	0	29	—	0	0.0	0.0	0.0	0	—
20176	Drink, fruit punch, non carbonated	12 fl-oz	360	200	0	50	0	0	0.0	0.0	0.0	0	—
20761	Drink, Island Punch	1 cup	252	110	0	27	—	0	0.0	0.0	0.0	0	—
20045	Drink, lemonade, prep f/pwd	1 cup	266	112	0	29	0	0	0.0	0.0	0.0	0	0
20746	Drink, pink lemonade	8 fl-oz	252	110	0	26	—	0	0.0	0.0	0.0	0	—
20123	Juice Drink, citrus fruit, calc fort	1 cup	240	112	1	28	0	0	0.0	0.0	0.0	0	1
20744	Juice Drink, raspberry peach	1 cup	252	120	0	29	—	0	0.0	0.0	0.0	0	—
793	Juice, apple	8 fl-oz	236	110	0	29	0	0	0.0	0.0	0.0	0	—
1853	Juice, grape	8 fl-oz	236	150	0	38	0	0	0.0	0.0	0.0	0	—
794	Juice, grapefruit	8 fl-oz	236	120	0	29	0	0	0.0	0.0	0.0	0	—
1854	Juice, orange	8 fl-oz	236	120	0	29	0	0	0.0	0.0	0.0	0	—
3128	Juice, prune, cnd	1 cup	256	182	2	45	3	0	0.0	0.1	0.0	0	1
6504	Juice, tomato, cnd	1 cup	243	50	2	10	2	0	0.0	0.0	0.0	0	100
6507	Juice, vegetable, cnd	1 cup	243	50	2	10	2	0	0.0	0.0	0.0	0	400
OTHER BEVERAGES													
38405	Drink, atole, cornmeal	1 cup	245	206	4	40	1	4	2.2	1.1	0.3	14	33
38362	Drink, horchata de arroz, rice beverage, Mexican	1 cup	245	100	0	25	0	0	0.0	0.0	0.0	0	0
20589	Drink, sugar cane, Puerto Rico	1 cup	240	164	0	42	0	0	0.0	0.0	0.0	0	0
Teas													
20495	Tea, bag	1 ea	2	0	0	0	0	0	0.0	0.0	0.0	0	0
20014	Tea, brewed w/tap water	1 cup	237	2	0	1	0	0	0.0	0.0	0.0	0	0
20538	Tea, Cool Drink, can/btl	1 cup	248	82	0	22	0	0	0.0	0.0	0.0	0	0
20681	Tea, green, sweetened, btl	1 cup	252	100	0	25	—	0	0.0	0.0	0.0	0	—
20894	Tea, herbal, Cranberry Cove, brewed	1 cup	237	0	0	0	0	0	0.0	0.0	0.0	0	0
20853	Tea, herbal, Echinacea Complete Care, brewed	1 cup	237	0	0	0	0	0	0.0	0.0	0.0	0	0
20899	Tea, herbal, Sleepytime, brewed	1 cup	237	0	0	0	0	0	0.0	0.0	0.0	0	0
30451	Tea, iced, 100%, inst, pwd	2 tsp	1	0	0	0	0	0	0.0	0.0	0.0	0	0
20724	Tea, iced, w/lemonade	8 fl-oz	252	110	0	28	0	0	0.0	0.0	0.0	0	—
Water													
20051	Water, btld	1 cup	237	0	0	0	0	0	0.0	0.0	0.0	0	0
20041	Water, municipal	1 cup	237	0	0	0	0	0	0.0	0.0	0.0	0	0
BEVERAGES, ALCOHOLIC													
34066	Beer, amber ale	12 fl-oz	356	169	2	14	—	0	0.0	0.0	0.0	0	—
22500	Beer, can/btl, 12 fl oz	12 fl-oz	356	139	1	11	0	0	0.0	0.0	0.0	0	0
34053	Beer, Light	12 fl-oz	353	105	1	5	0	0	0.0	0.0	0.0	0	—
22685	Beer, non alcoholic, Near	12 fl-oz	356	32	1	5	0	0	0.0	0.0	0.0	0	0
22671	Bourbon, 80 proof	1 fl-oz	28	64	0	0	0	0	0.0	0.0	0.0	0	0
22513	Brandy, 80 proof	1 fl-oz	28	64	0	0	0	0	0.0	0.0	0.0	0	0
22514	Gin, 80 proof	1 fl-oz	28	64	0	0	0	0	0.0	0.0	0.0	0	0
22547	Liqueur, Amaretto, 1 shot	1 ea	30	106	0	13	0	0	0.0	0.0	0.0	0	0
34052	Malt Beverage, Zima	12 fl-oz	353	185	0	21	0	0	0.0	0.0	0.0	0	—
22555	Mixed Drink, Bacardi cocktail	1 ea	63	117	0	6	0	0	0.0	0.0	0.0	0	0

Thia (mg)	Ribo (mg)	Niac (mg NE)	Vit B6 (mg)	Vit B12 (µg)	Fol (µg)	Vit C (mg)	Vit D (IU)	Vit E (mg AT)	Cal (mg)	Iron (mg)	Magn (mg)	Phos (mg)	Pota (mg)	Sodi (mg)	Zinc (mg)	Wat (%)	Alco (g)	Caff (mg)
0.00	0.21	2.53	0.25	0.00	0.0	73.2	—	0.0	126	0.01	2.5	47	60	10	0.0	87	0.00	0.00
—	—	—	—	0.00	—	6.0	—	—	0	0.00	—	0	0	0	—	94	0.00	0.00
—	—	—	—	—	—	0.0	—	—	—	—	—	—	—	10	—	88	0.00	0.00
—	—	—	—	0.00	—	65.0	—	—	—	—	—	0	0	45	—		0.00	0.00
—	—	—	—	—	—	—	—	—	—	—	—	—	—	10	—	89	0.00	0.00
0.00	0.00	0.00	0.00	0.00	0.0	34.0	—	0.0	29	0.05	2.7	3	3	19	0.1	89	0.00	0.00
—	—	—	—	—	—	0.0	—	—	—	—	—	—	—	10	—	90	0.00	0.00
0.05	0.02	0.31	0.05	0.00	5.2	79.8	0.0	0.1	316	0.21	16.7	20	196	4	0.1	88	0.00	0.00
—	—	—	—	—	—	0.0	—	—	—	—	—	—	—	10	—	88	0.00	0.00
—	—	—	—	—	—	—	—	—	—	—	—	—	—	10	—	88	0.00	0.00
—	—	—	—	—	—	—	—	—	—	—	—	—	—	10	—	84	0.00	0.00
—	—	—	—	—	—	—	—	—	—	—	—	—	—	0	—	87	0.00	0.00
—	—	—	—	—	—	—	—	—	—	—	—	—	—	0	—	—	0.00	0.00
0.03	0.18	2.00	0.56	0.00	0.0	10.5	—	0.3	31	3.01	35.8	64	707	10	0.5	81	0.00	0.00
—	—	—	—	—	—	72.0	—	—	20	0.72	—	—	430	750	—	94	0.00	0.00
—	—	—	—	—	—	60.0	—	—	40	0.72	—	—	520	620	—	94	0.00	0.00
0.12	0.23	0.81	0.07	0.36	6.4	0.9	—	0.1	140	0.67	24.2	117	185	55	0.6	80	0.00	0.00
0.00	0.00	0.14	0.00	0.00	0.4	0.1	—	0.0	12	0.34	3.5	5	6	7	0.1	89	0.00	0.00
0.07	0.03	0.05	0.00	0.00	0.0	0.0	—	0.0	12	2.25	8.0	5	39	42	0.2	81	0.00	0.00
—	—	—	—	—	—	0.0	—	—	0	0.00	—	—	25	0	—	—	0.00	55.00
0.00	0.02	0.00	0.00	0.00	11.8	0.0	—	0.0	0	0.05	7.1	2	88	7	0.0	100	0.00	47.36
—	—	—	—	—	—	0.0	—	—	0	0.00	—	73	38	33	—	—	0.00	11.00
—	—	—	—	—	—	0.0	—	—	—	—	—	—	—	10	—	90	0.00	18.00
—	—	—	—	—	—	0.0	—	—	0	0.00	—	—	30	0	—	100	0.00	0.00
—	—	—	—	—	—	35.0	—	—	0	0.00	—	—	—	0	7.5	100	0.00	0.00
—	—	—	—	—	—	0.0	—	—	0	0.00	—	—	30	0	—	100	0.00	0.00
—	—	—	—	—	—	0.0	—	—	0	0.00	—	—	45	0	—	—	0.00	40.00
—	—	—	—	—	—	0.0	—	—	—	—	—	—	—	10	—	89	0.00	18.00
0.00	0.00	0.00	0.00	0.00	0.0	0.0	—	0.0	2	0.01	2.4	0	0	2	0.0	100	0.00	0.00
0.00	0.00	0.00	0.00	0.00	0.0	0.0	—	0.0	5	0.00	2.4	0	0	5	0.0	100	0.00	0.00
—	—	—	—	—	—	—	—	—	—	—	—	—	44	—	—	18.65	0.00
0.01	0.09	1.83	0.15	0.07	21.4	0.0	—	0.0	14	0.07	21.4	50	96	14	0.0	93	12.82	0.00
0.03	0.03	1.40	—	—	—	—	—	—	11	—	—	—	59	11	—	98	14.11	0.00
0.01	0.09	1.61	0.18	0.07	21.4	0.0	—	0.0	25	0.03	32.1	110	89	18	0.0	98	1.07	0.00
0.00	0.00	0.00	0.00	0.00	0.0	0.0	—	0.0	0	0.00	0.0	1	1	0	0.0	67	9.28	0.00
0.00	0.00	0.00	0.00	0.00	0.0	0.0	—	0.0	0	0.00	0.0	1	1	0	0.0	67	9.28	0.00
0.00	0.00	0.00	0.00	0.00	0.0	0.0	—	0.0	0	0.00	0.0	1	1	0	0.0	67	9.28	0.00
0.00	0.00	0.01	0.00	0.00	0.0	0.0	0.0	0.0	0	0.01	0.5	1	4	2	0.0	30	7.73	0.00
0.03	0.03	0.87	—	—	—	—	—	—	38	—	—	—	51	20	—	—	16.94	0.00
0.00	0.00	0.02	0.00	0.00	1.2	1.0	0.0	0.0	2	0.05	1.2	3	12	11	0.0	68	13.72	0.00

6

PAGE KEY: 2 Beverage and Beverage Mixes   4 Other Beverages   4 Beverages, Alcoholic   6 Candies and Confections, Gum   10 Cereals, Breakfast Type
14 Cheese and Cheese Substitutes   16 Dairy Products and Substitutes   18 Desserts   24 Dessert Toppings   24 Eggs, Substitutes, and Egg Dishes   26 Ethnic Foods
30 Fast Foods/Restaurants   44 Fats, Oils, Margarines, Shortenings, and Substitutes   44 Fish, Seafood, and Shellfish   46 Food Additives
46 Fruit, Vegetable, or Blended Juices   48 Grains, Flours, and Fractions   48 Grain Products, Prepared and Baked Goods

Code	Food Name	Unit/ Amt	Wt (g)	Energy (kcal)	Prot (g)	Carb (g)	Fiber (g)	Fat (g)	Sat (g)	Mono (g)	Poly (g)	Chol (mg)	Vit A (RE)
34057	Mixed Drink, bloody mary, prep f/recipe	1 ea	209	46	1	7	1	0	0.0	—	—	0	117
22538	Mixed Drink, daiquiri, 6.8 fl oz can	1 ea	207	259	0	33	0	0	0.0	0.0	0.0	0	0
34058	Mixed Drink, gin & tonic, prep f/recipe	1 ea	232	160	0	8	0	0	0.0	0.0	0.0	0	0
22556	Mixed Drink, high ball	1 ea	160	105	0	0	0	0	0.0	0.0	0.0	0	0
22569	Mixed Drink, Irish coffee, 1 fl oz	1 ea	26	26	0	1	0	1	0.8	0.4	0.0	5	15
22568	Mixed Drink, Long Island iced tea	1 ea	125	119	0	9	0	0	0.0	0.0	0.0	0	0
22566	Mixed Drink, Mai Tai	1 ea	126	305	0	29	0	0	0.0	0.0	0.1	0	0
22557	Mixed Drink, margarita	1 ea	77	170	0	11	0	0	0.0	0.0	0.0	0	0
22571	Mixed Drink, Mexican eggnog/rompope	4 fl-oz	122	203	5	19	0	7	2.8	2.3	0.7	184	102
22561	Mixed Drink, pina colada	1 ea	141	245	1	32	0	3	2.3	0.1	0.0	0	0
22683	Mixed Drink, screwdriver cocktail	1 ea	213	182	1	18	0	0	0.0	0.0	0.0	0	14
22567	Mixed Drink, tequila sunrise	1 ea	172	189	1	15	0	0	0.0	0.0	0.0	0	17
22534	Mixed Drink, whiskey sour mix, btld	4 fl-oz	124	108	0	26	0	0	0.0	0.0	0.0	0	0
22593	Rum, 80 proof	1 fl-oz	28	64	0	0	0	0	0.0	0.0	0.0	0	0
22515	Tequila, 80 proof	1 fl-oz	28	64	0	0	0	0	0.0	0.0	0.0	0	0
22594	Vodka, 80 proof	1 fl-oz	28	64	0	0	0	0	0.0	0.0	0.0	0	0
22670	Whiskey, 80 proof	1 fl-oz	28	64	0	0	0	0	0.0	0.0	0.0	0	0
22577	Wine, all table types	6 fl-oz	177	136	0	6	0	0	0.0	0.0	0.0	0	0
22608	Wine, cooking, red	1 fl-oz	30	20	0	3	0	0	0.0	0.0	0.0	0	0
22609	Wine, cooking, white	1 fl-oz	30	20	0	3	0	0	0.0	0.0	0.0	0	0
22681	Wine, cooler	1 cup	227	113	0	13	0	0	0.0	0.0	0.0	0	0
22509	Wine, dry, sherry	1 fl-oz	29	20	0	0	—	0	0.0	0.0	0.0	0	0
20076	Wine, non alcoholic	4 fl-oz	116	7	1	1	0	0	0.0	0.0	0.0	0	0
22501	Wine, red	6 fl-oz	177	127	0	3	0	0	0.0	0.0	0.0	0	0
22600	Wine, rice, Japanese	1 fl-oz	29	39	0	1	0	0	0.0	0.0	0.0	0	0
22511	Wine, Sweet Vermouth	1 fl-oz	30	46	0	4	—	0	0.0	0.0	0.0	0	0
CANDIES AND CONFECTIONS, GUM													
23017	Baking Chips, milk chocolate	1.5 oz	43	228	3	25	1	13	6.1	5.6	0.3	10	21
90704	Candy Bar, 3 Musketeers, 0.8 oz bar	1 ea	23	94	1	17	0	3	1.5	1.0	0.1	2	3
23125	Candy Bar, 5th Avenue, 2 oz bar	1 ea	57	273	5	36	2	14	3.8	6.0	1.9	3	8
23049	Candy Bar, Almond Joy, 1.7 oz	1 ea	48	231	2	29	2	13	8.5	2.5	0.6	2	4
90678	Candy Bar, Baby Ruth, 1.2 oz bar	1 ea	34	158	2	21	1	9	4.2	2.2	1.1	1	1
90653	Candy Bar, Butterfinger, 1.6 oz bar	1 ea	45	216	3	33	1	9	4.6	2.2	1.1	0	0
23116	Candy Bar, Caramello, 1.6 oz bar	1 ea	45	210	3	29	1	10	5.8	2.4	0.3	12	28
23118	Candy Bar, carob, 3 oz bar	1 ea	85	459	7	48	3	27	24.7	0.4	0.3	3	0
23099	Candy Bar, crisped rice, chocolate chip, 1 oz bar	1 ea	28	115	1	21	1	4	1.5	1.1	1.0	0	100
4196	Candy Bar, dark chocolate, 1.5 oz bar	0.5 ea	42	230	2	25	4	14	9.0	—	—	3	0
4198	Candy Bar, dark chocolate, w/almonds, 1.5 oz bar	0.5 ea	42	230	3	23	4	15	8.0	—	—	3	0
91519	Candy Bar, Heath, bites	15 pce	39	207	2	25	1	12	6.1	3.4	1.0	7	18
23060	Candy Bar, Kit Kat, 1.5 oz bar	1 ea	43	220	3	27	0	11	7.6	2.5	0.4	5	10
23061	Candy Bar, Krackel, 1.5 oz bar	1 ea	43	218	3	27	1	11	6.8	2.7	0.2	5	9
23037	Candy Bar, Mars almond, 1.76 oz bar	1 ea	50	234	4	31	1	12	3.6	5.3	2.0	8	8
92633	Candy Bar, milk chocolate, 0.6 oz bar	1 ea	17	90	1	10	0	5	3.5	—	—	5	0
90687	Candy Bar, Milky Way, 1.9 oz bar	1 ea	54	228	2	39	1	9	4.2	3.2	0.3	8	10
23035	Candy Bar, Mounds, 1.9 oz bar	1 ea	54	262	2	32	2	14	11.1	0.2	0.1	1	0
23062	Candy Bar, Mr. Goodbar, 1.75 oz bar	1 ea	50	267	5	27	2	16	7.0	4.1	2.2	5	17
23133	Candy Bar, Nestle Crunch, 1.4 oz bar	1 ea	40	207	2	26	1	10	6.0	3.4	0.3	5	6

Thia (mg)	Ribo (mg)	Niac (mg NE)	Vit B6 (mg)	Vit B12 (µg)	Fol (µg)	Vit C (mg)	Vit D (IU)	Vit E (mg AT)	Cal (mg)	Iron (mg)	Magn (mg)	Phos (mg)	Pota (mg)	Sodi (mg)	Zinc (mg)	Wat (%)	Alco (g)	Caff (mg)
0.00	0.00	0.03	0.00	0.00	2.4	23.6	0.0	0.0	19	1.07	2.2	4	52	558	0.0	94	1.38	0.00
0.00	0.00	0.02	0.00	0.00	2.1	2.7	0.0	0.0	0	0.01	2.1	4	23	83	0.1	75	19.90	0.00
0.00	0.00	0.00	0.00	0.00	0.0	0.0	0.0	0.0	3	0.03	0.9	2	1	7	0.1	88	18.56	0.00
0.00	0.00	0.00	0.00	0.00	0.0	0.0	0.0	0.0	6	0.02	1.2	2	3	25	0.1	90	15.09	0.00
0.00	0.00	0.03	0.00	0.00	0.1	0.0	1.8	0.0	3	0.00	1.1	3	12	2	0.0	86	1.63	—
0.00	0.00	0.02	0.00	0.00	1.3	3.2	0.0	0.0	4	0.05	1.8	12	14	6	0.0	83	12.14	0.00
0.00	0.00	0.05	0.00	0.00	1.2	1.0	0.0	0.0	3	0.09	2.4	6	24	11	0.1	54	27.56	0.00
0.00	0.00	0.03	0.00	0.00	1.2	1.0	0.0	0.0	2	0.05	1.4	4	15	4	0.0	62	18.50	0.00
0.03	0.20	0.07	0.07	0.55	18.0	0.6	43.7	0.5	106	0.54	11.1	136	125	42	0.7	69	7.48	0.00
0.03	0.02	0.17	0.05	0.00	16.5	6.9	0.0	0.1	11	0.27	10.6	10	100	9	0.2	65	13.89	0.00
0.14	0.02	0.34	0.07	0.00	74.9	66.5	0.0	0.3	15	0.18	17.1	29	326	2	0.1	83	15.10	0.00
0.07	0.02	0.33	0.09	0.00	18.2	33.3	0.0	0.1	10	0.46	11.7	17	179	7	0.1	80	18.68	0.00
0.01	0.00	0.00	0.00	0.00	0.0	3.3	—	0.0	2	0.14	1.2	7	35	126	0.1	78	0.00	0.00
0.00	0.00	0.00	0.00	0.00	0.0	0.0	—	0.0	0	0.02	0.0	1	1	0	0.0	67	9.28	0.00
0.00	0.00	0.00	0.00	0.00	0.0	0.0	—	0.0	0	0.00	0.0	1	1	0	0.0	67	9.28	0.00
0.00	0.00	0.00	0.00	0.00	0.0	0.0	—	0.0	0	0.00	0.0	1	0	0	0.0	67	9.28	0.00
0.00	0.00	0.00	0.00	0.00	0.0	0.0	—	0.0	0	0.00	0.0	1	1	0	0.0	67	9.28	0.00
0.00	0.02	0.12	0.03	0.01	1.8	0.0	0.0	0.0	14	0.62	15.9	23	149	11	0.1	87	16.45	0.00
0.30	0.30	0.30	—	0.00	—	0.3	—	—	2	0.30	—	4	24	180	—	88	3.59	0.00
0.30	0.30	0.30	—	0.00	—	0.3	—	—	2	0.30	—	4	26	180	—	88	3.59	0.00
0.00	0.01	0.10	0.02	0.00	2.7	4.1	0.0	0.0	13	0.62	11.9	15	102	19	0.1	90	8.81	0.00
0.00	0.00	0.01	0.00	0.00	0.3	0.0	—	0.0	2	0.11	2.9	4	26	2	0.0	89	2.72	0.00
0.00	0.00	0.11	0.01	0.00	1.2	0.0	—	0.0	10	0.46	11.6	17	102	8	0.1	98	0.00	0.00
0.00	0.05	0.14	0.05	0.01	3.5	0.0	—	0.0	14	0.75	23.0	25	198	9	0.2	88	16.45	0.00
0.00	0.00	0.00	0.00	0.00	0.0	0.0	—	0.0	1	0.02	1.7	2	7	1	0.0	78	4.69	0.00
0.00	0.00	0.05	0.00	0.00	0.1	0.0	—	0.0	2	0.07	2.7	3	28	3	0.0	72	4.59	0.00
0.05	0.12	0.15	0.01	0.25	5.1	0.0	—	0.9	80	1.00	26.8	88	158	34	0.9	2	0.00	8.51
0.00	0.02	0.05	0.00	0.03	0.0	0.1	—	0.2	19	0.17	6.6	21	30	44	0.1	6	0.00	1.80
0.07	0.05	2.21	0.05	0.10	20.4	0.2	—	1.5	41	0.68	35.2	80	197	128	0.6	2	0.00	2.83
0.00	0.07	0.23	0.02	0.05	—	0.3	—	0.0	31	0.61	31.8	54	122	68	0.4	8	0.00	—
0.02	0.02	0.94	0.01	0.00	10.5	0.0	—	0.6	15	0.23	24.8	47	121	73	0.4	5	0.00	1.36
0.05	0.02	1.39	0.05	0.00	15.0	0.0	—	0.8	16	0.34	37.6	61	179	97	0.5	1	0.00	2.26
0.01	0.18	0.51	0.01	0.28	—	0.8	0.0	0.1	97	0.49	19.1	68	155	55	0.4	7	0.00	1.80
0.09	0.15	0.87	0.10	0.85	17.9	0.4	—	1.0	258	1.10	30.6	107	538	91	3.0	2	0.00	0.00
0.15	0.17	2.00	0.20	0.00	39.7	0.0	—	0.0	6	1.78	13.6	38	48	79	0.2	7	0.00	—
—	—	—	—	—	—	0.0	—	—	0	1.08	—	—	—	0	—	—	0.00	—
—	—	—	—	—	—	0.0	—	—	20	1.08	—	—	—	0	—	—	0.00	—
0.00	0.03	0.03	0.00	—	0.4	0.3	—	0.0	34	0.30	2.3	28	82	96	0.0	1	0.00	0.00
0.05	0.09	0.20	0.00	0.23	6.0	0.0	—	0.1	53	0.43	15.7	57	98	23	0.0	2	0.00	5.94
0.01	0.07	0.10	0.01	0.25	2.6	0.3	—	0.0	67	0.44	5.5	52	138	83	0.2	1	0.00	—
0.01	0.15	0.46	0.02	0.18	4.5	0.3	—	3.9	84	0.55	36.0	117	162	85	0.6	4	0.00	2.00
—	—	—	—	—	—	0.0	—	—	32	0.14	—	—	—	15	—	5	0.00	3.96
0.01	0.11	0.18	0.02	0.17	3.2	0.5	—	0.7	70	0.40	18.3	78	130	129	0.4	6	0.00	4.30
0.00	0.00	0.00	0.00	0.00	0.0	0.4	—	0.1	11	1.12	0.0	0	173	78	0.0	9	0.00	9.15
0.07	0.07	1.71	0.02	0.15	18.9	0.4	—	1.6	55	0.68	23.3	81	195	20	0.5	0	0.00	8.93
0.12	0.21	1.57	0.15	0.15	31.4	0.1	—	0.4	67	0.20	23.0	80	137	53	0.6	1	0.00	9.52

8

PAGE KEY: 2 Beverage and Beverage Mixes   4 Other Beverages   4 Beverages, Alcoholic   6 Candies and Confections, Gum   10 Cereals, Breakfast Type
14 Cheese and Cheese Substitutes   16 Dairy Products and Substitutes   18 Desserts   24 Dessert Toppings   24 Eggs, Substitutes, and Egg Dishes   26 Ethnic Foods
30 Fast Foods/Restaurants   44 Fats, Oils, Margarines, Shortenings, and Substitutes   44 Fish, Seafood, and Shellfish   46 Food Additives
46 Fruit, Vegetable, or Blended Juices   48 Grains, Flours, and Fractions   48 Grain Products, Prepared and Baked Goods

Code	Food Name	Unit/ Amt	Wt (g)	Energy (kcal)	Prot (g)	Carb (g)	Fiber (g)	Fat (g)	Sat (g)	Mono (g)	Poly (g)	Chol (mg)	Vit A (RE)
92654	Candy Bar, Payday, snack size, 0.7 oz bar	1 ea	20	90	2	10	—	5	0.5	—	—	0	—
23137	Candy Bar, peanut, 1.4 oz bar	1 ea	40	207	6	19	2	13	1.9	6.6	4.2	0	0
91513	Candy Bar, Reese's Nutrageous, 0.6 oz bar	2 ea	34	176	4	18	1	11	3.0	4.3	2.8	1	2
23036	Candy Bar, Skor, toffee bar, 1.4 oz bar	1 ea	40	212	1	24	1	13	7.5	3.7	0.5	21	57
23040	Candy Bar, Snickers, 2 oz bar	1 ea	57	265	5	37	1	11	4.2	4.7	1.5	8	22
23146	Candy Bar, Symphony, milk chocolate, 1.5 oz bar	1 ea	43	226	4	25	1	13	7.8	3.4	0.3	10	20
90705	Candy Bar, Twix, caramel, 2.06 oz two bar pkg	1 ea	58	291	3	38	1	14	5.2	7.8	0.5	3	15
92221	Candy Bar, Twix, chocolate fudge cookie bar, 3.6 oz bar	1 ea	100	550	7	56	3	33	5.0	14.3	12.5	6	11
23151	Candy Bar, Whatchamacallit, 1.7 oz bar	1 ea	48	238	4	30	1	11	8.2	1.8	0.4	6	19
92658	Candy Bar, Zero, 0.6 oz bar	1 ea	17	70	1	12	—	2	1.5	—	—	0	—
23085	Candy, Almond Roca	1 pce	11	48	1	7	0	2	1.1	0.6	0.2	1	2
4148	Candy, Bit O Honey, Nestle	6 pce	40	160	1	32	0	3	2.0	0.8	0.2	0	0
92707	Candy, caramel, Sugar Daddy, lrg	1 ea	48	200	1	43	0	2	1.0	—	—	0	0
23015	Candy, caramels	1 pce	10	39	0	8	0	1	0.7	0.1	0.0	1	0
92374	Candy, cotton	2.1 oz	60	220	3	56	—	0	0.0	0.0	0.0	0	—
23078	Candy, fondant, chocolate cvrd	2 pce	28	102	1	22	0	3	1.5	0.9	0.1	0	1
92647	Candy, Good N Plenty, snack size box	1 ea	17	60	0	14	0	0	0.0	0.0	0.0	0	0
23409	Candy, gumdrops	1.5 oz	43	168	0	42	0	0	0.0	0.0	0.0	0	0
23412	Candy, gummy worms, pces	10 pce	74	293	0	73	0	0	0.0	0.0	0.0	0	0
23031	Candy, hard, all flvrs	1 pce	6	24	0	6	0	0	0.0	0.0	0.0	0	0
92653	Candy, hard, lollipop	1 ea	17	60	0	16	0	0	0.0	0.0	0.0	0	0
23472	Candy, jawbreakers, Everlasting Gobstoppers, Willy Wonka	6 pce	16	59	0	15	—	0	0.0	0.0	0.0	—	—
23033	Candy, jellybeans, sml	10 pce	11	41	0	10	0	0	0.0	0.0	0.0	0	0
23063	Candy, Kisses, milk chocolate	6 pce	28	145	2	17	1	9	5.2	2.8	0.3	6	16
52154	Candy, licorice, black, vines/ropes	4 pce	40	140	1	33	0	0	0.0	0.0	0.0	0	0
52155	Candy, licorice, red, vines/ropes	4 pce	40	140	1	34	0	0	0.0	0.0	0.0	0	0
92644	Candy, malt choc, Whoppers	9 ea	20	90	1	15	0	4	3.0	—	—	0	0
23047	Candy, milk chocolate peanut	1.5 oz	43	219	4	26	1	11	4.4	4.7	1.8	4	11
92642	Candy, Milk Duds	7 ea	21	90	1	15	0	4	1.0	—	—	0	—
23193	Candy, mints, After Eight	5 pce	41	147	1	31	1	6	3.4	1.8	0.2	0	1
23225	Candy, mints, peppermint, Breath Saver	1 pce	2	10	0	2	0	0	0.0	0.0	0.0	0	—
92657	Candy, Nibs, licorice	9 ea	12	35	0	9	—	0	0.0	0.0	0.0	0	—
92201	Candy, nougat, 0.5 oz pce	1 ea	14	56	0	13	0	0	0.2	0.0	0.0	0	0
23021	Candy, peanuts, milk chocolate cvrd	1.5 oz	43	221	6	21	2	14	6.2	5.5	1.8	4	14
23088	Candy, peanuts, yogurt cvrd	1.5 oz	43	230	6	18	2	16	6.9	4.8	3.1	0	0
90803	Candy, pralines, prep f/recipe	1 pce	40	174	1	22	1	10	2.7	—	—	10	30
23517	Candy, raisins, chocolate cvrd	35 pce	40	160	1	27	2	7	4.0	—	—	0	2
23089	Candy, raisins, yogurt cvrd	1.5 oz	43	167	2	31	1	5	4.3	0.1	0.1	0	0
92643	Candy, Sixlets	6 ea	38	170	1	29	0	7	5.0	—	—	0	0
23485	Candy, Skittles, original bite size candies, 2.17 oz pkg	1 ea	62	249	0	56	0	3	0.5	1.8	0.1	0	0
23144	Candy, Starburst, fruit chews	1 pce	5	20	0	4	0	0	0.1	0.2	0.2	0	0
92705	Candy, Sugar Babies	30 ea	44	180	0	41	0	2	0.0	—	—	0	0
4149	Candy, SweeTarts, reg	8 pce	15	60	0	14	0	0	0.0	0.0	0.0	0	0
90806	Candy, taffy, prep f/recipe	1 pce	34	99	1	17	0	3	1.0	—	—	4	—
92769	Candy, Tootsie Roll	6 pce	40	155	1	35	0	1	0.4	0.8	0.1	1	0

Thia (mg)	Ribo (mg)	Niac (mg NE)	Vit B6 (mg)	Vit B12 (µg)	Fol (µg)	Vit C (mg)	Vit D (IU)	Vit E (mg AT)	Cal (mg)	Iron (mg)	Magn (mg)	Phos (mg)	Pota (mg)	Sodi (mg)	Zinc (mg)	Wat (%)	Alco (g)	Caff (mg)
—	—	—	—	—	—	—	—	—	—	—	—	—	—	65	—	13	0.00	0.00
0.03	0.05	3.14	0.05	0.00	29.8	0.0	—	1.6	31	0.37	43.7	122	162	62	1.6	2	0.00	0.00
0.05	0.02	1.77	0.02	—	19.0	0.2	—	0.4	23	0.41	23.1	60	124	48	0.4	2	0.00	—
0.00	0.03	0.05	0.00	0.10	1.2	0.2	—	0.0	52	0.23	4.0	24	61	126	0.1	2	0.00	—
0.02	0.07	2.03	0.05	0.09	15.3	0.0	—	0.9	60	0.68	40.8	108	183	129	1.4	6	0.00	4.53
0.03	0.15	0.14	0.01	0.17	—	0.9	0.0	0.1	107	0.38	23.4	88	186	43	0.5	1	0.00	28.06
0.07	0.10	0.43	0.00	0.17	11.1	0.2	—	1.1	53	0.46	18.7	64	110	113	0.6	4	0.00	1.75
0.14	0.20	1.11	0.03	0.33	9.0	1.0	—	2.7	130	1.30	46.0	147	309	266	0.9	2	0.00	10.00
0.05	0.10	1.19	0.01	0.18	8.7	0.4	—	0.6	57	0.54	13.5	67	146	144	0.2	3	0.00	4.82
—	—	—	—	—	—	—	—	—	—	—	—	—	—	35	—	—	0.00	—
0.00	0.01	0.15	0.00	0.00	3.3	0.0	—	0.2	16	0.10	4.9	19	34	20	0.1	5	0.00	—
0.00	0.10	0.01	0.00	0.07	1.6	0.0	—	0.4	20	0.11	2.8	18	50	120	0.1	8	0.00	0.00
—	—	—	—	—	—	0.0	—	—	20	0.00	—	—	—	65	—	—	0.00	0.00
0.00	0.02	0.02	0.00	0.00	0.5	0.1	—	0.3	14	0.00	1.7	12	22	25	0.0	8	0.00	0.00
—	—	—	—	—	—	—	—	—	—	—	—	—	—	0	—	—	0.00	0.00
0.00	0.01	0.15	0.00	0.00	0.3	0.0	—	0.1	5	0.43	17.6	27	47	7	0.1	8	0.00	1.12
—	—	—	—	—	—	0.0	—	—	0	0.11	—	—	—	40	—	—	0.00	0.00
0.00	0.00	0.00	0.00	0.00	0.0	0.0	—	0.0	1	0.17	0.4	0	2	19	0.0	1	0.00	0.00
0.00	0.00	0.00	0.00	0.00	0.0	0.0	—	0.0	2	0.30	0.7	1	4	33	0.0	1	0.00	0.00
0.00	0.00	0.00	0.00	0.00	0.0	0.0	—	0.0	0	0.01	0.2	0	0	2	0.0	1	0.00	0.00
—	—	—	—	—	—	0.0	—	—	0	0.00	—	—	—	10	—	5	0.00	0.00
—	—	—	—	—	—	—	—	—	—	—	—	—	—	1	—	8	0.00	0.00
0.00	0.00	0.00	0.00	0.00	0.0	0.0	—	0.0	0	0.00	0.2	0	4	6	0.0	6	0.00	0.00
0.01	0.09	0.09	0.00	0.10	2.3	0.1	—	0.4	54	0.38	17.0	61	109	23	0.4	1	0.00	6.96
—	—	—	—	—	—	0.0	—	—	0	0.00	—	—	—	60	—	15	0.00	0.00
—	—	—	—	—	—	0.0	—	—	0	0.00	—	—	—	20	—	12	0.00	0.00
—	—	—	—	—	—	0.0	—	—	40	0.18	—	—	—	65	—	—	0.00	—
0.03	0.07	1.74	0.03	0.07	16.2	0.2	—	1.1	43	0.49	32.3	99	148	20	1.0	2	0.00	4.67
—	—	—	—	—	—	—	—	—	—	—	—	—	—	40	—	6	0.00	—
0.01	0.01	0.11	0.00	0.00	0.4	0.0	—	0.2	9	0.62	18.5	23	69	5	0.2	6	0.00	8.19
—	—	—	—	—	—	—	—	—	—	—	—	—	0	0	—	0	0.00	0.00
—	—	—	—	—	—	0.0	—	—	0	0.00	—	—	—	60	—	25	0.00	0.00
0.00	0.01	0.07	0.00	0.00	0.7	0.0	—	0.4	4	0.07	4.5	8	15	5	0.1	2	0.00	0.00
0.05	0.07	1.80	0.09	0.18	3.4	0.0	—	1.5	44	0.56	40.8	90	213	17	1.0	2	0.00	9.35
0.14	0.09	2.48	0.07	0.18	49.9	0.1	—	2.3	64	0.93	35.0	113	202	24	0.8	4	0.00	0.00
0.05	0.02	0.11	0.01	0.02	2.5	0.2	4.8	0.4	20	0.34	13.4	33	67	40	0.4	17	0.00	0.00
—	—	—	—	—	—	1.0	—	—	16	3.00	—	—	—	40	—	10	0.00	—
0.05	0.07	0.33	0.07	0.12	3.9	0.9	—	0.6	48	0.56	10.3	55	236	19	0.2	10	0.00	0.00
—	—	—	—	—	—	0.0	—	—	40	0.00	—	—	—	55	—	1	0.00	—
0.00	0.00	0.00	0.00	0.00	0.0	41.2	—	0.3	0	0.00	0.6	1	6	10	0.0	4	0.00	0.00
0.00	0.00	0.00	0.00	0.00	0.0	2.6	—	0.0	0	0.00	0.1	0	0	3	0.0	7	0.00	0.00
—	—	—	—	—	—	0.0	—	—	20	0.00	—	—	—	40	—	—	0.00	0.00
—	—	—	—	—	—	0.0	—	—	0	0.00	—	—	—	0	—	—	0.00	0.00
0.00	0.01	0.10	0.00	0.00	1.3	0.0	1.0	0.6	9	0.01	9.1	16	19	152	0.1	34	0.00	0.00
0.01	0.02	0.07	0.00	0.00	3.6	0.0	—	0.3	14	0.31	8.8	23	46	18	0.2	7	0.00	2.79

Code	Food Name	Unit/ Amt	Wt (g)	Energy (kcal)	Prot (g)	Carb (g)	Fiber (g)	Fat (g)	Sat (g)	Mono (g)	Poly (g)	Chol (mg)	Vit A (RE)
4144	Candy, Treasures, peanut butter	4 pce	43	240	3	22	1	16	7.0	—	—	5	0
4143	Candy, Treasures, w/caramel	3 pce	35	170	1	22	0	9	5.0	—	—	5	0
23082	Chewing Gum, stick	1 pce	3	7	0	2	0	0	0.0	0.0	0.0	0	0
23369	Fruit Leather, cherry	1 oz	28	105	0	23	0	2	0.7	0.9	0.0	0	—
91256	Fudge, plain	1.5 oz	43	188	0	27	0	9	6.0	—	—	11	10
23007	Marshmallows	4 ea	29	92	1	23	0	0	0.0	0.0	0.0	0	0
92226	Snack, crisped rice, peanut butter, 3.6 oz bar	1 ea	100	443	6	71	2	16	5.3	6.0	3.0	3	250

CEREALS, BREAKFAST TYPE
Cereals, Cooked and Dry

Code	Food Name	Unit/ Amt	Wt (g)	Energy (kcal)	Prot (g)	Carb (g)	Fiber (g)	Fat (g)	Sat (g)	Mono (g)	Poly (g)	Chol (mg)	Vit A (RE)
40055	Cereal, hot, breakfast pilaf, ckd	0.5 cup	140	170	6	30	6	3	—	—	—	0	0
40179	Cereal, hot, Cream Of Rice, ckd w/water & salt	1 cup	244	127	2	28	0	0	0.0	0.1	0.1	0	0
38497	Cereal, hot, Farina, enrich, prep w/water & salt	1 cup	233	119	4	26	1	0	0.0	0.1	0.0	0	0
40186	Cereal, hot, Maltex, ckd w/water & salt	1 cup	249	189	6	39	2	1	0.2	0.1	0.4	0	0
40239	Cereal, hot, Maypo, ckd w/water & salt	1 cup	240	170	6	32	5	2	0.4	0.6	0.5	0	701
40138	Cereal, hot, multigrain, ckd	1 cup	246	202	7	40	4	2	0.3	0.5	1.1	0	116
38500	Cereal, hot, oat bran, prep w/water & salt	1 cup	219	94	4	16	4	2	0.4	0.7	0.8	0	4
40072	Cereal, hot, oatmeal, plain, inst, fort, prep w/water	0.75 cup	177	97	4	17	3	2	0.3	0.5	0.6	0	285
40190	Cereal, hot, Roman Meal, plain, ckd w/water & salt	1 cup	241	147	7	33	8	1	0.1	0.1	0.4	0	0
40188	Cereal, hot, wheat, plain, ckd w/water & salt	1 cup	240	122	4	26	1	0	0.0	0.1	0.0	0	0
40191	Cereal, hot, Wheatena, ckd w/water & salt	1 cup	243	143	5	29	5	1	0.2	0.2	0.6	0	1
40089	Grits, corn, inst, plain, prep w/water f/pkt	1 ea	137	93	2	21	1	0	0.0	0.0	0.1	0	0
38455	Grits, corn, white, dry	0.25 cup	42	150	3	33	1	0	0.0	0.0	0.0	0	20
38571	Grits, hominy, yellow, quick, dry	0.25 cup	37	125	3	29	2	1	0.2	0.2	0.3	0	21

Cereals, Ready To Eat

Code	Food Name	Unit/ Amt	Wt (g)	Energy (kcal)	Prot (g)	Carb (g)	Fiber (g)	Fat (g)	Sat (g)	Mono (g)	Poly (g)	Chol (mg)	Vit A (RE)
54234	Cereal, 100% Bran	0.33 cup	29	83	4	23	8	1	0.1	—	—	0	150
40095	Cereal, All-Bran	0.5 cup	30	78	4	22	9	1	0.2	0.2	0.6	0	158
40258	Cereal, Alpha-Bits, 1.1 oz svg	1 ea	32	130	3	27	1	2	0.0	—	—	0	150
40098	Cereal, Apple Jacks	1 cup	30	117	1	27	1	1	0.1	0.2	0.3	0	42
40278	Cereal, Banana Nut Crunch	1 cup	59	249	5	44	4	6	0.8	—	—	0	150
40394	Cereal, Basic 4	1 cup	55	202	4	42	3	3	0.4	1.0	1.1	0	118
61203	Cereal, bran flakes	0.75 cup	30	96	3	24	5	1	0.1	0.1	0.3	0	225
40032	Cereal, Cap'N Crunch	0.75 cup	27	108	1	23	1	2	0.4	0.3	0.2	0	4
40297	Cereal, Cheerios	1 cup	30	111	4	22	4	2	0.4	0.6	0.2	0	150
40325	Cereal, Chex, corn	1 cup	30	112	2	26	1	0	0.1	0.1	0.1	0	140
40333	Cereal, Chex, rice	1.25 cup	31	117	2	27	0	0	0.1	0.1	0.1	0	155
40335	Cereal, Chex, wheat	1 cup	30	104	3	24	3	1	0.1	0.1	0.2	0	90
40414	Cereal, Cinnamon Grahams	0.75 cup	30	113	2	26	1	1	0.2	0.3	0.3	0	150
40126	Cereal, Cinnamon Toast Crunch	0.75 cup	30	127	2	24	1	3	0.5	1.5	1.0	0	150
61272	Cereal, Coco Roos, chocolate	0.75 cup	30	122	1	26	1	1	0.3	0.6	0.1	0	397
40102	Cereal, Cocoa Krispies	0.75 cup	31	118	2	27	1	1	0.6	0.1	0.1	0	153
40257	Cereal, Cocoa Pebbles	0.75 cup	29	115	1	25	0	1	1.1	—	—	0	150
40425	Cereal, Cocoa Puffs	1 cup	30	117	1	26	1	1	0.2	0.5	0.2	0	0
40103	Cereal, Complete Oat Bran Flakes	0.75 cup	30	105	3	23	4	1	0.2	0.5	0.3	0	235
40324	Cereal, Cookie Crisp	1 cup	30	117	1	26	0	1	0.2	0.4	0.2	0	145
61214	Cereal, corn flakes, plain	1 cup	28	101	2	24	1	0	0.0	0.0	0.0	0	216
40206	Cereal, Corn Pops	1 cup	31	118	1	28	0	0	0.1	0.1	0.1	0	144

Thia (mg)	Ribo (mg)	Niac (mg NE)	Vit B6 (mg)	Vit B12 (µg)	Fol (µg)	Vit C (mg)	Vit D (IU)	Vit E (mg AT)	Cal (mg)	Iron (mg)	Magn (mg)	Phos (mg)	Pota (mg)	Sodi (mg)	Zinc (mg)	Wat (%)	Alco (g)	Caff (mg)
—	—	—	—	—	—	0.0	—	—	40	0.36	—	—	—	80	—	—	0.00	—
—	—	—	—	—	—	0.0	—	—	40	0.00	—	—	—	60	—	—	0.00	—
0.00	0.00	0.00	0.00	0.00	0.0	0.0	0.0	0.0	0	0.00	0.0	0	0	0	0.0	3	0.00	0.00
0.00	0.00	0.00	—	—	—	—	—	—	7	0.07	—	—	46	56	—	—	0.00	0.00
—	—	—	—	—	—	0.0	—	—	0	0.18	—	—	—	42	—	—	0.00	0.00
0.00	0.00	0.01	0.00	0.00	0.3	0.0	—	0.0	1	0.07	0.6	2	1	23	0.0	16	0.00	0.00
0.43	0.44	6.90	0.52	—	119.0	14.9	—	—	344	5.17	28.0	102	185	406	0.5	4	0.00	0.00
—	—	—	—	—	—	0.0	—	—	20	1.44	—	—	—	15	—	—	0.00	0.00
0.00	0.00	0.98	0.07	0.00	7.3	0.0	0.0	0.0	7	0.49	7.3	41	49	422	0.4	88	0.00	0.00
0.15	0.10	1.80	0.01	0.00	53.6	0.0	0.0	0.0	9	11.00	7.0	30	33	128	0.2	87	0.00	0.00
0.25	0.10	2.36	0.07	0.00	29.9	0.0	0.0	1.1	22	1.78	57.3	177	266	189	1.9	81	0.00	0.00
0.70	0.79	9.35	0.93	2.77	12.0	28.3	0.0	0.2	130	8.38	52.8	247	211	259	1.5	83	0.00	0.00
0.38	0.46	4.42	0.46	0.00	17.2	0.0	0.0	3.4	69	5.40	66.4	184	138	2	0.9	79	0.00	0.00
0.25	0.07	0.20	0.02	0.00	11.0	0.0	0.0	0.1	24	2.11	65.7	180	151	101	1.2	89	0.00	0.00
0.25	0.31	3.59	0.37	0.00	76.1	0.0	0.0	0.2	99	7.67	40.7	96	94	80	0.8	86	0.00	0.00
0.23	0.11	3.07	0.10	0.00	24.1	0.0	0.0	0.4	29	2.11	108.5	214	301	198	1.8	83	0.00	0.00
0.47	0.23	5.76	0.01	0.00	4.8	0.0	0.0	0.0	5	9.60	4.8	24	31	324	0.2	88	0.00	2.40
0.02	0.05	1.33	0.05	0.00	21.9	0.0	0.0	1.3	15	1.36	51.0	146	187	578	1.7	85	0.00	0.00
0.15	0.18	2.21	0.05	0.00	46.6	0.0	0.0	0.0	8	7.96	9.6	29	38	288	0.2	82	0.00	0.00
—	—	—	—	—	—	0.0	—	—	0	0.36	—	—	35	0	—	14	0.00	0.00
0.18	0.14	1.59	0.09	0.00	57.0	0.0	—	0.1	1	1.51	14.8	46	62	1	0.3	12	0.00	0.00
0.37	0.43	5.00	0.50	0.00	100.0	0.0	0.0	—	22	8.10	80.6	236	275	121	3.7	3	0.00	0.00
0.68	0.81	4.44	3.59	5.63	393.0	6.0	51.0	0.4	117	5.28	108.6	345	306	73	3.7	2	0.00	0.00
—	—	—	—	—	—	0.0	—	—	100	2.70	—	—	—	210	—	—	0.00	0.00
0.50	0.38	4.61	0.44	1.37	93.0	13.8	38.1	0.0	8	4.17	16.5	38	36	142	1.5	3	0.00	0.00
0.37	0.41	5.00	0.50	1.50	99.7	0.1	40.1	—	21	16.20	48.4	183	171	253	1.5	4	0.00	0.00
0.30	0.34	3.90	0.38	1.14	78.7	0.0	31.4	0.6	196	3.51	40.2	232	155	316	3.0	7	0.00	0.00
0.37	0.43	5.00	0.50	1.50	99.9	0.0	39.9	0.3	17	8.10	64.2	152	185	220	1.5	4	0.00	0.00
0.43	0.47	5.71	0.56	0.00	420.1	0.0	0.0	0.2	4	5.15	15.1	45	54	202	4.3	2	0.00	0.00
0.54	0.50	5.76	0.66	1.42	200.1	6.0	39.9	0.1	122	10.31	39.3	132	209	213	4.6	4	0.00	0.00
0.37	0.43	5.01	0.50	1.50	200.1	6.0	0.0	0.1	100	9.00	8.4	22	25	288	3.8	2	0.00	0.00
0.38	0.43	5.17	0.51	1.54	206.8	6.2	41.2	0.0	103	9.30	9.3	35	30	292	3.9	3	0.00	0.00
0.23	0.25	3.00	0.30	0.89	240.0	3.6	24.0	0.2	60	8.69	24.0	90	113	267	2.4	2	0.00	0.00
0.37	0.43	5.01	0.50	1.50	99.9	6.0	39.9	0.1	100	4.50	8.1	20	44	237	3.8	3	0.00	0.00
0.37	0.43	5.01	0.50	1.50	99.9	6.0	39.9	0.3	100	4.50	8.1	80	43	206	3.8	3	0.00	0.00
0.40	0.44	5.28	0.52	1.59	105.9	15.9	—	0.1	21	4.76	10.8	42	53	201	0.2	3	0.00	1.20
0.46	0.69	4.96	1.01	2.15	197.5	15.0	40.3	0.1	40	6.88	11.8	32	61	197	1.5	3	0.00	1.54
0.37	0.43	5.00	0.50	1.50	100.0	0.0	40.0	—	3	1.79	10.7	23	42	157	1.5	3	0.00	—
0.37	0.43	5.01	0.50	1.50	99.9	6.0	0.0	0.1	100	4.50	8.1	20	50	171	3.8	3	0.00	0.60
1.64	1.79	21.00	2.09	6.03	403.5	63.0	42.0	12.7	16	18.89	45.0	105	120	210	15.6	3	0.00	0.00
0.37	0.43	5.01	0.50	1.50	99.9	6.0	39.9	0.1	100	4.50	8.4	40	27	178	3.8	2	0.00	0.60
0.37	0.43	5.00	0.50	1.50	100.0	0.0	40.0	0.1	1	5.40	4.5	15	33	266	0.1	4	0.00	0.00
0.37	0.43	4.98	0.50	1.51	102.0	6.0	50.2	0.0	5	1.91	2.2	10	26	120	1.5	3	0.00	0.00

PAGE KEY: 2 Beverage and Beverage Mixes   4 Other Beverages   4 Beverages, Alcoholic   6 Candies and Confections, Gum   10 Cereals, Breakfast Type
14 Cheese and Cheese Substitutes   16 Dairy Products and Substitutes   18 Desserts   24 Dessert Toppings   24 Eggs, Substitutes, and Egg Dishes   26 Ethnic Foods
30 Fast Foods/Restaurants   44 Fats, Oils, Margarines, Shortenings, and Substitutes   44 Fish, Seafood, and Shellfish   46 Food Additives
46 Fruit, Vegetable, or Blended Juices   48 Grains, Flours, and Fractions   48 Grain Products, Prepared and Baked Goods

Code	Food Name	Unit/ Amt	Wt (g)	Energy (kcal)	Prot (g)	Carb (g)	Fiber (g)	Fat (g)	Sat (g)	Mono (g)	Poly (g)	Chol (mg)	Vit A (RE)
40205	Cereal, Cracklin' Oat Bran	0.75 cup	55	225	5	39	6	8	2.3	4.6	1.2	0	252
4354	Cereal, Cranberry Almond Crunch	1 cup	55	210	4	43	3	3	0.0	—	—	0	150
40017	Cereal, crispy rice	1 cup	28	111	2	25	0	0	0.0	0.0	0.0	0	372
40040	Cereal, Crispy Wheaties 'N Raisins	1 cup	55	183	4	45	5	1	0.2	0.1	0.4	0	150
61179	Cereal, Familia	1 cup	122	473	12	90	10	8	0.9	3.9	2.0	0	2
61303	Cereal, Fiber 7	3.6 oz	100	353	14	78	14	1	0.3	0.2	0.6	0	106
40130	Cereal, Fiber One	0.5 cup	30	59	2	24	14	1	0.1	0.1	0.4	0	0
40218	Cereal, Froot Loops	1 cup	30	118	2	26	1	1	0.5	0.1	0.2	0	142
61306	Cereal, frosted flakes	0.75 cup	30	116	1	27	1	0	0.1	0.0	0.1	0	218
40043	Cereal, Frosted Mini Wheats	1 cup	51	173	5	41	5	1	0.2	0.1	0.5	0	0
60932	Cereal, Frosted Oats	0.75 cup	28	111	2	23	1	2	0.4	0.5	0.3	0	178
40256	Cereal, Fruit & Bran, peaches raisins & almonds, svg	1 cup	55	190	4	42	6	3	0.0	—	—	0	150
40266	Cereal, Fruity Pebbles	0.75 cup	27	108	1	24	0	1	0.2	—	—	0	150
60964	Cereal, Go Lean	0.75 cup	40	114	10	23	8	1	0.2	0.2	0.4	0	1
40245	Cereal, Golden Crisp	0.75 cup	27	107	1	25	0	0	0.1	—	—	0	150
40299	Cereal, Golden Grahams	0.75 cup	30	112	2	25	1	1	0.2	0.4	0.4	0	150
40009	Cereal, granola, 100% Natural, honey raisin oats	0.5 cup	51	225	5	34	3	9	3.6	3.8	1.1	1	1
40048	Cereal, granola, homemade, w/oats & wheat germ	0.5 cup	61	299	9	32	5	15	2.8	4.7	6.5	0	1
40277	Cereal, Grape Nuts	0.5 cup	58	208	6	47	5	1	0.2	0.2	0.7	0	150
40265	Cereal, Grape Nuts Flakes	0.75 cup	29	106	3	24	3	1	0.2	0.2	0.5	0	150
60969	Cereal, Harmony	3.6 oz	100	365	11	79	4	2	0.5	0.8	0.6	0	273
40004	Cereal, Harvest Oat Flakes	0.75 cup	29	109	3	23	2	1	0.2	0.4	0.4	0	2
61344	Cereal, Healthy Fiber, multigrain flakes	0.75 cup	28	100	3	23	4	0	0.0	0.0	0.0	0	20
60958	Cereal, Heart to Heart	1 oz	28	99	4	22	4	1	0.3	0.3	0.3	0	323
40293	Cereal, Honey Bunches Of Oats, almond	0.75 cup	31	126	2	24	1	3	0.3	—	—	0	150
40427	Cereal, Honey Graham Oh!s	0.75 cup	27	111	1	23	1	2	0.5	0.4	0.2	0	177
40264	Cereal, Honeycomb	1.33 cup	29	115	2	26	1	1	0.2	—	—	0	150
40134	Cereal, Just Right	1 cup	43	160	3	36	2	1	0.1	0.2	0.8	0	294
40410	Cereal, Kaboom	1.25 cup	30	115	3	24	2	1	0.3	0.3	0.4	0	150
40010	Cereal, Kix	1.33 cup	30	113	2	26	1	1	0.2	0.2	0.2	0	154
40011	Cereal, Life, plain	0.75 cup	32	120	3	25	2	1	0.3	0.5	0.5	0	1
40300	Cereal, Lucky Charms	1 cup	30	114	2	25	2	1	0.2	0.3	0.3	0	150
40124	Cereal, Mueslix, five grain muesli	1 cup	82	289	6	63	6	5	0.7	2.0	1.8	0	747
40449	Cereal, Oat Bran O's	0.75 cup	28	100	3	23	3	0	0.0	0.0	0.0	0	20
40302	Cereal, Oatmeal Raisin Crisp	1 cup	55	204	5	45	4	2	0.4	0.7	0.6	0	0
54233	Cereal, Oreo O's	0.75 cup	27	112	1	22	1	2	0.4	—	—	0	150
40216	Cereal, Product 19	1 cup	30	100	2	25	1	0	0.1	0.1	0.2	0	216
40018	Cereal, puffed rice	1 cup	14	54	1	12	0	0	0.0	0.0	0.0	0	0
40209	Cereal, raisin bran	1 cup	61	195	5	47	7	2	0.3	0.3	0.9	0	155
40210	Cereal, Rice Krispies	1.25 cup	33	119	2	28	0	0	0.1	0.1	0.1	0	153
40420	Cereal, Rice Krispies Treats	0.75 cup	30	122	1	26	0	2	0.4	0.9	0.2	0	152
40020	Cereal, Shredded Wheat, biscuits	1 ea	21	72	2	17	2	0	0.1	0.1	0.2	0	0
40068	Cereal, Smacks	0.75 cup	27	104	2	24	1	0	0.1	0.2	0.2	0	153
40211	Cereal, Special K	1 cup	31	117	7	22	1	0	0.1	0.1	0.2	0	230
40413	Cereal, Toasty O's	1 cup	30	112	3	22	3	2	0.4	0.7	0.6	0	375
40412	Cereal, Tootie Fruities	1 cup	32	125	2	28	1	1	0.3	0.3	0.2	0	218

PAGE KEY: 52 Granola Bars, Cereal Bars, Diet Bars, Scones, and Tarts   52 Meals and Dishes   56 Meats   62 Nuts, Seeds, and Products   64 Poultry   66 Salad Dressings, Dips, and Mayonnaise   66 Salads   68 Sandwiches   70 Sauces and Gravies   70 Snack Foods—Chips, Pretzels, Popcorn   72 Soups, Stews, and Chilis   74 Spices, Flavors, and Seasonings   76 Sports Bars and Drinks   76 Supplemental Foods and Formulas   78 Sweeteners and Sweet Substitutes   78 Vegetables and Legumes   92 Weight Loss Bars and Drinks   94 Miscellaneous

Thia (mg)	Ribo (mg)	Niac (mg NE)	Vit B6 (mg)	Vit B12 (µg)	Fol (µg)	Vit C (mg)	Vit D (IU)	Vit E (mg AT)	Cal (mg)	Iron (mg)	Magn (mg)	Phos (mg)	Pota (mg)	Sodi (mg)	Zinc (mg)	Wat (%)	Alco (g)	Caff (mg)
0.41	0.47	5.67	0.56	1.71	112.8	17.6	45.0	0.8	23	2.03	67.7	179	248	157	1.7	3	0.00	0.00
—	—	—	—	—	—	0.0	—	—	0	1.79	—	—	—	190	—	—	0.00	0.00
0.51	0.58	6.92	0.68	0.07	88.2	14.8	—	0.0	5	0.69	11.8	31	27	206	0.5	2	0.00	0.00
0.75	0.85	10.01	1.00	3.02	200.2	0.0	40.2	0.3	0	7.48	42.4	140	227	251	7.5	7	0.00	0.00
0.38	0.67	2.20	0.11	0.34	19.5	0.7	—	1.4	211	3.39	386.7	411	603	61	2.3	2	0.00	0.00
0.52	0.60	7.05	0.69	2.11	141.0	4.2	—	1.0	71	2.53	144.0	327	460	53	2.9	3	0.00	0.00
0.37	0.43	5.01	0.50	1.50	99.9	6.0	0.0	0.2	100	4.50	60.0	150	232	129	3.8	4	0.00	0.00
0.68	0.57	7.26	1.10	2.11	105.6	14.1	37.5	0.1	4	6.11	9.9	34	36	150	5.7	3	0.00	0.00
0.73	0.81	9.68	0.97	1.45	96.9	14.5	38.7	0.0	0	4.36	2.4	10	20	194	0.1	3	0.00	0.00
0.37	0.41	5.00	0.50	1.50	100.0	0.0	0.0	0.3	16	14.78	60.2	150	173	5	1.6	6	0.00	0.00
0.28	0.50	5.90	0.58	0.00	448.0	7.1	0.0	0.1	7	5.32	17.4	68	52	242	4.4	2	0.00	0.00
—	—	—	—	—	—	0.0	—	—	20	5.40	—	—	—	260	—	—	0.00	0.00
0.37	0.41	5.00	0.50	1.50	99.9	0.0	40.0	—	1	1.79	5.1	16	30	158	1.5	3	0.00	0.00
0.14	0.05	1.29	0.12	0.00	25.6	0.0	—	0.2	56	2.00	66.0	190	370	66	0.3	2	0.00	0.00
0.37	0.41	5.00	0.50	1.50	99.9	0.0	40.0	—	4	1.79	16.5	37	34	40	1.5	3	0.00	0.00
0.37	0.43	5.01	0.50	1.50	99.9	6.0	39.9	0.1	350	4.50	8.1	200	50	268	3.8	3	0.00	0.00
0.12	0.11	0.80	0.07	0.10	14.1	0.4	0.0	0.5	59	1.24	48.9	152	250	19	1.0	4	0.00	0.00
0.44	0.18	1.28	0.18	0.00	50.6	0.7	0.0	3.6	48	2.58	106.8	279	328	13	2.5	5	0.00	0.00
0.37	0.41	5.00	0.50	1.50	99.8	0.0	40.0	—	20	16.20	58.0	139	178	354	1.2	4	0.00	0.00
0.37	0.43	5.00	0.50	1.50	100.0	0.0	40.0	0.1	11	8.10	29.9	88	99	140	1.2	3	0.00	0.00
2.73	1.54	18.20	1.82	7.59	727.0	55.0	73.0	24.5	1091	16.39	44.0	182	166	645	13.6	3	0.00	0.00
0.07	0.10	0.69	0.05	0.00	11.1	0.0	0.0	0.5	16	0.87	32.4	102	99	204	0.8	2	0.00	0.00
0.15	0.17	2.00	0.20	0.60	40.0	0.0	—	—	0	0.72	—	—	100	15	—	5	0.00	0.00
0.15	0.05	0.51	1.73	5.15	343.6	25.8	—	11.6	15	1.84	85.1	25	85	1	1.3	3	0.00	0.00
0.37	0.41	5.00	0.50	1.50	100.1	0.0	40.0	—	11	8.10	21.4	60	70	187	0.3	3	0.00	0.00
0.43	0.50	5.90	0.58	0.00	420.1	7.1	0.0	0.2	3	5.30	0.0	38	42	162	4.4	3	0.00	0.00
0.37	0.43	5.00	0.50	1.50	100.0	0.0	40.0	—	5	2.70	10.7	27	35	215	1.5	2	0.00	0.00
0.30	0.34	3.91	0.38	1.15	80.0	0.0	—	1.8	11	12.68	26.7	83	95	264	0.7	3	0.00	0.00
0.37	0.43	5.01	0.50	1.50	200.1	6.0	39.9	0.1	100	8.10	15.9	80	63	285	3.8	2	0.00	0.00
0.37	0.43	5.01	0.50	1.50	200.1	6.3	42.3	0.1	150	8.10	8.1	40	35	267	3.8	2	0.00	0.00
0.40	0.46	5.50	0.55	0.00	416.0	0.0	0.0	0.2	112	8.94	30.7	133	91	164	4.1	4	0.00	0.00
0.37	0.43	5.01	0.50	1.50	200.1	6.0	39.9	0.1	100	4.50	15.9	60	57	203	3.8	2	0.00	0.00
0.75	0.83	9.84	0.99	3.27	196.8	0.8	0.0	8.9	67	8.93	82.0	215	369	107	7.5	8	0.00	0.00
0.15	0.17	2.00	0.20	0.60	40.0	0.0	—	—	0	0.72	—	—	90	90	—	3	0.00	0.00
0.37	0.41	5.01	0.50	1.49	100.1	6.1	0.0	1.4	20	4.51	40.2	100	200	216	3.8	6	0.00	0.00
0.37	0.41	5.00	0.50	1.50	99.9	0.0	40.0	—	5	1.79	14.9	32	49	128	1.5	2	0.00	
1.50	1.71	20.01	2.06	6.00	399.9	61.2	39.3	13.5	5	18.09	15.9	40	50	207	15.3	3	0.00	0.00
0.05	0.03	0.49	0.00	0.00	21.6	0.0	0.0	0.0	1	0.40	4.2	17	16	1	0.2	4	0.00	0.00
0.38	0.43	5.17	0.51	1.54	103.7	0.4	41.5	0.4	29	4.63	83.0	259	372	362	1.5	8	0.00	0.00
0.87	0.79	7.09	0.92	2.00	151.1	6.4	40.9	0.0	5	2.65	9.6	39	39	319	0.5	4	0.00	0.00
0.38	0.41	5.09	0.50	1.50	204.0	6.0	40.5	0.1	3	1.86	6.9	24	24	189	0.2	3	0.00	0.00
0.05	0.01	1.09	0.05	—	10.5	0.0	0.0	—	9	0.68	35.7	75	74	1	0.5	5	0.00	0.00
0.37	0.43	5.00	0.50	1.50	101.3	6.1	40.0	0.1	6	0.34	15.9	46	41	50	0.4	2	0.00	0.00
0.52	0.58	7.13	1.98	6.05	399.9	21.0	50.0	4.7	9	8.36	19.2	68	61	224	0.9	3	0.00	0.00
0.37	0.43	5.00	0.50	0.00	99.9	15.0	40.0	0.2	40	8.10	32.1	100	94	284	3.8	4	0.00	0.00
0.37	0.43	5.00	0.50	1.50	99.8	15.0	40.0	0.3	100	4.50	8.0	20	39	149	3.8	3	0.00	0.00

Code	Food Name	Unit/ Amt	Wt (g)	Energy (kcal)	Prot (g)	Carb (g)	Fiber (g)	Fat (g)	Sat (g)	Mono (g)	Poly (g)	Chol (mg)	Vit A (RE)
40021	Cereal, Total, wheat	0.75 cup	30	97	3	22	3	1	0.2	0.1	0.3	0	150
40128	Cereal, Uncle Sam	1 cup	55	237	9	36	11	6	0.7	1.1	4.6	0	0
40307	Cereal, Wheaties	1 cup	30	107	3	24	3	1	0.2	0.3	0.3	0	150
40362	Cereal, whole grain, w/raisins, all nat	0.5 cup	50	195	4	41	3	3	0.7	0.8	0.5	0	1

CHEESE AND CHEESE SUBSTITUTES

Natural Cheeses

Code	Food Name	Unit/ Amt	Wt (g)	Energy (kcal)	Prot (g)	Carb (g)	Fiber (g)	Fat (g)	Sat (g)	Mono (g)	Poly (g)	Chol (mg)	Vit A (RE)
47855	Cheese, blue, 1" cube	1 ea	17	61	4	0	0	5	3.2	1.3	0.1	13	35
47859	Cheese, brie, 1" cube	1 ea	17	57	4	0	0	5	3.0	1.4	0.1	17	30
47861	Cheese, camembert, 1" cube	1 ea	17	51	3	0	0	4	2.6	1.2	0.1	12	41
47863	Cheese, cheddar, 1" cube	1 ea	17	69	4	0	0	6	3.6	1.6	0.2	18	46
1551	Cheese, cheddar, fat free, 1" cube	1 ea	28	40	8	1	0	0	0.0	0.0	0.0	3	60
1525	Cheese, cheddar, five peppercorn, 1" cube	1 ea	28	110	7	1	0	9	5.0	—	—	30	60
1008	Cheese, cheddar, shredded	0.25 cup	28	114	7	0	0	9	6.0	2.7	0.3	30	77
47864	Cheese, cheddar, slice, 1 oz	1 ea	28	114	7	0	0	9	6.0	2.7	0.3	30	77
47865	Cheese, colby, 1" cube	1 ea	17	68	4	0	0	6	3.5	1.6	0.2	16	47
1010	Cheese, colby, shredded	0.25 cup	28	111	7	1	0	9	5.7	2.6	0.3	27	77
47866	Cheese, colby, slice, 1 oz	1 ea	28	112	7	1	0	9	5.7	2.6	0.3	27	77
47871	Cheese, feta, 1" cube	1 ea	17	45	2	1	0	4	2.5	0.8	0.1	15	21
47873	Cheese, fontina, 1" cube	1 ea	15	58	4	0	0	5	2.9	1.3	0.2	17	40
1078	Cheese, goat, hard	3.6 oz	100	452	31	2	0	36	24.6	8.1	0.8	105	494
1080	Cheese, goat, soft	3.6 oz	100	268	19	1	0	21	14.6	4.8	0.5	46	293
1054	Cheese, gouda	1 oz	28	101	7	1	0	8	5.0	2.2	0.2	32	47
47881	Cheese, limburger, 1" cube	1 ea	18	59	4	0	0	5	3.0	1.5	0.1	16	61
47884	Cheese, monterey jack, 1" cube	1 ea	17	64	4	0	0	5	3.3	1.5	0.2	15	35
1017	Cheese, monterey jack, shredded	0.25 cup	28	105	7	0	0	9	5.4	2.5	0.3	25	58
47885	Cheese, monterey jack, slice, 1 oz	1 ea	28	106	7	0	0	9	5.4	2.5	0.3	25	58
1553	Cheese, mozzarella, fat free, 1" cube	1 ea	28	40	8	1	0	0	0.0	0.0	0.0	3	60
47891	Cheese, muenster, 1" cube	1 ea	18	64	4	0	0	5	3.3	1.5	0.1	17	52
1021	Cheese, muenster, shredded	0.25 cup	28	104	7	0	0	8	5.4	2.5	0.2	27	84
1075	Cheese, parmesan, grated	1 Tbs	5	22	2	0	0	1	0.9	0.4	0.1	4	6
1061	Cheese, parmesan, hard, 1" cube	1 ea	10	40	4	0	0	3	1.7	0.8	0.1	7	11
1510	Cheese, pepper jack, 1" cube	1 ea	28	110	7	1	0	9	5.0	—	—	30	60
47899	Cheese, provolone, 1" cube	1 ea	17	60	4	0	0	5	2.9	1.3	0.1	12	41
47900	Cheese, provolone, slice, 1 oz	1 ea	28	100	7	1	0	8	4.8	2.1	0.2	20	69
1064	Cheese, ricotta, whole milk	0.25 cup	62	108	7	2	0	8	5.1	2.2	0.2	32	76
13348	Cheese, string, mozzarella, sticks, 1 oz	1 ea	28	50	8	1	0	2	1.0	—	—	5	40
47911	Cheese, sweitzer, 1" cube	1 ea	15	57	4	1	0	4	2.7	1.1	0.1	14	34
47908	Cheese, Swiss, 1" cube	1 ea	15	57	4	1	0	4	2.7	1.1	0.1	14	34
1027	Cheese, Swiss, shredded	0.25 cup	27	103	7	1	0	8	4.8	2.0	0.3	25	61
47912	Cheese, Swiss, slice, 1 oz	1 ea	28	108	8	2	0	8	5.0	2.1	0.3	26	64
1508	Cottage Cheese	0.5 cup	114	100	13	4	0	4	3.0	—	—	15	60
1047	Cottage Cheese, 1% fat	0.5 cup	113	81	14	3	0	1	0.7	0.3	0.0	5	12
1014	Cottage Cheese, 2% fat	0.5 cup	113	102	16	4	0	2	1.4	0.6	0.1	9	25
47848	Cottage Cheese, fat free, small curd	0.5 cup	126	90	12	8	0	0	0.0	0.0	0.0	10	40
1015	Cream Cheese	2 Tbs	29	101	2	1	0	10	6.4	2.9	0.4	32	108
1452	Cream Cheese, fat free	2 Tbs	29	28	4	2	0	0	0.3	0.1	0.0	2	81
1083	Cream Cheese, soft	2 Tbs	30	100	2	1	0	10	7.0	—	—	30	60

Thia (mg)	Ribo (mg)	Niac (mg NE)	Vit B6 (mg)	Vit B12 (μg)	Fol (μg)	Vit C (mg)	Vit D (IU)	Vit E (mg AT)	Cal (mg)	Iron (mg)	Magn (mg)	Phos (mg)	Pota (mg)	Sodi (mg)	Zinc (mg)	Wat (%)	Alco (g)	Caff (mg)
2.10	2.42	26.43	2.81	6.42	477.0	60.0	39.9	13.5	1104	22.35	39.3	89	103	192	17.5	3	0.00	0.00
1.25	1.45	8.97	0.52	0.00	29.2	33.8	—	0.4	52	2.22	113.3	206	245	113	2.1	4	0.00	0.00
0.75	0.85	9.98	1.00	3.00	200.1	6.0	39.9	0.2	0	8.10	32.1	100	111	218	7.5	3	0.00	0.00
0.15	0.09	0.93	0.07	0.05	12.0	0.3	0.0	0.9	30	1.32	42.5	134	204	118	1.0	4	0.00	0.00
0.00	0.07	0.18	0.02	0.20	6.2	0.0	—	0.0	91	0.05	4.0	67	44	241	0.5	42	0.00	0.00
0.00	0.09	0.05	0.03	0.28	11.1	0.0	—	0.0	31	0.09	3.4	32	26	107	0.4	48	0.00	0.00
0.00	0.07	0.10	0.03	0.21	10.5	0.0	2.0	0.0	66	0.05	3.4	59	32	143	0.4	52	0.00	0.00
0.00	0.05	0.00	0.00	0.14	3.1	0.0	2.0	0.0	123	0.11	4.8	87	17	106	0.5	37	0.00	0.00
—	—	—	—	—	—	—	—	—	400	—	—	—	—	220	—	63	0.00	0.00
—	—	—	—	—	—	0.0	—	—	200	0.00	—	—	—	180	—	36	0.00	0.00
0.00	0.10	0.01	0.01	0.23	5.1	0.0	3.4	0.1	204	0.18	7.9	145	28	175	0.9	37	0.00	0.00
0.00	0.10	0.01	0.01	0.23	5.1	0.0	3.4	0.1	204	0.18	7.9	145	28	176	0.9	37	0.00	0.00
0.00	0.05	0.01	0.00	0.14	3.1	0.0	—	0.0	118	0.12	4.5	79	22	104	0.5	38	0.00	0.00
0.00	0.10	0.02	0.01	0.23	5.1	0.0	—	0.1	194	0.20	7.3	129	36	171	0.9	38	0.00	0.00
0.00	0.10	0.02	0.01	0.23	5.1	0.0	—	0.1	194	0.21	7.4	130	36	171	0.9	38	0.00	0.00
0.02	0.14	0.17	0.07	0.28	5.4	0.0	—	0.0	84	0.10	3.2	57	11	190	0.5	55	0.00	0.00
0.00	0.02	0.01	0.00	0.25	0.9	0.0	—	0.0	82	0.02	2.1	52	10	120	0.5	38	0.00	0.00
0.14	1.19	2.40	0.07	0.11	4.0	0.0	—	0.3	895	1.87	54.0	729	48	346	1.6	29	0.00	0.00
0.07	0.37	0.43	0.25	0.18	12.0	0.0	—	0.2	140	1.89	16.0	256	26	368	0.9	61	0.00	0.00
0.00	0.09	0.01	0.01	0.43	6.0	0.0	2.7	0.1	198	0.07	8.2	155	34	232	1.1	41	0.00	0.00
0.00	0.09	0.02	0.01	0.18	10.4	0.0	—	0.0	89	0.01	3.8	71	23	144	0.4	48	0.00	0.00
0.00	0.07	0.01	0.00	0.14	3.1	0.0	—	0.0	128	0.11	4.6	76	14	92	0.5	41	0.00	0.00
0.00	0.10	0.02	0.01	0.23	5.1	0.0	—	0.1	211	0.20	7.6	125	23	151	0.8	41	0.00	0.00
0.00	0.10	0.02	0.01	0.23	5.1	0.0	—	0.1	211	0.20	7.7	126	23	152	0.9	41	0.00	0.00
—	—	—	—	—	—	—	—	—	400	—	—	—	—	220	—	63	0.00	0.00
0.00	0.05	0.01	0.00	0.25	2.1	0.0	—	0.0	125	0.07	4.7	82	23	110	0.5	42	0.00	0.00
0.00	0.09	0.02	0.01	0.41	3.4	0.0	—	0.1	203	0.11	7.6	132	38	177	0.8	42	0.00	0.00
0.00	0.01	0.00	0.00	0.10	0.5	0.0	—	0.0	55	0.03	1.9	36	6	76	0.2	21	0.00	0.00
0.00	0.02	0.02	0.00	0.11	0.7	0.0	2.9	0.0	122	0.07	4.5	71	9	165	0.3	29	0.00	0.00
—	—	—	—	—	—	0.0	—	—	200	0.00	—	—	—	170	—	36	0.00	0.00
0.00	0.05	0.01	0.00	0.25	1.7	0.0	—	0.0	129	0.09	4.8	84	23	149	0.5	41	0.00	0.00
0.00	0.09	0.03	0.01	0.40	2.8	0.0	—	0.1	214	0.15	7.9	141	39	248	0.9	41	0.00	0.00
0.00	0.11	0.05	0.02	0.20	7.4	0.0	—	0.1	128	0.23	6.8	98	65	52	0.7	72	0.00	0.00
—	—	—	—	—	—	0.0	—	—	200	0.00	—	—	—	220	—	58	0.00	0.00
0.00	0.03	0.00	0.00	0.50	0.9	0.0	6.6	0.1	119	0.02	5.7	85	12	29	0.7	37	0.00	0.00
0.00	0.03	0.00	0.00	0.50	0.9	0.0	6.6	0.1	119	0.02	5.7	85	12	29	0.7	37	0.00	0.00
0.01	0.07	0.01	0.01	0.89	1.6	0.0	11.9	0.1	214	0.05	10.3	153	21	52	1.2	37	0.00	0.00
0.01	0.07	0.02	0.01	0.94	1.7	0.0	12.5	0.1	224	0.05	10.8	161	22	54	1.2	37	0.00	0.00
—	—	—	—	—	—	0.0	—	—	100	0.00	—	—	—	400	—	80	0.00	0.00
0.01	0.18	0.14	0.07	0.70	13.6	0.0	—	0.0	69	0.15	5.7	151	97	459	0.4	82	0.00	0.00
0.02	0.20	0.15	0.09	0.80	14.7	0.0	—	0.0	78	0.18	6.8	171	108	459	0.5	79	0.00	0.00
—	—	—	—	—	—	0.0	—	—	80	0.00	—	—	—	450	—	—	0.00	0.00
0.00	0.05	0.02	0.00	0.11	3.8	0.0	—	0.1	23	0.34	1.7	30	35	86	0.2	54	0.00	0.00
0.00	0.05	0.05	0.00	0.15	10.7	0.0	—	0.0	54	0.05	4.1	126	47	158	0.3	76	0.00	0.00
—	0.02	—	—	0.00	—	0.0	—	—	20	0.00	0.0	40	40	100	0.0	56	0.00	0.00

16

PAGE KEY: 2 Beverage and Beverage Mixes 4 Other Beverages 4 Beverages, Alcoholic 6 Candies and Confections, Gum 10 Cereals, Breakfast Type
14 Cheese and Cheese Substitutes 16 Dairy Products and Substitutes 18 Desserts 24 Dessert Toppings 24 Eggs, Substitutes, and Egg Dishes 26 Ethnic Foods
30 Fast Foods/Restaurants 44 Fats, Oils, Margarines, Shortenings, and Substitutes 44 Fish, Seafood, and Shellfish 46 Food Additives
46 Fruit, Vegetable, or Blended Juices 48 Grains, Flours, and Fractions 48 Grain Products, Prepared and Baked Goods

Code	Food Name	Unit/ Amt	Wt (g)	Energy (kcal)	Prot (g)	Carb (g)	Fiber (g)	Fat (g)	Sat (g)	Mono (g)	Poly (g)	Chol (mg)	Vit A (RE)
Process Cheese and Cheese Substitutes													
1001	Cheese Product, American, cold pack	1 oz	28	94	6	2	0	7	4.4	2.0	0.2	18	48
1376	Cheese Product, monterey, past, proc, slice	1 pce	21	70	4	1	0	5	3.0	—	—	20	20
48288	Cheese Substitute	3.6 oz	100	141	22	9	0	1	0.8	0.4	0.0	6	10
48332	Cheese, American, past, proc, fat free, 1" cube	1 ea	16	24	4	2	0	0	0.1	0.0	0.0	2	70
48314	Cheese, American, past, proc, low fat, 1" cube	1 ea	18	32	4	1	0	1	0.8	0.4	0.0	6	11
1096	Cheese, American, past, proc, low fat, shredded	1 cup	113	203	28	4	0	8	5.0	2.3	0.3	40	67
1092	Cheese, mozzarella, imit	0.25 cup	28	70	3	7	0	3	1.0	1.8	0.5	0	123
47918	Cheese, pimento, past, proc, 1" cube	1 ea	18	66	4	0	0	5	3.4	1.6	0.2	16	46
48311	Cottage Cheese Substitute, soy	1 cup	225	340	28	16	0	18	2.6	4.0	10.3	0	9
DAIRY PRODUCTS AND SUBSTITUTES													
Creams and Substitutes													
54390	Cream Substitute, light	1 cup	242	167	2	22	0	8	2.2	4.9	1.0	0	1
506	Cream Substitute, pwd	1 tsp	2	11	0	1	0	1	0.6	0.0	0.0	0	0
500	Cream, half & half	2 Tbs	30	39	1	1	0	3	2.1	1.0	0.1	11	30
54384	Cream, half & half, fat free	1 Tbs	15	9	0	1	0	0	0.1	0.1	0.0	1	2
501	Cream, light	1 Tbs	15	29	0	1	0	3	1.8	0.8	0.1	10	28
502	Cream, whipping, heavy	2 Tbs	30	103	1	1	0	11	6.9	3.2	0.4	41	124
503	Cream, whipping, heavy, whipped	2 Tbs	15	52	0	0	0	6	3.4	1.6	0.2	20	62
54262	Creamer, non-dairy	1 Tbs	17	20	0	2	0	1	0.0	0.5	0.0	0	0
54315	Creamer, soy milk, plain	1 Tbs	15	15	0	1	0	1	0.0	—	—	0	0
504	Sour Cream, cultured	2 Tbs	29	62	1	1	0	6	3.8	1.7	0.2	13	52
54383	Sour Cream, fat free	3.6 oz	100	74	3	16	0	0	0.0	0.0	0.0	9	74
505	Sour Cream, imitation, cultured	2 Tbs	29	60	1	2	0	6	5.1	0.2	0.0	0	0
Milks and Non-Dairy Milks													
7	Buttermilk, low fat, cultured	1 cup	245	98	8	12	0	2	1.3	0.6	0.1	10	17
17	Eggnog	1 cup	254	343	10	34	0	19	11.3	5.7	0.9	150	117
81	Milk Substitute, fluid, w/hydrog veg oil	1 cup	244	149	4	15	0	8	1.9	4.9	1.2	0	0
4	Milk, 1%, w/add vit A & D	1 cup	244	102	8	12	0	2	1.5	0.7	0.1	12	142
2	Milk, 2%, w/add vit A & D	1 cup	244	122	8	11	0	5	3.1	1.4	0.2	20	134
18	Milk, chocolate, 2%, cmrcl	1 cup	250	180	8	26	1	5	3.1	1.5	0.2	18	138
59	Milk, chocolate, nonfat/skim	1 cup	250	144	9	27	1	1	0.7	0.3	0.0	4	142
173	Milk, evaporated	2 Tbs	32	40	2	3	0	2	1.5	0.4	0.1	10	0
23	Milk, goat	1 cup	244	168	9	11	0	10	6.5	2.7	0.4	27	142
1	Milk, whole, 3.25%	1 cup	244	146	8	11	0	8	4.6	2.0	0.5	24	70
66	Milk, whole, dry pwd	1 Tbs	8	40	2	3	0	2	1.3	0.6	0.1	8	21
20584	Rice Milk	1 cup	245	144	3	28	2	2	0.3	0.5	1.1	0	0
20033	Soy Milk	1 cup	245	127	11	12	3	5	0.6	0.9	1.9	0	152
20920	Soy Milk, chocolate	1 cup	250	140	5	23	0	4	0.0	—	—	0	100
20493	Tea, rice	1 cup	245	144	3	28	2	2	0.3	0.5	1.1	0	0
Yogurt													
2425	Yogurt, banana creme, lowfat, 6 oz ctn	1 ea	170	170	5	33	0	2	1.0	—	—	10	150
2836	Yogurt, cherry, fruit on the bottom, 8 oz ctn	1 ea	227	220	9	42	1	2	1.0	—	—	10	0
2574	Yogurt, coffee, nonfat, 8 oz ctn	1 ea	227	207	12	40	0	0	0.2	0.1	0.0	4	4
72088	Yogurt, fruit, nonfat	1 cup	245	230	11	47	0	0	0.3	0.1	0.0	5	7
2426	Yogurt, plain custard	1 cup	227	130	15	19	0	0	0.0	0.0	0.0	5	0

PAGE KEY: 52 Granola Bars, Cereal Bars, Diet Bars, Scones, and Tarts 52 Meals and Dishes 56 Meats 62 Nuts, Seeds, and Products 64 Poultry 66 Salad Dressings, Dips, and Mayonnaise 66 Salads 68 Sandwiches 70 Sauces and Gravies 70 Snack Foods—Chips, Pretzels, Popcorn 72 Soups, Stews, and Chilis 74 Spices, Flavors, and Seasonings 76 Sports Bars and Drinks 76 Supplemental Foods and Formulas 78 Sweeteners and Sweet Substitutes 78 Vegetables and Legumes 92 Weight Loss Bars and Drinks 94 Miscellaneous

Thia (mg)	Ribo (mg)	Niac (mg NE)	Vit B6 (mg)	Vit B12 (μg)	Fol (μg)	Vit C (mg)	Vit D (IU)	Vit E (mg AT)	Cal (mg)	Iron (mg)	Magn (mg)	Phos (mg)	Pota (mg)	Sodi (mg)	Zinc (mg)	Wat (%)	Alco (g)	Caff (mg)
0.00	0.12	0.01	0.03	0.36	1.4	0.0	—	0.2	141	0.23	8.5	113	103	274	0.9	43	0.00	0.00
—	—	—	—	—	—	0.0	—	—	100	0.00	—	—	—	280	—	—	0.00	0.00
0.02	0.47	0.15	0.12	1.23	8.0	0.0	—	0.0	552	0.91	35.0	499	336	1239	3.3	64	0.00	0.00
0.00	0.07	0.02	0.00	0.18	4.3	0.0	—	0.0	110	0.03	5.8	150	46	244	0.5	57	0.00	0.00
0.00	0.07	0.00	0.00	0.14	1.6	0.0	—	0.0	123	0.07	4.3	149	32	257	0.6	59	0.00	0.00
0.02	0.43	0.09	0.09	0.87	10.2	0.0	—	0.3	773	0.49	27.1	935	203	1616	3.8	59	0.00	0.00
0.00	0.12	0.09	0.00	0.23	3.1	0.0	0.6	0.6	172	0.10	11.6	165	129	194	0.5	47	0.00	0.00
0.00	0.05	0.00	0.00	0.11	1.4	0.4	—	0.1	107	0.07	3.8	130	28	250	0.5	39	0.00	0.00
0.00	0.31	1.12	0.15	0.00	49.5	0.0	—	1.4	423	12.60	513.0	500	448	45	3.9	71	0.00	0.00
0.00	0.00	0.00	0.00	0.00	0.0	0.0	—	0.7	2	1.36	0.0	182	428	145	0.1	86	0.00	0.00
0.00	0.00	0.00	0.00	0.00	0.0	0.0	—	0.0	0	0.01	0.1	8	16	4	0.0	2	0.00	0.00
0.00	0.03	0.01	0.00	0.10	0.9	0.3	—	0.1	32	0.01	3.0	29	39	12	0.2	81	0.00	0.00
0.00	0.03	0.01	0.00	0.07	0.6	0.1	—	0.0	14	0.00	2.4	23	31	22	0.1	86	0.00	0.00
0.00	0.01	0.00	0.00	0.02	0.3	0.1	—	0.1	14	0.00	1.4	12	18	6	0.0	74	0.00	0.00
0.00	0.02	0.00	0.00	0.05	1.2	0.2	15.5	0.3	19	0.00	2.1	18	22	11	0.1	58	0.00	0.00
0.00	0.01	0.00	0.00	0.02	0.6	0.1	7.8	0.2	10	0.00	1.0	9	11	6	0.0	58	0.00	0.00
—	—	—	—	—	—	0.0	—	—	0	0.00	—	—	25	0	—	82	0.00	0.00
—	—	—	—	—	—	0.0	—	—	0	0.00	—	—	—	5	—	—	0.00	0.00
0.00	0.03	0.01	0.00	0.09	3.2	0.3	—	0.2	33	0.01	3.2	24	41	15	0.1	71	0.00	0.00
0.03	0.15	0.07	0.01	0.30	11.0	0.0	—	0.0	125	0.00	10.0	95	129	141	0.5	81	0.00	0.00
0.00	0.00	0.00	0.00	0.00	0.0	0.0	—	0.2	1	0.10	1.7	13	46	29	0.3	71	0.00	0.00
0.07	0.37	0.14	0.07	0.54	12.2	2.5	—	0.1	284	0.11	27.0	218	370	257	1.0	90	0.00	0.00
0.09	0.47	0.27	0.12	1.13	2.5	3.8	—	0.5	330	0.50	48.3	277	419	137	1.2	74	0.00	0.00
0.02	0.20	0.00	0.00	0.00	0.0	0.0	—	0.7	81	0.94	14.6	181	278	190	2.9	88	0.00	0.00
0.05	0.44	0.23	0.09	1.07	12.2	0.0	126.8	0.0	290	0.07	26.8	232	366	107	1.0	90	0.00	0.00
0.10	0.44	0.21	0.09	1.12	12.2	0.5	104.8	0.1	285	0.07	26.8	229	366	100	1.0	89	0.00	0.00
0.09	0.40	0.31	0.10	0.85	12.5	2.2	100.0	0.1	285	0.60	32.5	255	422	150	1.0	84	0.00	5.00
0.09	0.34	0.28	0.10	0.87	13.6	2.3	100.0	0.1	292	0.68	45.5	265	486	121	1.2	85	0.00	7.50
0.00	0.10	0.05	0.01	0.05	2.5	0.0	25.0	0.0	80	0.00	7.6	60	95	30	0.2	76	0.00	0.00
0.11	0.34	0.68	0.10	0.17	2.4	3.2	29.3	0.2	327	0.11	34.2	271	498	122	0.7	87	0.00	0.00
0.10	0.44	0.25	0.09	1.07	12.2	0.0	98.7	0.1	276	0.07	24.4	222	349	98	1.0	88	0.00	0.00
0.01	0.10	0.05	0.01	0.25	3.0	0.7	25.0	0.0	73	0.03	6.8	62	106	30	0.3	2	0.00	0.00
0.09	0.02	1.86	0.17	0.00	3.4	0.0	—	1.3	15	0.50	53.6	96	50	86	0.8	86	0.00	—
0.15	0.11	0.70	0.23	2.99	39.2	0.0	39.2	3.3	93	2.70	61.2	135	304	135	1.1	88	0.00	0.00
—	0.50	—	—	3.00	24.0	0.0	120.0	—	300	1.44	—	—	350	75	0.6	—	0.00	—
0.09	0.02	1.86	0.17	0.00	3.4	0.0	—	1.3	15	0.50	53.6	96	50	86	0.8	86	0.00	—
—	—	—	—	—	—	0.0	80.0	—	200	0.00	—	150	260	80	—	76	0.00	0.00
—	—	—	—	—	—	0.0	—	—	300	0.00	—	—	480	150	—	77	0.00	0.00
0.10	0.47	0.25	0.10	1.24	24.7	1.8	2.3	0.0	404	0.20	38.7	318	518	155	2.0	76	0.00	0.00
0.10	0.43	0.25	0.10	1.14	22.1	1.7	—	0.1	372	0.17	36.8	292	475	142	1.8	75	0.00	0.00
0.15	0.50	—	—	—	—	0.0	—	—	400	0.00	32.0	300	550	220	—	84	0.00	0.00

PAGE KEY: 2 Beverage and Beverage Mixes 4 Other Beverages 4 Beverages, Alcoholic 6 Candies and Confections, Gum 10 Cereals, Breakfast Type 14 Cheese and Cheese Substitutes 16 Dairy Products and Substitutes 18 Desserts 24 Dessert Toppings 24 Eggs, Substitutes, and Egg Dishes 26 Ethnic Foods 30 Fast Foods/Restaurants 44 Fats, Oils, Margarines, Shortenings, and Substitutes 44 Fish, Seafood, and Shellfish 46 Food Additives 46 Fruit, Vegetable, or Blended Juices 48 Grains, Flours, and Fractions 48 Grain Products, Prepared and Baked Goods

Code	Food Name	Unit/ Amt	Wt (g)	Energy (kcal)	Prot (g)	Carb (g)	Fiber (g)	Fat (g)	Sat (g)	Mono (g)	Poly (g)	Chol (mg)	Vit A (RE)
2000	Yogurt, plain, low fat, 12g prot/8 oz	1 cup	245	154	13	17	0	4	2.5	1.0	0.1	15	34
71587	Yogurt, soy, vanilla, 6 oz ctn	1 ea	170	120	4	23	1	2	0.0	—	—	0	10
7546	Yogurt, tofu	1 cup	262	246	9	42	1	5	0.7	1.0	2.7	0	10
2015	Yogurt, vanilla, low fat	1 cup	245	208	12	34	0	3	2.0	0.8	0.1	12	29

DESSERTS

Brownies and Bars

Code	Food Name	Unit/ Amt	Wt (g)	Energy (kcal)	Prot (g)	Carb (g)	Fiber (g)	Fat (g)	Sat (g)	Mono (g)	Poly (g)	Chol (mg)	Vit A (RE)
47100	Bar, apple cinnamon, fruit & oatmeal, 1.3 oz pce	1 ea	37	136	2	26	1	3	0.4	1.0	0.2	0	261
23171	Bar, Rice Krispie, 1 oz pce	1 ea	28	107	1	20	0	3	0.6	1.3	0.8	0	85
62904	Brownie, cmrcl prep, square, lrg, 2 3/4" x 7/8"	1 ea	56	227	3	36	1	9	2.4	5.0	1.3	10	11
47019	Brownie, prep f/recipe, 2" square	1 ea	24	112	1	12	1	7	1.8	2.6	2.3	18	46

Cakes & Cheesecakes

Code	Food Name	Unit/ Amt	Wt (g)	Energy (kcal)	Prot (g)	Carb (g)	Fiber (g)	Fat (g)	Sat (g)	Mono (g)	Poly (g)	Chol (mg)	Vit A (RE)
46004	Cake, angel food, cmrcl prep, 1/12 pce	1 pce	28	73	2	16	0	0	0.0	0.0	0.1	0	0
46102	Cake, applesauce, w/icing	1 pce	108	399	3	69	1	13	2.7	5.9	4.0	20	39
46103	Cake, banana, w/o icing	1 pce	87	262	3	46	1	8	1.6	3.6	2.1	32	83
46262	Cake, carrot, buttercream frosted	1 pce	71	280	2	36	1	15	3.5	—	—	35	100
46062	Cake, chocolate, prep f/rec, w/o frosting 9" whl or 1/12 pce	1 pce	95	340	5	51	2	14	5.2	5.7	2.6	55	39
46120	Cake, chocolate, w/fluffy white icing, prep f/recipe, slice	1 pce	91	280	3	43	1	11	2.7	—	—	23	50
46118	Cake, chocolate, w/vanilla icing, 1/12 piece	1 pce	103	367	3	53	1	17	4.3	—	—	23	52
46005	Cake, coffee, cinnamon, w/crumb topping prep f/mix, 1/8 pce	1 pce	56	178	3	30	1	5	1.0	2.2	1.8	27	20
42721	Cake, Ding Dongs, w/cream filling, Hostess	1 ea	80	368	3	45	2	19	11.0	4.0	1.2	14	—
46205	Cake, fruit, cmrcl prep	1 pce	43	139	1	26	2	4	0.5	1.8	1.4	2	3
45562	Cake, funnel	1 pce	90	278	7	29	1	14	2.7	4.4	6.3	63	58
46000	Cake, gingerbread, prep f/rec, 1/9 of 8" square	1 pce	74	263	3	36	1	12	3.1	5.3	3.1	24	10
46108	Cake, graham cracker	1 pce	45	159	3	22	0	7	1.6	3.2	1.6	33	66
46111	Cake, lemon, w/icing	1 pce	109	385	3	71	1	11	1.9	4.8	3.4	34	62
46070	Cake, pineapple upside down, prep f/rec, 1/9th of 8" square	1 pce	115	367	4	58	1	14	3.4	6.0	3.8	25	75
71261	Cake, pound, w/butter, cmrcl prep, 1/10 pce	1 pce	30	116	2	15	0	6	3.5	1.8	0.3	66	47
46077	Cake, shortcake, biscuit type, prep f/recipe	3.6 oz	100	346	6	48	1	14	3.8	6.0	3.6	3	19
46116	Cake, spice, w/icing	1 pce	109	368	5	62	1	12	3.2	5.9	1.9	50	39
46115	Cake, sponge, chocolate, w/o icing	1 pce	66	197	5	36	1	4	1.4	1.5	0.5	139	62
46455	Cake, yellow, prep f/dry mix, 2" x 3" pce	1 pce	55	150	2	27	0	4	1.0	2.5	0.0	0	0
46012	Cake, yellow, w/chocolate icing, cmrcl prep, 1/8 of 18 oz	1 pce	64	243	2	35	1	11	3.0	6.1	1.4	35	21
62352	Cheesecake, cherry	1 ea	113	330	6	27	1	22	13.0	—	—	100	300
49001	Cheesecake, no bake, prep f/dry mix, 1/12 of 9"	1 pce	99	271	5	35	2	13	6.6	4.5	0.8	29	99
46426	Cupcake, chocolate, w/frosting, low fat	1 ea	43	131	2	29	2	2	0.5	0.8	0.2	0	0

Cookies

Code	Food Name	Unit/ Amt	Wt (g)	Energy (kcal)	Prot (g)	Carb (g)	Fiber (g)	Fat (g)	Sat (g)	Mono (g)	Poly (g)	Chol (mg)	Vit A (RE)
90634	Cookie Crumbs, chocolate wafer	1 cup	112	485	7	81	4	16	4.7	5.4	4.7	2	3
62910	Cookie Crumbs, vanilla wafer, lower fat	1 cup	80	353	4	59	2	12	3.1	5.2	3.1	41	6
47073	Cookie, almond	2 ea	20	103	2	10	1	6	1.0	3.4	1.6	9	41
47074	Cookie, applesauce	2 ea	36	132	2	23	1	4	0.9	2.0	1.2	9	42
47746	Cookie, biscotti, chocolate	1 ea	30	120	1	15	2	6	3.0	—	—	20	0
90163	Cookie, biscuit, arrowroot	1 ea	5	22	0	4	0	1	0.2	0.4	0.1	0	0
90164	Cookie, biscuit, tea	1 ea	5	22	0	4	0	1	0.2	0.4	0.1	0	0
90637	Cookie, chocolate chip bar, prep w/marg f/recipe, 2" square	1 ea	32	156	2	19	1	9	2.6	3.3	2.7	10	50
47031	Cookie, chocolate chip, enrich, higher fat, cmrcl, med 2.25"	1 ea	10	49	1	6	0	2	0.8	1.3	0.1	0	0
42726	Cookie, chocolate chip, refrig dough	1 ea	28	127	1	18	1	6	1.8	2.5	0.5	—	—

PAGE KEY: 52 Granola Bars, Cereal Bars, Diet Bars, Scones, and Tarts   52 Meals and Dishes   56 Meats   62 Nuts, Seeds, and Products   64 Poultry 66 Salad Dressings, Dips, and Mayonnaise   66 Salads   68 Sandwiches   70 Sauces and Gravies   70 Snack Foods—Chips, Pretzels, Popcorn 72 Soups, Stews, and Chilis   74 Spices, Flavors, and Seasonings   76 Sports Bars and Drinks   76 Supplemental Foods and Formulas 78 Sweeteners and Sweet Substitutes   78 Vegetables and Legumes   92 Weight Loss Bars and Drinks   94 Miscellaneous

Thia (mg)	Ribo (mg)	Niac (mg NE)	Vit B6 (mg)	Vit B12 (µg)	Fol (µg)	Vit C (mg)	Vit D (IU)	Vit E (mg AT)	Cal (mg)	Iron (mg)	Magn (mg)	Phos (mg)	Pota (mg)	Sodi (mg)	Zinc (mg)	Wat (%)	Alco (g)	Caff (mg)
0.10	0.51	0.28	0.11	1.37	27.0	2.0	—	0.1	448	0.20	41.7	353	573	172	2.2	85	0.00	0.00
—	—	—	—	—	—	0.0	—	—	500	0.72	—	—	—	20	—	—	0.00	0.00
0.15	0.05	0.62	0.05	0.00	15.7	6.5	—	0.8	309	2.77	104.8	100	123	92	0.8	78	0.00	0.00
0.10	0.49	0.25	0.10	1.29	27.0	2.0	—	0.0	419	0.17	39.2	331	537	162	2.0	79	0.00	0.00
0.23	0.49	5.80	0.57	0.00	116.1	0.2	0.0	0.0	10	0.46	8.2	34	49	85	0.2	15	0.00	0.00
0.10	0.10	1.30	0.12	0.00	27.5	3.9	0.0	0.4	2	0.50	4.2	12	12	123	0.1	13	0.00	0.00
0.14	0.11	0.95	0.01	0.03	26.3	0.0	—	0.1	16	1.25	17.4	57	83	175	0.4	14	0.00	1.12
0.02	0.05	0.23	0.01	0.03	7.0	0.1	—	0.7	14	0.43	12.7	32	42	82	0.2	13	0.00	—
0.02	0.14	0.25	0.00	0.01	9.9	0.0	—	0.0	40	0.15	3.4	9	26	212	0.0	33	0.00	0.00
0.11	0.11	0.99	0.05	0.05	5.2	0.9	3.5	1.8	20	1.28	10.1	45	137	163	0.2	20	0.07	0.00
0.14	0.17	1.16	0.20	0.07	11.5	2.9	3.1	1.2	26	1.11	15.5	50	168	181	0.3	33	0.10	0.00
0.05	0.07	0.40	—	—	8.0	0.0	—	—	20	0.72	—	—	—	230	—	—	0.00	0.00
0.12	0.20	1.08	0.03	0.15	25.6	0.2	—	1.5	57	1.52	30.4	101	133	299	0.7	24	0.00	—
0.10	0.12	0.82	0.01	0.07	29.3	0.1	2.9	0.9	18	0.93	10.8	41	64	207	0.3	36	0.00	—
0.12	0.12	0.94	0.01	0.09	33.4	0.2	4.6	0.9	23	1.02	11.3	47	61	232	0.3	28	0.00	—
0.09	0.10	0.85	0.02	0.07	26.9	0.1	—	0.1	76	0.80	10.1	120	63	236	0.3	30	0.00	0.00
—	—	—	—	—	—	—	—	—	3	1.84	—	—	—	241	—	12	0.00	—
0.01	0.03	0.34	0.01	0.00	8.6	0.2	—	0.4	14	0.88	6.9	22	66	116	0.1	25	0.00	0.00
0.23	0.31	1.86	0.05	0.23	13.6	0.4	—	2.4	128	1.86	17.7	137	155	117	0.6	42	0.00	0.00
0.14	0.11	1.28	0.14	0.03	24.4	0.1	—	1.8	53	2.13	51.8	40	325	242	0.3	28	0.00	0.00
0.05	0.10	0.61	0.01	0.09	5.2	0.1	7.2	1.0	51	0.75	6.9	52	50	189	0.3	28	0.07	0.00
0.07	0.11	0.73	0.03	0.11	6.0	1.5	4.4	1.6	67	0.81	5.9	154	53	359	0.2	22	0.00	0.00
0.18	0.18	1.37	0.03	0.09	29.9	1.4	—	1.5	138	1.70	14.9	94	129	367	0.4	32	0.00	0.00
0.03	0.07	0.38	0.00	0.07	12.3	0.0	—	0.2	10	0.40	3.3	41	36	119	0.1	25	0.00	0.00
0.31	0.27	2.56	0.02	0.07	53.0	0.2	—	2.0	205	2.53	16.0	143	106	506	0.5	28	0.00	0.00
0.12	0.18	1.12	0.03	0.11	9.1	0.1	8.7	2.2	76	1.50	13.4	209	136	281	0.4	27	0.17	0.00
0.10	0.20	0.73	0.05	0.25	14.2	0.9	15.8	0.4	21	1.66	19.7	89	98	42	0.6	30	0.00	4.59
—	—	—	—	—	—	0.0	—	—	12	0.54	—	90	45	240	—	—	0.00	0.00
0.07	0.10	0.80	0.01	0.10	14.1	0.0	—	1.5	24	1.33	19.2	103	114	216	0.4	22	0.00	—
—	—	—	—	—	—	1.2	—	—	60	1.08	—	—	—	250	—	—	0.00	0.00
0.11	0.25	0.49	0.05	0.31	29.7	0.5	—	1.1	170	0.46	18.8	232	209	376	0.5	44	0.00	0.00
0.01	0.05	0.31	0.00	0.00	6.5	0.0	—	0.8	15	0.66	10.8	79	96	178	0.2	23	0.00	0.86
0.23	0.30	3.20	0.05	0.10	68.3	0.0	—	0.8	35	4.48	59.4	148	235	650	1.2	4	0.00	7.84
0.21	0.25	2.48	0.05	0.10	48.0	0.0	—	0.2	38	1.89	11.2	83	78	250	0.3	5	0.00	0.00
0.05	0.07	0.50	0.00	0.01	4.1	0.0	0.8	1.6	15	0.51	14.9	35	44	47	0.2	6	0.00	0.00
0.07	0.05	0.37	0.02	0.01	3.1	0.4	1.0	0.7	27	0.72	11.4	47	74	78	0.2	19	0.00	0.00
—	—	—	—	—	—	0.0	—	—	0	0.72	—	—	—	30	—	—	0.00	—
0.01	0.01	0.17	0.00	0.00	5.0	0.0	—	0.0	2	0.12	0.9	6	5	19	0.0	4	0.00	0.00
0.01	0.01	0.17	0.00	0.00	5.0	0.0	—	0.0	2	0.12	0.9	6	5	19	0.0	4	0.00	0.00
0.05	0.05	0.43	0.02	0.02	10.6	0.1	—	0.9	12	0.79	17.6	32	72	116	0.3	6	0.00	5.11
0.01	0.01	0.23	0.00	0.00	6.3	0.0	—	0.2	4	0.36	4.8	12	15	30	0.1	4	0.00	1.10
—	—	—	—	—	—	—	—	—	—	—	—	—	—	88	—	10	0.00	—

PAGE KEY: 2 Beverage and Beverage Mixes 4 Other Beverages 4 Beverages, Alcoholic 6 Candies and Confections, Gum 10 Cereals, Breakfast Type 14 Cheese and Cheese Substitutes 16 Dairy Products and Substitutes 18 Desserts 24 Dessert Toppings 24 Eggs, Substitutes, and Egg Dishes 26 Ethnic Foods 30 Fast Foods/Restaurants 44 Fats, Oils, Margarines, Shortenings, and Substitutes 44 Fish, Seafood, and Shellfish 46 Food Additives 46 Fruit, Vegetable, or Blended Juices 48 Grains, Flours, and Fractions 48 Grain Products, Prepared and Baked Goods

Code	Food Name	Unit/ Amt	Wt (g)	Energy (kcal)	Prot (g)	Carb (g)	Fiber (g)	Fat (g)	Sat (g)	Mono (g)	Poly (g)	Chol (mg)	Vit A (RE)
43660	Cookie, chocolate sandwich	3 ea	33	150	2	23	2	6	0.5	3.5	2.0	0	0
47041	Cookie, chocolate wafer	2 ea	12	52	1	9	0	2	0.5	0.6	0.5	0	0
50962	Cookie, chocolate, fudge stripes	3 ea	32	159	2	21	1	8	5.1	—	—	2	5
47183	Cookie, cinnamon, Teddy Grahams	22 ea	28	120	2	22	—	4	1.0	—	—	—	—
50971	Cookie, creme sandwich, sug free	3 ea	28	120	1	21	2	6	1.3	—	—	1	0
47733	Cookie, Do-Si-Dos	3 ea	36	170	3	22	1	8	1.0	—	—	0	0
47012	Cookie, fig bar	2 ea	32	111	1	23	1	2	0.4	1.0	0.9	0	3
47043	Cookie, fortune	3 ea	24	91	1	20	0	1	0.2	0.3	0.1	0	0
47324	Cookie, fudge brownie, sugar free	1 ea	24	79	1	18	0	0	0.1	0.1	0.0	0	0
47044	Cookie, fudge, cake type	1 ea	21	73	1	16	1	1	0.2	0.4	0.1	0	0
47045	Cookie, gingersnap	4 ea	28	116	2	22	1	3	0.7	1.5	0.4	0	0
47077	Cookie, granola	1 ea	13	60	1	9	1	2	1.6	0.2	0.2	0	0
47737	Cookie, lemon drop	3 ea	33	160	2	20	0	8	2.0	—	—	0	0
43676	Cookie, lemon sandwich	3 ea	33	469	2	23	2	6	0.5	3.5	2.0	0	0
47109	Cookie, molasses, med	1 ea	15	64	1	11	0	2	0.5	1.1	0.3	0	0
47161	Cookie, newton, fig	2 ea	31	116	2	19	2	3	1.0	1.0	0.0	0	—
47252	Cookie, Nutter Butter sandwich	2 ea	28	130	3	19	1	6	1.0	2.5	1.0	5	—
47496	Cookie, oatmeal raisin, home style	1 ea	26	107	1	17	1	4	0.8	1.3	0.3	3	1
47052	Cookie, oatmeal, refrig dough	2 ea	32	136	2	19	1	6	1.5	3.4	0.8	8	3
50948	Cookie, peanut butter	2 ea	28	134	2	16	1	7	1.5	—	—	0	0
47079	Cookie, pecan sandies	1 ea	15	75	1	10	0	4	0.9	2.0	0.5	3	2
47061	Cookie, raisin, soft type	2 ea	30	120	1	20	0	4	1.0	2.3	0.5	1	2
47734	Cookie, Samoas	2 ea	28	160	2	17	2	9	6.0	—	—	0	0
47665	Cookie, shortbread	1 ea	15	75	1	10	0	4	0.9	2.0	0.5	3	2
47011	Cookie, snickerdoodle, prep f/recipe	1 ea	20	80	1	12	0	3	2.1	—	—	9	25
50941	Cookie, sugar	2 ea	28	127	1	18	0	6	1.2	—	—	0	0
47738	Cookie, Tagalongs	2 ea	28	150	3	13	2	10	4.0	—	—	0	0
47739	Cookie, Thin Mints	4 ea	28	140	1	18	1	8	2.0	—	—	0	0
47740	Cookie, Trefoils	5 ea	32	160	2	20	0	8	1.0	—	—	0	0
47715	Cookie, vanilla sandwich	5 ea	43	210	2	30	1	10	2.5	—	—	5	0
47513	Cookie, wedding cake	1 ea	10	53	0	7	0	3	0.5	—	—	0	0
47026	Crackers, animal	10 ea	12	56	1	9	0	2	0.4	1.0	0.2	0	0
50966	Crackers, animal, frosted	1 ea	56	282	2	38	1	14	8.3	—	—	0	0
Doughnuts													
45630	Doughnut, buttermilk, glazed	1 ea	64	270	3	35	0	13	3.0	—	—	15	0
71335	Doughnut, cake, holes	1 ea	14	59	1	7	0	3	0.5	1.3	1.1	5	5
62914	Doughnut, cream puff, choc, custard filled, prep f/rec 3.5 x 2	1 ea	112	293	7	27	1	18	4.6	7.3	4.4	142	234
45508	Doughnut, eclair, chocolate, custard filled, prep f/rec, 5 x 2	1 ea	100	262	6	24	1	16	4.1	6.5	3.9	127	209
71343	Doughnut, glazed, enrich, lrg, 4 1/4"	1 ea	75	302	5	33	1	17	4.4	9.6	2.2	4	3
45507	Doughnut, jelly filled, 3 1/2" oval	1 ea	85	289	5	33	1	16	4.1	8.7	2.0	22	15
71856	Doughnut, plain, wheat free	1 ea	54	154	8	19	0	5	1.5	—	—	33	4
Frozen Desserts													
46110	Cake, ice cream, chocolate roll, 12 oz whl or 1/10 pce	1 pce	34	101	1	14	0	5	2.1	1.8	0.8	15	22
90721	Frozen Dessert Pop, 1.75 fl oz bar	1 ea	52	37	0	10	0	0	0.0	0.0	0.0	0	0
23050	Frozen Dessert Pop, double stick	1 ea	128	92	0	24	0	0	0.0	0.0	0.0	0	0
23051	Frozen Dessert, slushy	1 cup	193	247	1	63	0	0	0.0	0.0	0.0	0	0
23114	Frozen Dessert, snow cone	1 ea	190	243	1	62	0	0	0.0	0.0	0.0	0	0

Thia (mg)	Ribo (mg)	Niac (mg NE)	Vit B6 (mg)	Vit B12 (μg)	Fol (μg)	Vit C (mg)	Vit D (IU)	Vit E (mg AT)	Cal (mg)	Iron (mg)	Magn (mg)	Phos (mg)	Pota (mg)	Sodi (mg)	Zinc (mg)	Wat (%)	Alco (g)	Caff (mg)
—	—	—	—	—	—	0.0	—	—	40	1.08	—	—	—	105	—	—	0.00	—
0.01	0.02	0.34	0.00	0.00	7.3	0.0	—	0.1	4	0.47	6.4	16	25	70	0.1	4	0.00	0.83
—	—	—	—	—	—	0.0	—	—	14	0.61	—	—	—	128	—	—	0.00	—
—	—	—	—	—	—	—	—	—	—	—	—	—	—	170	—	—	0.00	—
0.07	0.07	0.75	—	—	16.5	0.0	—	—	4	0.38	—	—	—	67	—	1	0.00	0.00
—	—	—	—	—	—	0.0	—	—	0	0.36	—	—	—	105	—	—	0.00	0.00
0.05	0.07	0.60	0.01	0.02	11.2	0.1	—	0.2	20	0.93	8.6	20	66	112	0.1	16	0.00	0.00
0.03	0.02	0.43	0.00	0.00	15.8	0.0	—	0.0	3	0.34	1.7	8	10	66	0.0	8	0.00	0.00
0.01	0.02	0.38	0.00	0.00	—	0.0	—	0.0	4	0.43	7.3	17	40	106	0.1	14	0.00	—
0.05	0.03	0.25	0.00	0.01	9.0	0.0	—	0.1	7	0.51	6.7	17	29	40	0.1	12	0.00	0.00
0.05	0.07	0.91	0.02	0.00	24.4	0.0	—	0.3	22	1.78	13.7	23	97	183	0.2	5	0.00	0.00
0.07	0.02	0.23	0.05	0.00	10.5	0.1	—	0.0	9	0.37	13.1	46	47	43	0.2	3	0.00	0.00
—	—	—	—	—	—	0.0	—	—	0	0.72	—	—	—	150	—	8	0.00	0.00
—	—	—	—	—	—	0.0	—	—	40	1.08	—	—	—	80	—	5	0.00	0.00
0.05	0.03	0.44	0.01	0.00	13.4	0.0	—	0.0	11	0.95	7.8	14	52	69	0.1	6	0.00	0.00
—	—	—	—	—	—	—	—	—	—	0.69	—	—	78	116	—	—	0.00	0.00
—	—	—	—	—	—	—	—	—	—	0.72	—	—	55	110	—	0	0.00	0.00
0.07	0.03	0.44	—	—	—	0.0	—	—	8	0.58	—	—	60	98	—	11	0.00	0.00
0.07	0.05	0.60	0.00	0.00	11.2	0.0	—	0.8	10	0.68	9.0	33	47	94	0.2	15	0.00	0.00
0.05	0.05	1.20	—	—	17.4	0.0	—	—	10	0.62	—	—	—	114	—	8	0.00	0.00
0.05	0.05	0.50	0.00	0.00	1.4	0.0	0.9	0.5	5	0.40	2.6	16	15	68	0.1	4	0.00	0.00
0.05	0.05	0.58	0.01	0.00	9.6	0.1	—	0.7	14	0.68	6.3	25	42	101	0.1	13	0.00	0.00
—	—	—	—	—	—	2.4	—	—	0	0.72	—	—	—	45	—	—	0.00	0.00
0.05	0.05	0.50	0.00	0.00	1.4	0.0	0.9	0.5	5	0.40	2.6	16	15	68	0.1	4	0.00	0.00
0.05	0.03	0.40	0.00	0.00	13.6	0.1	2.7	0.1	8	0.46	2.1	10	23	75	0.1	18	0.00	0.00
0.05	0.02	0.67	—	—	14.8	0.0	—	—	12	0.63	—	—	—	86	—	9	0.00	0.00
—	—	—	—	—	—	0.0	—	—	0	0.72	—	—	—	85	—	—	0.00	0.00
—	—	—	—	—	—	0.0	—	—	200	—	—	—	—	80	—	—	0.00	0.00
—	—	—	—	—	—	0.0	—	—	0	0.36	—	—	—	90	—	—	0.00	0.00
—	—	—	—	—	—	0.0	—	—	20	1.08	—	—	—	125	—	1	0.00	0.00
—	—	—	—	—	—	0.0	—	—	0	0.23	—	—	—	15	—	—	0.00	0.00
0.03	0.03	0.43	0.00	0.00	12.9	0.0	—	0.0	5	0.34	2.2	14	12	49	0.1	4	0.00	0.00
—	—	—	—	—	—	0.0	—	—	5	0.62	—	—	—	141	—	—	0.00	0.00
—	—	—	—	—	—	0.0	—	—	60	1.08	—	—	—	290	—	19	0.00	0.00
0.02	0.02	0.25	0.00	0.03	7.3	0.0	—	0.3	6	0.27	2.8	38	18	76	0.1	21	0.00	0.00
0.12	0.30	0.88	0.07	0.37	48.2	0.3	—	2.3	71	1.32	16.8	120	131	377	0.7	52	0.00	2.24
0.11	0.27	0.80	0.05	0.34	43.0	0.3	—	2.0	63	1.17	15.0	107	117	337	0.6	52	0.00	2.00
0.27	0.15	2.14	0.03	0.07	36.8	0.1	—	0.3	32	1.52	16.5	70	81	256	0.6	25	0.00	0.00
0.27	0.11	1.82	0.09	0.18	57.8	0.0	—	0.4	21	1.50	17.0	72	67	249	0.6	36	0.00	0.00
0.02	133.86	0.10	0.02	0.00	19.9	9.6	0.0	0.0	57	0.40	8.2	84	132	—	—	—	0.00	0.00
0.03	0.07	0.30	0.00	0.07	2.3	0.1	3.5	0.3	42	0.50	9.1	40	57	45	0.2	39	0.02	—
0.00	0.00	0.00	0.00	0.00	0.0	0.0	—	0.0	0	0.00	0.5	0	2	6	0.0	80	0.00	0.00
0.00	0.00	0.00	0.00	0.00	0.0	0.0	—	0.0	0	0.00	1.3	0	5	15	0.0	80	0.00	0.00
0.00	0.00	0.00	0.00	0.00	0.0	1.9	—	0.0	4	0.31	1.9	2	6	42	0.0	67	0.00	0.00
0.00	0.00	0.00	0.00	0.00	0.0	1.9	—	0.0	4	0.30	1.9	2	6	42	0.0	67	0.00	0.00

PAGE KEY: 2 Beverage and Beverage Mixes   4 Other Beverages   4 Beverages, Alcoholic   6 Candies and Confections, Gum   10 Cereals, Breakfast Type
14 Cheese and Cheese Substitutes   16 Dairy Products and Substitutes   18 Desserts   24 Dessert Toppings   24 Eggs, Substitutes, and Egg Dishes   26 Ethnic Foods
30 Fast Foods/Restaurants   44 Fats, Oils, Margarines, Shortenings, and Substitutes   44 Fish, Seafood, and Shellfish   46 Food Additives
46 Fruit, Vegetable, or Blended Juices   48 Grains, Flours, and Fractions   48 Grain Products, Prepared and Baked Goods

Code	Food Name	Unit/ Amt	Wt (g)	Energy (kcal)	Prot (g)	Carb (g)	Fiber (g)	Fat (g)	Sat (g)	Mono (g)	Poly (g)	Chol (mg)	Vit A (RE)
2032	Frozen Dessert, sundae, hot fudge	1 ea	158	284	6	48	0	9	5.0	2.3	0.8	21	62
2045	Frozen Yogurt Cone, chocolate, sml	1 ea	78	168	4	24	1	7	4.2	2.3	0.4	1	37
2044	Frozen Yogurt Sandwich	1 ea	85	181	4	32	0	4	2.3	1.3	0.4	1	37
72125	Frozen Yogurt, chocolate	1 cup	174	221	5	38	4	6	4.0	1.7	0.2	23	70
625	Frozen Yogurt, vanilla, lowfat	0.5 cup	106	200	9	31	0	4	2.5	—	—	65	40
72188	Ice Cream Bar, Fudgsicle	1 ea	61	90	3	16	1	2	1.0	—	—	5	0
72187	Ice Cream Bar, Fudgsicle, fat free	1 ea	51	65	3	14	1	0	0.2	—	—	2	0
2113	Ice Cream Cone, chocolate, small	1 ea	78	173	3	25	1	7	4.4	2.2	0.4	18	62
2092	Ice Cream Cone, chocolate dipped	1 ea	78	187	3	24	1	10	5.7	2.9	0.5	29	77
2093	Ice Cream Cone, vanilla, small	1 ea	78	166	3	21	0	8	5.0	2.4	0.4	32	86
2087	Ice Cream Sandwich	1 ea	59	144	3	22	1	6	3.2	1.7	0.4	20	53
2051	Ice Cream, chocolate, soft serve	1 cup	173	355	6	48	1	17	10.3	4.8	0.6	43	147
71814	Ice Cream, neapolitan	0.5 cup	65	130	2	16	0	7	4.0	—	—	25	40
71810	Ice Cream, rocky road	0.5 cup	65	160	3	19	1	8	4.5	—	—	25	40
2053	Ice Cream, strawberry, imit	0.5 cup	66	132	2	16	0	7	5.9	0.4	0.1	0	0
2004	Ice Cream, vanilla	0.5 cup	66	133	2	16	0	7	4.5	2.0	0.3	29	79
72119	Ice Cream, vanilla, fat free	3.6 oz	100	138	4	30	1	0	0.0	0.0	0.0	0	202
2052	Ice Cream, vanilla, imit	0.5 cup	66	132	2	16	0	7	5.9	0.4	0.1	0	0
2020	Milk Shake, chocolate, fast food	1 cup	166	211	6	34	3	6	3.8	1.8	0.2	22	45
2482	Milk Shake, vanilla, fountain type	1 cup	166	224	5	35	0	8	4.9	2.3	0.3	32	80
2011	Sherbet, orange	0.5 cup	74	107	1	22	2	1	0.9	0.4	0.1	0	8
Fruit Desserts													
49005	Apple Brown Betty	0.75 cup	155	268	4	47	3	8	4.2	—	—	16	53
49019	Cobbler, berry	1 cup	217	507	6	94	4	13	2.9	5.6	4.1	2	23
49023	Crisp, cherry	1 cup	246	704	6	113	3	27	4.7	12.3	8.6	2	250
49015	Strudel, apple	1 pce	71	195	2	29	2	8	1.5	2.3	3.8	4	5
Gelatin Desserts													
23052	Gelatin, prep f/dry mix w/water	0.5 cup	135	84	2	19	0	0	0.0	0.0	0.0	0	0
Pastries and Sweet Rolls													
42363	Buns, honey	1 ea	65	270	3	35	1	13	3.0	—	—	0	0
45523	Croissant, cheese, med	1 ea	57	236	5	27	1	12	6.1	3.7	1.4	32	120
71042	Danish, cinnamon nut, 4 1/4"	1 ea	65	280	5	30	1	16	3.8	8.9	2.8	30	6
71041	Danish, raisin nut, 4 1/4"	1 ea	65	280	5	30	1	16	3.8	8.9	2.8	30	6
42746	Danish, strawberry swirl	1 ea	62	254	3	37	1	11	3.0	3.6	4.4	0	0
45549	Dumpling, apple	1 ea	190	672	7	85	3	35	6.9	15.2	10.7	0	8
45515	Fritter, apple	1 ea	24	87	1	8	0	6	1.2	2.4	1.6	20	13
45593	Pastry, apple cinnamon	1 ea	52	205	2	37	1	5	0.9	3.1	1.4	0	100
45594	Pastry, brown sugar cinnamon	1 ea	50	219	3	32	1	9	1.0	3.6	4.6	0	100
45572	Pastry, cheese danish	1 ea	71	266	6	26	1	16	4.8	8.0	1.8	11	26
45595	Pastry, cherry	1 ea	52	204	2	37	1	5	0.9	3.0	1.6	0	100
45601	Pastry, chocolate fudge, frosted	1 ea	52	201	3	37	1	5	1.0	2.7	1.1	0	100
45782	Pastry, s'mores	1 ea	52	204	3	36	1	5	1.5	3.1	0.9	0	100
Pastry, Pie, Dessert Crusts, and Cones													
45500	Crust, pie, graham cracker, prep f/rec, bkd, 9" or 1/8 pce	1 pce	30	148	1	19	0	7	1.6	3.4	2.1	0	61
45535	Crust, pie, rtb, enrich, fzn, 9" whl or 1/8 pce	1 pce	18	82	1	8	0	5	0.8	2.2	2.0	0	0

Thia (mg)	Ribo (mg)	Niac (mg NE)	Vit B6 (mg)	Vit B12 (µg)	Fol (µg)	Vit C (mg)	Vit D (IU)	Vit E (mg AT)	Cal (mg)	Iron (mg)	Magn (mg)	Phos (mg)	Pota (mg)	Sodi (mg)	Zinc (mg)	Wat (%)	Alco (g)	Caff (mg)
0.05	0.30	1.07	0.12	0.64	9.5	2.4	19.0	0.7	207	0.57	33.2	228	395	182	0.9	60	0.00	1.58
0.07	0.18	0.68	0.05	0.18	4.7	0.5	—	0.2	99	0.97	30.8	116	197	84	0.6	53	0.00	—
0.03	0.15	0.34	0.05	0.18	7.3	0.5	—	0.1	95	0.34	12.0	98	151	57	0.4	52	0.00	0.00
0.07	0.31	0.23	0.07	0.11	20.9	11.7	—	0.2	174	0.80	43.5	155	407	110	0.5	71	0.00	5.21
—	—	—	—	—	—	0.0	—	—	250	0.00	—	—	—	55	—	—	0.00	0.00
—	—	—	—	—	—	0.0	—	—	80	0.36	—	—	—	65	—	65	0.00	—
—	—	—	—	—	—	0.5	—	—	81	0.46	—	—	—	48	—	66	0.00	—
0.03	0.12	0.36	0.02	0.27	4.3	0.4	6.2	0.3	88	0.49	17.3	83	168	46	0.4	54	0.00	2.33
0.03	0.18	0.34	0.03	0.25	3.8	0.4	3.7	0.2	88	0.46	18.2	83	161	61	0.6	52	0.00	2.33
0.03	0.18	0.28	0.03	0.28	3.9	0.4	3.7	0.1	95	0.23	11.5	82	151	65	0.5	58	0.00	0.00
0.02	0.11	0.18	0.02	0.18	4.8	0.3	2.4	0.1	60	0.28	12.7	64	122	36	0.4	48	0.00	—
0.07	0.27	0.21	0.05	0.63	9.4	1.1	6.9	0.5	206	0.66	37.3	184	384	89	1.0	58	0.00	5.19
—	—	—	—	—	—	2.0	0.0	—	60	0.00	—	—	—	55	—	61	0.00	—
—	—	—	—	—	—	0.0	0.0	—	60	0.36	—	—	—	65	—	—	0.00	—
0.02	0.15	0.07	0.03	0.38	1.3	0.3	0.0	0.1	90	0.07	10.0	71	144	49	0.7	61	0.00	0.00
0.02	0.15	0.07	0.02	0.25	3.3	0.4	22.9	0.2	84	0.05	9.2	69	131	53	0.5	61	0.00	0.00
0.05	0.25	0.14	0.05	0.44	7.0	0.0	—	0.0	149	0.00	21.0	150	302	97	1.1	64	0.00	0.00
0.02	0.15	0.07	0.03	0.38	1.3	0.3	0.0	0.1	90	0.07	10.0	71	144	49	0.7	61	0.00	0.00
0.10	0.40	0.27	0.07	0.56	8.3	0.7	57.7	0.2	188	0.51	28.3	170	333	161	0.7	72	0.00	1.65
0.05	0.25	0.20	0.05	0.49	7.4	9.0	—	0.1	172	0.38	19.6	135	247	86	0.8	70	0.00	—
0.01	0.07	0.05	0.01	0.09	5.2	4.3	—	0.0	40	0.10	5.9	30	71	34	0.4	66	0.00	0.00
0.23	0.14	2.01	0.07	0.01	32.4	0.3	8.2	0.3	74	1.98	16.4	51	150	309	0.4	61	0.00	0.00
0.31	0.28	2.55	0.07	0.05	12.8	12.4	—	2.8	181	2.39	19.7	134	189	260	0.5	47	0.00	0.00
0.20	0.25	1.98	0.14	0.14	16.1	2.7	—	4.3	153	3.50	19.7	323	219	836	0.4	40	0.00	0.00
0.02	0.01	0.23	0.02	0.15	19.9	1.2	—	1.0	11	0.30	6.4	23	106	191	0.1	44	0.00	0.00
0.00	0.00	0.00	0.00	0.00	1.4	0.0	—	0.0	4	0.02	1.4	30	1	101	0.0	84	0.00	0.00
—	—	—	—	—	—	0.0	—	—	0	0.36	—	—	—	160	—	—	0.00	0.00
0.30	0.18	1.23	0.03	0.18	42.2	0.1	—	0.8	30	1.23	13.7	74	75	316	0.5	21	0.00	0.00
0.14	0.15	1.49	0.07	0.14	53.9	1.1	—	0.5	61	1.16	20.8	72	62	236	0.6	20	0.00	0.00
0.14	0.15	1.49	0.07	0.14	53.9	1.1	—	0.5	61	1.16	20.8	72	62	236	0.6	20	0.00	0.00
—	—	—	—	—	—	0.0	—	—	20	1.08	—	—	—	170	—	16	0.00	0.00
0.40	0.30	3.53	0.05	0.00	11.2	1.6	—	4.5	13	3.11	16.6	76	130	10	0.5	33	0.00	0.00
0.03	0.05	0.31	0.01	0.05	2.9	0.3	—	0.7	13	0.34	3.0	22	34	10	0.1	37	0.00	0.00
0.15	0.17	1.98	0.20	0.00	41.6	0.0	—	0.0	12	1.82	5.7	28	47	174	0.3	12	0.00	0.00
0.15	0.17	2.00	0.20	0.00	40.0	0.0	—	0.0	16	1.79	8.0	32	68	214	0.6	10	0.00	0.00
0.12	0.18	1.41	0.02	0.11	42.6	0.1	—	0.2	25	1.13	10.6	77	70	320	0.5	31	0.00	0.00
0.15	0.17	1.98	0.20	0.00	41.6	0.0	—	0.0	15	1.82	8.3	44	59	220	0.6	12	0.00	0.00
0.15	0.15	1.98	0.20	0.00	52.0	0.0	—	0.0	20	1.82	15.1	44	82	203	0.3	12	0.00	—
0.15	0.15	1.98	0.20	0.00	52.0	0.0	—	0.0	15	1.82	10.9	39	65	199	0.2	12	0.00	—
0.02	0.05	0.63	0.00	0.00	7.2	0.0	—	0.7	6	0.64	5.4	19	26	171	0.1	4	0.00	0.00
0.05	0.07	0.43	0.00	0.00	12.6	0.0	—	0.4	3	0.36	2.9	10	18	104	0.1	21	0.00	0.00

Code	Food Name	Unit/ Amt	Wt (g)	Energy (kcal)	Prot (g)	Carb (g)	Fiber (g)	Fat (g)	Sat (g)	Mono (g)	Poly (g)	Chol (mg)	Vit A (RE)
Pies													
48004	Pie, apple, cmrcl prep, w/enrich flour, 8" whl or 1/6 pce	1 pce	117	277	2	40	2	13	4.4	5.1	2.6	0	39
48023	Pie, banana cream, no bake, prep f/mix, 9" whl or 1/8 pce	1 pce	92	231	3	29	1	12	6.4	4.2	0.7	27	92
48025	Pie, blueberry, cmrcl prep, 8" whl or 1/6 pce	1 pce	117	271	2	41	1	12	2.0	5.0	4.1	0	55
48005	Pie, cherry, cmrcl prep, 8" whl or 1/6 pce	1 pce	117	304	2	47	1	13	3.0	6.8	2.4	0	68
48031	Pie, chocolate cream, cmrcl prep, 8" whl or 1/6 pce	1 pce	113	344	3	38	2	22	5.6	12.6	2.7	6	0
71646	Pie, key lime, w/o topping, 10" whl or 1/8 pce	1 pce	113	420	6	55		20	12.0	—	—	20	40
48177	Pie, lemon, 4 oz svg	1 ea	113	320	3	50	2	12	3.0	—	—	40	0
48040	Pie, peach, 8" whl or 1/6 pce	1 pce	117	261	2	38	1	12	1.8	5.0	4.4	0	19
48012	Pie, pecan, cmrcl prep, 8" whl or 1/6 pce	1 pce	113	452	5	65	4	21	4.0	12.1	3.6	36	59
48000	Pie, pumpkin, cmrcl prep, 8" whl or 1/6 pce	1 pce	109	229	4	30	3	10	1.9	4.4	3.4	22	613
48130	Pie, rhubarb, 9" or 1/8 pce	1 pce	118	316	3	48	2	13	3.6	—	—	3	18
48185	Pie, strawberry, 3.7 oz svg	1 ea	106	310	2	50	1	12	3.0	—	—	0	0
Puddings, Custards, and Pie Fillings													
2659	Custard, chocolate, prep f/dry mix w/2% milk	0.5 cup	136	116	4	18	1	3	1.7	0.8	0.1	10	68
48001	Pie Filling, apple, cnd	0.5 cup	128	129	0	33	1	0	0.0	0.0	0.0	0	0
48015	Pie Filling, cherry, cnd	0.5 cup	132	152	0	37	1	0	0.0	0.0	0.0	0	26
48017	Pie Filling, lemon	0.5 cup	133	463	6	93	1	9	2.2	3.8	1.9	175	125
48044	Pie Filling, pumpkin, cnd	0.5 cup	135	140	1	36	11	0	0.1	0.0	0.0	0	1120
58203	Pudding, all flvrs, not choc, inst, low cal, dry mix	3.6 oz	100	342	1	82	1	1	0.2	0.2	0.3	0	0
2649	Pudding, rice, prep f/dry mix w/2% milk	0.5 cup	144	160	5	30	0	2	1.4	0.6	0.1	9	68
2653	Pudding, tapioca, prep f/dry mix w/2% milk	0.5 cup	141	148	4	28	0	2	1.4	0.6	0.1	8	68
2764	Pudding, vanilla, fat free, 4 oz snack cup	1 ea	113	104	2	23	0	0	0.2	0.0	0.0	2	35
56331	Roll, yorkshire pudding, prep f/recipe, 1.5 oz svg	1 pce	42	87	3	10	0	4	1.8	1.7	0.3	32	27
DESSERT TOPPINGS													
46037	Frosting, chocolate, creamy, 16 oz can	1.328 oz	38	149	0	24	0	7	2.1	3.4	0.8	0	0
46038	Frosting, coconut nut, rte, 16 oz can	1.328 oz	38	155	1	20	1	9	2.6	4.6	1.3	0	0
46323	Frosting, cream cheese, rte	2 Tbs	35	150	0	24	0	6	1.5	—	—	0	0
46330	Frosting, lemon creme, rte	2 Tbs	35	150	0	24	0	6	1.5	—	—	0	0
46336	Frosting, strawberry creme, rte	2 Tbs	35	150	0	24	0	6	1.5	—	—	0	0
54308	Syrup, caramel	2 Tbs	39	100	1	25	0	0	0.0	0.0	0.0	0	0
23437	Syrup, chocolate	2 Tbs	39	100	1	24	—	0	0.0	0.0	0.0	0	0
54312	Syrup, raspberry	2 Tbs	38	100	0	25	0	0	0.0	0.0	0.0	0	0
23069	Topping, butterscotch	2 Tbs	41	103	1	27	0	0	0.0	0.0	0.0	0	11
23070	Topping, caramel	2 Tbs	41	103	1	27	0	0	0.0	0.0	0.0	0	11
23014	Topping, chocolate fudge	2 Tbs	38	133	2	24	1	3	1.5	1.5	0.1	1	2
92528	Topping, hot fudge	1 Tbs	19	70	1	10	—	2	1.0	—	—	5	—
23071	Topping, marshmallow cream, 7 oz jar	1 ea	198	639	2	157	0	1	0.1	0.2	0.1	0	0
23163	Topping, pineapple	2 Tbs	42	108	0	28	0	0	0.0	0.0	0.0	0	1
23164	Topping, strawberry	2 Tbs	42	108	0	28	0	0	0.0	0.0	0.0	0	1
510	Topping, whipped cream, pressurized	2 Tbs	8	19	0	1	0	2	1.0	0.5	0.1	6	14
565	Topping, whipped, lite, Cool Whip	2 Tbs	9	20	0	2	0	1	1.0	0.0	0.0	0	0
EGGS, SUBSTITUTES, AND EGG DISHES													
19525	Egg Substitute, liquid	0.25 cup	63	53	8	0	0	2	0.4	0.6	1.0	1	23
7736	Egg Substitute, Scramblers, fzn	0.25 cup	57	39	7	2	0	0	—	—	—	2	62
19507	Egg Whites, raw	0.625 cup	152	79	17	1	0	0	0.0	0.0	0.0	0	0

PAGE KEY: 52 Granola Bars, Cereal Bars, Diet Bars, Scones, and Tarts   52 Meals and Dishes   56 Meats   62 Nuts, Seeds, and Products   64 Poultry   66 Salad Dressings, Dips, and Mayonnaise   66 Salads   68 Sandwiches   70 Sauces and Gravies   70 Snack Foods—Chips, Pretzels, Popcorn   72 Soups, Stews, and Chilis   74 Spices, Flavors, and Seasonings   76 Sports Bars and Drinks   76 Supplemental Foods and Formulas   78 Sweeteners and Sweet Substitutes   78 Vegetables and Legumes   92 Weight Loss Bars and Drinks   94 Miscellaneous

Thia (mg)	Ribo (mg)	Niac (mg NE)	Vit B6 (mg)	Vit B12 (μg)	Fol (μg)	Vit C (mg)	Vit D (IU)	Vit E (mg AT)	Cal (mg)	Iron (mg)	Magn (mg)	Phos (mg)	Pota (mg)	Sodi (mg)	Zinc (mg)	Wat (%)	Alco (g)	Caff (mg)
0.02	0.02	0.31	0.03	0.00	31.6	3.7	—	1.8	13	0.52	8.2	28	76	311	0.2	52	0.00	0.00
0.09	0.12	0.64	0.02	0.18	19.3	0.5	—	1.5	67	0.41	11.0	154	104	267	0.3	51	0.00	0.00
0.00	0.03	0.34	0.03	0.00	31.6	3.2	—	1.2	9	0.34	5.8	27	58	380	0.2	52	0.00	0.00
0.02	0.02	0.23	0.05	0.00	31.6	1.1	—	0.9	14	0.56	9.4	34	95	288	0.2	46	0.00	0.00
0.03	0.11	0.76	0.01	0.00	14.7	0.0	—	3.1	41	1.21	23.7	77	144	154	0.3	44	0.00	0.00
—	—	—	—	—	—	0.0	—	—	150	0.72	—	—	—	200	—	—	0.00	0.00
—	—	—	—	—	—	0.0	—	—	20	0.72	—	—	—	330	—	—	0.00	0.00
0.07	0.03	0.23	0.02	0.00	33.9	1.1	—	1.1	9	0.57	7.0	26	146	316	0.1	54	0.00	0.00
0.10	0.14	0.28	0.01	0.10	38.4	1.2	—	0.4	19	1.17	20.3	87	84	479	0.6	19	0.00	0.00
0.05	0.17	0.20	0.05	0.28	26.2	1.1	—	1.1	65	0.86	16.4	77	168	307	0.5	58	0.00	0.00
0.18	0.14	1.53	0.01	0.00	36.3	3.8	0.8	1.1	46	1.30	11.4	35	166	197	0.2	45	0.00	0.00
—	—	—	—	—	—	9.0	—	—	20	1.08	—	—	—	300	—	—	0.00	0.00
0.05	0.20	0.15	0.05	0.44	6.8	1.2	49.0	0.1	171	0.40	27.2	133	248	71	0.7	80	0.00	1.36
0.01	0.00	0.03	0.01	0.00	0.0	0.1	—	0.0	5	0.37	2.5	9	57	56	0.1	73	0.00	0.00
0.02	0.01	0.18	0.05	0.00	5.3	4.8	—	0.3	15	0.31	9.2	20	139	24	0.1	71	0.00	0.00
0.09	0.25	0.56	0.07	0.34	18.9	14.1	—	1.2	29	1.12	8.3	88	99	108	0.6	18	0.00	0.00
0.01	0.15	0.50	0.20	0.00	47.2	4.7	—	1.1	50	1.42	21.6	61	186	281	0.4	71	0.00	0.00
0.00	0.00	0.00	0.00	0.00	0.0	0.0	—	0.1	19	0.23	7.0	2179	47	4232		4	0.00	0.00
0.10	0.20	0.63	0.05	0.34	5.8	1.0	48.3	0.1	151	0.52	18.7	125	187	157	0.5	73	0.00	0.00
0.03	0.20	0.10	0.05	0.34	5.6	1.0	48.5	0.1	148	0.07	16.9	116	188	171	0.5	75	0.00	0.00
—	—	—	—	—	—	0.3	—	—	86	0.05	—	115	123	241	—	76	0.00	0.00
0.03	0.07	—	0.02	0.41	3.8	0.4	—	—	55	0.37	—	—	67	248	0.3	57	0.00	0.00
0.00	0.00	0.03	0.00	0.00	0.4	0.0	—	0.6	3	0.52	7.9	30	74	69	0.1	17	0.00	0.75
0.00	0.00	0.07	0.01	0.00	0.8	0.1	—	0.6	5	0.20	7.2	24	70	73	0.2	21	0.00	0.00
—	—	—	—	—	—	0.0	—	—	0	0.00	—	—	—	70	—	14	0.00	0.00
—	—	—	—	—	—	0.0	—	—	0	0.00	—	—	—	70	—	14	0.00	0.00
—	—	—	—	—	—	0.0	—	—	0	0.00	—	—	—	70	—	14	0.00	0.00
—	—	—	—	—	—	0.0	—	—	20	0.00	—	—	—	105	—	33	0.00	0.00
—	—	—	—	—	—	0.0	—	—	0	0.36	—	—	—	25	—	35	0.00	7.00
—	—	—	—	—	—	0.0	—	—	0	0.00	—	—	—	5	—	31	0.00	0.00
0.00	0.03	0.01	0.00	0.03	0.8	0.1	—	0.0	22	0.07	2.9	19	34	143	0.1	32	0.00	0.00
0.00	0.03	0.01	0.00	0.03	0.8	0.1	—	0.0	22	0.07	2.9	19	34	143	0.1	32	0.00	0.00
0.02	0.10	0.14	0.02	0.10	1.9	0.0	—	0.9	38	0.60	24.3	64	171	131	0.3	22	0.00	2.66
—	—	—	—	—	—	—	—	—	—	—	—	—	—	80	—	25	0.00	—
0.00	0.00	0.15	0.00	0.00	2.0	0.0	—	0.0	6	0.43	4.0	16	10	159	0.1	20	0.00	0.00
0.01	0.00	0.03	0.00	0.00	0.9	1.3	—	0.0	3	0.05	2.6	1	18	18	0.0	33	0.00	0.00
0.00	0.00	0.07	0.00	0.00	2.6	5.8	—	0.0	3	0.11	1.7	2	22	9	0.0	33	0.00	0.00
0.00	0.00	0.00	0.00	0.01	0.2	0.0	—	0.0	8	0.00	0.8	7	11	10	0.0	61	0.00	0.00
—	—	—	—	—	—	0.0	—	—	0	0.00	—	0	0	0	—	66	0.00	0.00
0.07	0.18	0.07	0.00	0.18	9.4	0.0	—	0.2	33	1.32	5.6	76	207	111	0.8	83	0.00	0.00
0.17	0.40	0.00	0.12	1.76	—	0.0	—	—	19	0.62	—	59	95	122	0.7	83	0.00	0.00
0.00	0.67	0.15	0.00	0.14	6.1	0.0	0.0	0.0	11	0.11	16.7	23	248	252	0.0	88	0.00	0.00

PAGE KEY: 2 Beverage and Beverage Mixes   4 Other Beverages   4 Beverages, Alcoholic   6 Candies and Confections, Gum   10 Cereals, Breakfast Type
14 Cheese and Cheese Substitutes   16 Dairy Products and Substitutes   18 Desserts   24 Dessert Toppings   24 Eggs, Substitutes, and Egg Dishes   26 Ethnic Foods
30 Fast Foods/Restaurants   44 Fats, Oils, Margarines, Shortenings, and Substitutes   44 Fish, Seafood, and Shellfish   46 Food Additives
46 Fruit, Vegetable, or Blended Juices   48 Grains, Flours, and Fractions   48 Grain Products, Prepared and Baked Goods

Code	Food Name	Unit/ Amt	Wt (g)	Energy (kcal)	Prot (g)	Carb (g)	Fiber (g)	Fat (g)	Sat (g)	Mono (g)	Poly (g)	Chol (mg)	Vit A (RE)
19600	Egg Yolks, raw	0.25 cup	61	196	10	2	0	16	5.8	7.1	2.6	750	238
19539	Eggs, deviled	1 ea	31	63	4	0	0	5	1.2	1.7	1.5	122	50
19510	Eggs, hard bld, lrg	1 ea	50	78	6	1	0	5	1.6	2.0	0.7	212	85
19516	Eggs, scrambled, prep f/one lrg egg butter & milk	1 ea	61	101	7	1	0	7	2.2	2.9	1.3	215	89
19509	Eggs, whole, lrg, fried	1 ea	46	92	6	0	0	7	2.0	2.9	1.2	210	93
19501	Eggs, whole, raw, lrg	1 ea	50	74	6	0	0	5	1.5	1.9	0.7	212	70
19535	Omelette, one egg w/cheese & ham	1 ea	78	156	11	2	0	11	4.5	4.4	1.4	198	133
19536	Omelette, Spanish	1 ea	145	178	8	6	1	14	3.4	5.9	3.0	220	211
19544	Omelette, w/sausage, one egg	1 ea	95	167	11	2	0	13	3.9	5.2	1.9	267	149

ETHNIC FOODS

Italian Foods

Code	Food Name	Unit/ Amt	Wt (g)	Energy (kcal)	Prot (g)	Carb (g)	Fiber (g)	Fat (g)	Sat (g)	Mono (g)	Poly (g)	Chol (mg)	Vit A (RE)
16260	Dinner, chicken, alfredo, w/broccoli, fzn, Healthy Choice	1 ea	326	300	25	34	2	7	3.0	—	—	50	20
56128	Dish, ravioli, cheese, w/tomato sauce, svg	1 ea	250	341	15	38	2	15	6.4	5.0	1.9	162	236
53432	Sauce, marinara	0.5 cup	127	120	2	20	2	4	1.0	—	—	0	50

Mexican Foods

Code	Food Name	Unit/ Amt	Wt (g)	Energy (kcal)	Prot (g)	Carb (g)	Fiber (g)	Fat (g)	Sat (g)	Mono (g)	Poly (g)	Chol (mg)	Vit A (RE)
90856	Beans, refried, fat free, cnd	0.5 cup	130	110	7	21	6	0	0.0	0.0	0.0	0	0
9096	Beans, refried, original, cnd	0.5 cup	128	100	6	18	5	2	1.0	—	—	0	0
9095	Beans, refried, spicy, cnd	0.5 cup	128	100	6	18	6	2	1.0	—	—	0	0
82019	Burrito, bean & cheese, ckd	1 ea	142	300	9	46	4	9	4.5	—	—	15	40
3770	Chicle, fresh, pulp	1 cup	241	200	1	48	13	3	0.5	1.3	0.0	0	14
7931	Chili Peppers, jalapeno, fresh	1 ea	14	4	0	1	0	0	0.0	0.0	0.0	0	11
45777	Dessert, Churro	1 ea	26	116	1	12	0	7	2.0	4.1	0.9	2	6
70150	Dinner, burrito, beef & bean, w/salsa, fzn	1 ea	305	540	24	62	8	22	9.2	8.8	1.8	49	81
1753	Dinner, enchilada & tamale, beef, combination ckd f/fzn	1 ea	312	450	10	56	9	20	8.0	—	—	30	150
56124	Dish, fajitas, beef	1 ea	223	399	23	36	3	18	5.5	7.6	3.5	45	43
56123	Dish, fajitas, chicken	1 ea	223	363	20	44	5	12	2.3	5.5	3.1	39	65
3634	Guava, fresh	0.5 cup	82	56	2	12	4	1	0.2	0.1	0.3	0	51
5224	Jicama, fresh	1 cup	120	46	1	11	—	0	0.0	0.0	0.1	0	2
20122	Mixed Drink, pina colada, non alcoholic, mix	1 ea	30	32	0	7	0	1	0.5	0.0	0.0	0	0
3199	Passion Fruit, purple, fresh	1 ea	18	17	0	4	2	0	0.0	0.0	0.1	0	23
3745	Plantain, fresh, med	1 ea	179	218	2	57	4	1	0.3	0.1	0.1	0	200
56122	Quesadilla	1 ea	54	183	6	18	1	10	3.5	3.4	2.2	13	41
42185	Rolls, Mexican, bolillo	1 ea	117	307	10	61	2	2	0.5	0.2	0.6	1	4
53676	Salsa	2 Tbs	30	10	0	2	0	0	0.0	0.0	0.0	0	0
53207	Salsa, chunky, restaurant style	2 Tbs	30	10	0	1	0	0	0.0	0.0	0.0	0	0
27127	Salsa, garden pepper, med	2 Tbs	31	10	0	2	0	0	0.0	0.0	0.0	0	10
53642	Salsa, green chili, mild	2 Tbs	30	8	0	1	0	0	—	—	—	—	14
53584	Salsa, hot, cnd	2 Tbs	32	5	0	2	0	0	0.0	0.0	0.0	0	20
53645	Salsa, picante, med	2 Tbs	30	8	0	1	0	0	—	—	—	0	14
53647	Salsa, ranchera, hot	2 Tbs	30	9	0	2	0	0	—	—	—	0	36
53686	Salsa, restaurant style	62 g	62	30	2	6	2	0	0.0	0.0	0.0	0	20
4017	Salsa, rstd garlic	68 g	68	30	2	6	2	0	0.0	0.0	0.0	0	20
53643	Salsa, suprema, med	2 Tbs	30	8	0	1	0	0	—	—	—	0	10
27123	Salsa, thick 'n chunky, med	2 Tbs	30	10	0	3	0	0	0.0	0.0	0.0	0	20
53640	Salsa, thick 'n chunky, med	2 Tbs	30	8	0	1	0	0	—	—	—	0	18
53245	Salsa, verde, med	2 Tbs	29	10	0	2	—	0	0.0	0.0	0.0	0	0
53103	Sauce, enchilada, green	1 cup	250	187	4	13	4	14	8.1	3.9	1.2	43	156

PAGE KEY: 52 Granola Bars, Cereal Bars, Diet Bars, Scones, and Tarts   52 Meals and Dishes   56 Meats   62 Nuts, Seeds, and Products   64 Poultry
66 Salad Dressings, Dips, and Mayonnaise   66 Salads   68 Sandwiches   70 Sauces and Gravies   70 Snack Foods—Chips, Pretzels, Popcorn
72 Soups, Stews, and Chilis   74 Spices, Flavors, and Seasonings   76 Sports Bars and Drinks   76 Supplemental Foods and Formulas
78 Sweeteners and Sweet Substitutes   78 Vegetables and Legumes   92 Weight Loss Bars and Drinks   94 Miscellaneous

Thia (mg)	Ribo (mg)	Niac (mg NE)	Vit B6 (mg)	Vit B12 (µg)	Fol (µg)	Vit C (mg)	Vit D (IU)	Vit E (mg AT)	Cal (mg)	Iron (mg)	Magn (mg)	Phos (mg)	Pota (mg)	Sodi (mg)	Zinc (mg)	Wat (%)	Alco (g)	Caff (mg)
0.10	0.31	0.00	0.20	1.17	88.7	0.0	65.3	1.6	78	1.65	3.0	237	66	29	1.4	52	0.00	0.00
0.01	0.15	0.01	0.05	0.31	12.7	0.0	15.0	0.6	15	0.34	2.9	50	37	50	0.3	70	0.00	0.00
0.02	0.25	0.02	0.05	0.56	22.0	0.0	—	0.5	25	0.60	5.0	86	63	62	0.5	75	0.00	0.00
0.02	0.27	0.05	0.07	0.46	18.3	0.1	21.0	0.5	43	0.73	7.3	104	84	171	0.6	73	0.00	0.00
0.02	0.23	0.03	0.07	0.63	23.5	0.0	17.2	0.6	27	0.91	6.0	96	68	94	0.6	69	0.00	0.00
0.02	0.23	0.03	0.07	0.63	23.5	0.0	17.3	0.5	26	0.92	6.0	96	67	70	0.6	76	0.00	0.00
0.10	0.31	0.60	0.11	0.61	17.0	0.1	—	0.8	113	0.81	12.4	179	145	372	1.2	67	0.00	0.00
0.07	0.36	0.81	0.17	0.50	29.7	19.0	—	2.0	60	1.15	16.2	142	269	170	0.8	80	0.00	0.00
0.12	0.36	0.69	0.12	0.79	23.1	0.4	52.4	1.0	64	1.07	12.1	156	162	294	1.1	72	0.00	0.00
—	—	—	—	—	—	12.0	—	—	100	1.79	—	—	—	530	—	—	0.00	0.00
0.31	0.43	2.95	0.18	0.38	30.3	9.4	—	2.1	172	3.09	32.9	220	405	574	1.5	72	0.00	0.00
—	—	—	—	0.00	—	1.2	—	—	0	0.72	—	—	—	480	—	—	0.00	0.00
—	—	—	—	—	—	0.0	—	—	40	2.70	—	—	—	460	—	77	0.00	0.00
—	—	—	—	—	—	0.0	—	—	40	1.98	—	—	—	510	—	78	0.00	0.00
—	—	—	—	—	—	0.0	—	—	40	1.98	—	—	—	630	—	78	0.00	0.00
—	—	—	—	—	—	0.0	—	—	40	0.72	—	—	—	690	—	—	0.00	0.00
0.00	0.05	0.47	0.09	0.00	33.7	35.4	—	0.6	51	1.92	28.9	29	465	29	0.2	78	0.00	0.00
0.01	0.00	0.15	0.07	0.00	6.6	6.2	—	0.1	1	0.10	2.7	4	30	0	0.0	92	0.00	0.00
0.03	0.02	0.37	0.00	0.00	1.2	0.0	—	1.0	2	0.33	1.7	8	8	7	0.1	23	0.00	0.00
0.49	0.44	5.69	0.31	1.08	134.4	20.1	—	1.6	144	5.53	70.7	350	685	881	3.6	63	0.00	0.00
—	—	—	—	—	—	0.0	—	—	150	1.79	—	—	—	1530	—	—	0.00	0.00
0.38	0.30	5.40	0.37	2.05	23.0	26.8	—	1.7	84	3.75	37.6	238	479	316	3.5	65	0.00	0.00
0.43	0.33	6.11	0.37	0.10	41.8	36.8	—	1.7	101	3.31	48.2	188	534	343	1.6	65	0.00	0.00
0.05	0.02	0.88	0.09	0.00	40.4	188.3	—	0.6	15	0.20	18.1	33	344	2	0.2	81	0.00	0.00
0.01	0.02	0.23	0.05	0.00	14.4	24.2	—	0.5	14	0.72	14.4	22	180	5	0.2	90	0.00	0.00
0.00	0.00	0.03	0.00	0.00	3.5	1.5	0.0	0.0	3	0.05	2.3	2	21	2	0.0	75	0.00	0.00
0.00	0.01	0.27	0.01	0.00	2.5	5.4	—	0.0	2	0.28	5.2	12	63	5	0.0	73	0.00	0.00
0.09	0.10	1.23	0.54	0.00	39.4	32.9	—	0.3	5	1.07	66.2	61	893	7	0.3	65	0.00	0.00
0.12	0.14	1.09	0.03	0.05	5.8	14.7	—	1.0	132	1.21	13.4	107	77	230	0.6	35	0.00	0.00
0.69	0.46	6.59	0.03	0.00	41.1	0.0	0.3	0.1	14	3.80	22.1	90	98	7	0.8	37	0.00	0.00
—	—	—	—	—	—	2.4	—	—	0	0.00	—	—	55	115	—	92	0.00	0.00
—	—	—	—	—	—	0.0	—	—	0	0.00	—	—	—	140	—	95	0.00	0.00
—	—	—	—	—	—	0.0	—	—	0	0.00	—	—	—	240	—	91	0.00	0.00
—	—	—	—	—	—	4.1	—	—	5	0.28	—	—	—	175	—	92	0.00	0.00
—	—	—	—	—	—	2.4	—	—	0	0.00	—	—	95	170	—	92	0.00	0.00
—	—	—	—	—	—	2.5	—	—	4	0.01	—	—	—	150	—	92	0.00	0.00
—	—	—	—	—	—	1.3	—	—	5	0.03	—	—	—	171	—	91	0.00	0.00
—	—	—	—	—	—	1.2	—	—	0	0.36	—	—	—	420	—	85	0.00	0.00
—	—	—	—	—	—	1.2	—	—	20	0.00	—	—	—	460	—	—	0.00	0.00
—	—	—	—	—	—	1.5	—	—	3	0.01	—	—	—	166	—	92	0.00	0.00
—	—	—	—	—	—	0.0	—	—	0	0.00	—	—	—	230	—	88	0.00	0.00
—	—	—	—	—	—	4.4	—	—	6	0.05	—	—	—	160	—	92	0.00	0.00
—	—	—	—	—	—	0.0	—	—	0	0.00	—	—	—	95	—	91	0.00	0.00
0.09	0.15	2.92	0.18	0.14	13.3	23.1	0.0	0.9	77	1.17	41.4	118	540	30	0.6	87	0.00	0.00

PAGE KEY: 2 Beverage and Beverage Mixes 4 Other Beverages 4 Beverages, Alcoholic 6 Candies and Confections, Gum 10 Cereals, Breakfast Type
14 Cheese and Cheese Substitutes 16 Dairy Products and Substitutes 18 Desserts 24 Dessert Toppings 24 Eggs, Substitutes, and Egg Dishes 26 Ethnic Foods
30 Fast Foods/Restaurants 44 Fats, Oils, Margarines, Shortenings, and Substitutes 44 Fish, Seafood, and Shellfish 46 Food Additives
46 Fruit, Vegetable, or Blended Juices 48 Grains, Flours, and Fractions 48 Grain Products, Prepared and Baked Goods

Code	Food Name	Unit/ Amt	Wt (g)	Energy (kcal)	Prot (g)	Carb (g)	Fiber (g)	Fat (g)	Sat (g)	Mono (g)	Poly (g)	Chol (mg)	Vit A (RE)
53102	Sauce, enchilada, red	1 cup	250	321	3	10	2	31	16.7	10.1	2.8	91	349
53224	Sauce, taco, thick & smooth, med	1 Tbs	16	10	0	2	0	0	0.0	0.0	0.0	0	0
91932	Seasoning, fajita	0.25 tsp	1	0	0	0	0	0	0.0	0.0	0.0	0	—
57531	Taco, sml	1 ea	171	369	21	27	—	21	11.4	6.6	1.0	56	139
56113	Tamale, w/meat	1 ea	70	134	6	11	1	7	2.6	3.1	1.0	19	14
5445	Tomatillo, fresh, med	1 ea	34	11	0	2	1	0	0.0	0.1	0.1	0	4
42023	Tortilla, corn, med, 6″	1 ea	26	57	1	12	2	1	0.1	0.2	0.4	0	0
90646	Tortilla, flour, 6″	1 ea	32	100	3	16	1	2	0.6	1.2	0.5	0	0
66017	Tostada, bean & cheese	1 ea	144	223	10	27	—	10	5.4	3.1	0.7	30	73
56645	Tostada, beef & cheese	1 ea	163	315	19	23	—	16	10.4	3.3	1.0	41	83
Asian Foods													
7084	Bean Cakes, Japanese style	1 ea	32	130	2	16	1	7	1.0	2.9	2.6	0	0
6459	Bean Sprouts, cnd, svg	1 ea	83	12	1	2	1	0	0.0	—	—	0	0
5654	Broccoli, stir fried	1 cup	156	44	5	8	5	1	0.1	0.0	0.3	0	216
1717	Dinner, stir fry, chicken & veg, oriental, fzn, Healthy Choice	1 ea	337	360	19	57	5	6	2.0	—	—	25	350
70455	Dish, beef, oriental style	1 ea	227	300	10	45	2	7	3.0	—	—	51	100
56094	Dish, chop suey, beef, w/noodles	1 cup	220	421	22	31	—	24	4.7	8.3	9.2	43	103
56234	Dish, chop suey, pork, w/noodles	1 cup	220	448	22	31	4	27	4.8	7.7	12.8	48	19
57618	Dish, chow mein, pork, w/noodles	1 cup	220	448	22	31	4	27	4.8	7.7	12.8	48	19
56238	Dish, chow mein, shrimp, w/noodles	1 cup	220	272	17	24	3	13	1.9	3.1	6.9	82	15
2999	Dish, duck curry, Thai, prep f/recipe, svg	1 ea	277	316	17	5	1	25	8.3	—	—	72	77
56288	Dish, egg foo yung, pork	1 ea	86	124	8	4	1	8	2.1	3.0	2.3	167	86
1991	Dish, green curry chicken, Thai, prep f/recipe, svg	1 ea	386	614	23	18	5	54	42.6	—	—	53	846
1998	Dish, peanut chicken w/rice, Thai, prep f/recipe, svg	1 ea	309	272	19	26	3	11	2.3	—	—	36	351
2998	Dish, potstickers, veal, Thai, prep f/recipe, svg	1 ea	244	647	27	99	4	14	5.0	—	—	58	26
2995	Dish, spring roll, vegetable, Thai, prep f/recipe	1 pce	63	158	4	20	1	7	0.9	—	—	3	140
2996	Dish, sweet noodles, Thai, prep f/recipe, svg	1 ea	142	339	14	37	2	15	2.4	—	—	121	66
3249	Java Plum, fresh	3 ea	9	5	0	1	—	0	—	—	—	0	0
7503	Miso	1 cup	275	547	32	73	15	17	3.1	3.4	8.8	0	22
7508	Natto	1 cup	175	371	31	25	9	19	2.8	4.3	10.9	0	0
38048	Pasta, chow mein noodles, dry	1 cup	45	237	4	26	2	14	2.0	3.5	7.8	0	0
5121	Peas, edible pod, fresh	10 ea	34	14	1	3	1	0	0.0	0.0	0.0	0	37
5666	Peas, snow, pods, stir fried	1 cup	165	69	5	12	4	0	0.1	0.0	0.1	0	21
5665	Peas, snow, pods, stmd	1 cup	165	69	5	12	4	0	0.1	0.0	0.1	0	23
38082	Rice, brown, med grain, ckd	0.5 cup	98	109	2	23	2	1	0.2	0.3	0.3	0	0
38021	Rice, wild, ckd	1 cup	164	166	7	35	3	1	0.1	0.1	0.3	0	0
38289	Rice, wild, dry	1 cup	160	571	24	120	10	2	0.2	0.3	1.1	0	3
1985	Salad, chicken, broiled, Thai, prep f/recipe, svg	1 ea	403	257	24	25	2	7	1.9	—	—	60	139
1987	Sauce, coconut, Thai, prep f/recipe, svg	1 ea	126	65	2	13	2	1	0.1	—	—	0	207
1999	Sauce, peanut, Thai, prep f/recipe, svg	0.75 cup	199	412	18	19	4	33	6.6	—	—	0	37
53461	Sauce, plum, rts	2 Tbs	38	70	0	16	0	0	0.1	0.1	0.2	0	2
53357	Sauce, sweet & sour, rts	2 Tbs	33	40	0	8	0	1	0.1	0.2	0.4	0	5
53004	Sauce, teriyaki, rts	1 Tbs	18	15	1	3	0	0	0.0	0.0	0.0	0	0
5253	Seaweed, agar, fresh	0.5 cup	40	10	0	3	0	0	0.0	0.0	0.0	0	0
50181	Soup, won ton	1 cup	241	182	14	14	1	7	2.3	3.0	1.0	53	99
91818	Sushi, California roll	1 ea	198	292	8	49	3	3	1.0	—	—	3	90

Thia (mg)	Ribo (mg)	Niac (mg NE)	Vit B6 (mg)	Vit B12 (µg)	Fol (µg)	Vit C (mg)	Vit D (IU)	Vit E (mg AT)	Cal (mg)	Iron (mg)	Magn (mg)	Phos (mg)	Pota (mg)	Sodi (mg)	Zinc (mg)	Wat (%)	Alco (g)	Caff (mg)
0.07	0.12	0.74	0.14	0.10	17.0	20.3	0.0	1.6	55	0.62	20.0	76	336	36	0.3	82	0.00	0.00
—	—	—	—	—	—	0.0	—	—	0	0.36	—	—	40	125	—	85	0.00	0.00
—	—	—	—	—	—	—	—	—	—	—	—	—	—	130	—	—	0.00	0.00
0.15	0.43	3.21	0.23	1.03	68.4	2.2	—	1.9	221	2.41	70.1	203	474	802	3.9	58	0.00	0.00
0.17	0.14	2.49	0.09	0.17	4.5	1.0	—	0.3	24	1.41	20.7	67	140	84	0.9	64	0.00	0.00
0.00	0.00	0.62	0.01	0.00	2.4	4.0	—	0.1	2	0.20	6.8	13	91	0	0.1	92	0.00	0.00
0.01	0.01	0.38	0.05	0.00	1.3	0.0	—	0.1	21	0.31	18.7	82	48	12	0.3	46	0.00	0.00
0.17	0.09	1.13	0.01	0.00	33.3	0.0	—	0.1	41	1.07	7.0	40	50	204	0.2	30	0.00	0.00
0.10	0.33	1.32	0.15	0.68	43.2	1.3	—	1.2	210	1.88	59.0	117	403	543	1.9	66	0.00	0.00
0.10	0.55	3.15	0.23	1.16	75.0	2.6	—	—	217	2.86	63.6	179	572	896	3.7	62	0.00	0.00
0.07	0.05	0.55	0.01	0.00	9.1	0.0	0.0	1.2	3	0.67	6.1	21	58	1	0.2	23	0.00	0.00
—	—	—	—	0.00	—	14.2	—	—	10	0.25	—	—	—	20	—	96	0.00	0.00
0.09	0.18	0.93	0.23	0.00	88.5	123.4	0.0	0.7	75	1.37	39.0	103	505	42	0.6	91	0.00	0.00
—	—	—	—	—	—	4.8	—	—	40	2.70	—	—	—	600	—	—	0.00	0.00
—	—	—	—	—	—	18.0	—	—	60	2.70	—	—	—	1220	—	—	0.00	0.00
0.36	0.37	5.73	0.38	1.67	43.8	20.1	—	1.8	39	4.19	54.2	262	519	950	3.5	63	0.00	0.00
0.77	0.43	6.23	0.41	0.41	41.8	20.2	—	2.7	45	3.29	52.8	249	489	848	2.6	62	0.00	0.00
0.77	0.43	6.23	0.41	0.41	41.8	20.2	—	2.7	45	3.29	52.8	249	489	848	2.6	62	0.00	0.00
0.23	0.23	4.46	0.18	0.58	45.1	9.4	—	1.3	58	3.42	51.2	220	391	710	1.3	74	0.00	0.00
0.15	0.25	4.46	0.23	0.28	8.9	5.0	10.2	0.6	72	2.94	77.8	204	742	602	1.7	80	0.00	0.00
0.12	0.25	0.79	0.14	0.40	22.3	3.2	—	1.1	27	0.81	11.9	105	157	131	0.9	75	0.00	0.00
0.15	0.17	7.65	0.49	0.23	57.0	91.5	7.1	2.0	65	7.82	140.7	331	866	889	2.6	74	0.00	0.00
0.21	0.11	8.25	0.47	0.14	66.1	67.3	5.1	1.7	42	2.66	48.0	191	344	901	1.2	81	0.00	0.00
0.87	0.72	12.23	0.21	0.57	145.1	1.8	5.1	1.4	106	6.73	50.2	238	329	1020	2.9	41	0.00	0.00
0.18	0.14	1.87	0.02	0.00	31.7	0.9	8.2	1.3	58	1.77	11.9	42	75	263	0.4	49	0.00	0.00
0.07	0.09	1.01	0.14	0.56	15.2	4.6	50.8	1.6	277	2.92	40.1	170	176	377	1.3	50	0.00	0.00
0.00	0.00	0.01	0.00	0.00	—	1.3	—	—	2	0.01	1.4	2	7	1	0.0	83	0.00	0.00
0.27	0.63	2.49	0.55	0.21	52.2	0.0	—	0.0	157	6.84	132.0	437	578	10252	7.0	43	0.00	0.00
0.28	0.33	0.00	0.23	0.00	14.0	22.8	—	0.0	380	15.05	201.2	304	1276	12	5.3	55	0.00	0.00
0.25	0.18	2.68	0.05	0.00	40.5	0.0	—	1.6	9	2.13	23.4	72	54	198	0.6	1	0.00	0.00
0.05	0.02	0.20	0.05	0.00	14.3	20.4	—	0.1	15	0.70	8.2	18	68	1	0.1	89	0.00	0.00
0.21	0.12	0.93	0.25	0.00	55.1	84.2	0.0	0.6	71	3.43	39.6	87	330	7	0.4	89	0.00	0.00
0.21	0.12	0.93	0.23	0.00	58.4	84.2	0.0	0.6	71	3.43	39.6	87	330	7	0.4	89	0.00	0.00
0.10	0.00	1.29	0.15	0.00	3.9	0.0	—	0.2	10	0.51	42.9	75	77	1	0.6	73	0.00	0.00
0.09	0.14	2.10	0.21	0.00	42.6	0.0	—	0.4	5	0.98	52.5	134	166	5	2.2	74	0.00	0.00
0.18	0.41	10.77	0.62	0.00	152.0	0.0	—	1.3	34	3.14	283.2	693	683	11	9.5	8	0.00	0.00
0.15	0.15	10.36	0.56	0.25	29.1	27.3	8.6	0.7	38	2.00	48.7	208	511	1637	1.1	85	0.00	0.00
0.05	0.05	0.85	0.02	0.00	6.9	5.0	0.0	0.1	33	0.74	17.2	27	319	82	0.2	85	0.00	0.00
0.09	0.14	10.18	0.44	0.00	55.1	2.2	0.0	6.4	40	2.13	107.8	297	544	3376	2.1	60	0.00	0.00
0.00	0.02	0.38	0.02	0.00	2.3	0.2	—	0.1	5	0.55	4.6	8	99	205	0.1	54	0.00	0.00
0.00	0.00	0.07	0.00	0.00	0.7	0.0	—	0.1	6	0.28	2.3	3	22	116	0.0	71	0.00	0.00
0.00	0.00	0.23	0.01	0.00	3.6	0.0	—	0.0	4	0.31	11.0	28	40	690	0.0	68	0.00	0.00
0.00	0.00	0.01	0.00	0.00	34.0	0.0	—	0.3	22	0.74	26.8	2	90	4	0.2	91	0.00	0.00
0.40	0.25	4.59	0.20	0.40	18.8	3.4	—	0.4	31	1.75	20.6	153	316	543	1.1	84	0.00	0.00
—	—	—	—	—	—	4.8	—	—	20	1.08	—	—	—	952	—	—	0.00	0.00

Code	Food Name	Unit/ Amt	Wt (g)	Energy (kcal)	Prot (g)	Carb (g)	Fiber (g)	Fat (g)	Sat (g)	Mono (g)	Poly (g)	Chol (mg)	Vit A (RE)
91814	Sushi, cucumber roll	6 pce	85	120	3	25	2	1	0.0	—	—	0	50
92378	Sushi, krab roll	6 pce	112	150	7	30	2	1	0.0	—	—	3	60
56313	Sushi, w/veg & fish	3 oz	85	119	5	24	1	0	0.1	0.1	0.1	6	70
6880	Sweetpotatoes, fresh, cubes	1 cup	133	114	2	27	4	0	0.0	0.0	0.0	0	1886
6206	Vegetables, Japanese style, fzn	0.5 cup	127	78	2	8	2	5	2.3	—	—	12	96
6208	Vegetables, Japanese style, stir fry, fzn	0.5 cup	116	35	2	7	2	0	0.0	—	—	0	74
57294	Vegetables, oriental style, stir fry, fzn	0.5 cup	54	41	2	7	0	1	0.1	—	—	0	38
6646	Vegetables, pepper style, stir fry, fzn	0.5 cup	54	15	0	3	1	0	0.0	—	—	0	23
6592	Vegetables, teriyaki, marinated/seasoned, fzn	1.25 cup	110	100	2	7	2	7	1.0	—	—	0	500
6460	Waterchestnuts, slices, cnd	100 g	100	50	1	12	5	0	0.0	—	—	0	0
5222	Watercress, fresh, chpd	1 cup	34	4	1	0	0	0	0.0	0.0	0.0	0	160
49116	Wrappers, egg roll, 7" square	1 ea	32	93	3	19	1	0	0.1	0.1	0.2	3	1

FAST FOODS/RESTAURANTS

Generic Fast Food

Code	Food Name	Unit/ Amt	Wt (g)	Energy (kcal)	Prot (g)	Carb (g)	Fiber (g)	Fat (g)	Sat (g)	Mono (g)	Poly (g)	Chol (mg)	Vit A (RE)
56654	Cheeseburger, double, double bun, reg, w/condiments & veg	1 ea	228	650	30	53	—	35	12.8	12.6	6.4	93	84
56648	Cheeseburger, lrg, plain	1 ea	185	609	30	47	—	33	14.8	12.7	2.4	96	185
66015	Cheeseburger, reg, w/condiments & veg	1 ea	154	359	18	28	—	20	9.2	7.2	1.5	52	91
6175	Dish, corn, cob, w/butter	1 ea	146	155	4	32	—	3	1.6	1.0	0.6	6	51
6185	Dish, mashed potatoes	0.5 cup	121	100	3	20	—	1	0.6	0.4	0.4	2	15
17187	Fish, fillet, brd/batter fried	3 oz	85	197	12	14	0	10	2.4	2.2	5.3	29	9
42353	French Toast, w/butter	2 pce	135	356	10	36	0	19	7.7	7.1	2.4	116	138
66007	Hamburger, reg, plain	1 ea	90	274	12	31	—	12	4.1	5.5	0.9	35	0
2022	Milk Shake, strawberry, fast food	1 cup	283	320	10	53	1	8	4.9	2.2	0.3	31	74
2024	Milk Shake, vanilla, fast food	1 cup	166	185	6	30	0	5	3.1	1.4	0.2	18	63
56639	Nachos, w/cheese	7 pce	113	346	9	36	—	19	7.8	8.0	2.2	18	154
6176	Onion Rings, breaded, fried, svg	8 pce	78	259	3	29	—	15	6.5	6.3	0.6	13	2
45122	Pancakes, w/butter & syrup	1 ea	116	260	4	45	1	7	2.9	2.6	1.0	29	41
5463	Potatoes, hash browns	0.5 cup	72	151	2	16	—	9	4.3	3.9	0.5	9	3
6173	Salad, potato	0.333 cup	95	108	1	13	—	6	1.0	1.6	2.9	57	28
56623	Salad, tossed, veg, w/o dressing	1.5 cup	207	33	3	7	—	0	0.0	0.0	0.1	0	236
56601	Sandwich, breakfast, egg bacon, w/biscuit	1 ea	150	458	17	29	1	31	8.0	13.4	7.5	352	108
56602	Sandwich, breakfast, egg ham, w/biscuit	1 ea	192	442	20	30	1	27	5.9	11.0	7.7	300	240
56600	Sandwich, breakfast, egg, w/biscuit	1 ea	136	373	12	32	1	22	4.7	9.1	6.4	245	181
56606	Sandwich, croissant, w/egg & cheese	1 ea	127	368	13	24	—	25	14.1	7.5	1.4	216	282
56607	Sandwich, croissant, w/egg, cheese & bacon	1 ea	129	413	16	24	—	28	15.4	9.2	1.8	215	142
66031	Sandwich, english muffin, w/cheese & sausage	1 ea	115	393	15	29	1	24	9.9	10.1	2.7	59	104
56604	Sandwich, ham, w/biscuit	1 ea	113	386	13	44	1	18	11.4	4.8	1.0	25	33

A&W Restaurants

Code	Food Name	Unit/ Amt	Wt (g)	Energy (kcal)	Prot (g)	Carb (g)	Fiber (g)	Fat (g)	Sat (g)	Mono (g)	Poly (g)	Chol (mg)	Vit A (RE)
81303	Cheeseburger	1 ea	191	500	28	43	3	24	9.0	—	—	90	200
81305	Cheeseburger, deluxe, w/bacon	1 ea	278	600	32	44	4	33	12.0	—	—	110	250
81319	Dish, french fries, cheese, svg	1 ea	170	390	4	50	4	19	5.0	—	—	5	0
81352	Frozen Dessert, Oreo, med, A&W Polar Swirl	1 ea	397	833	16	125	2	30	11.7	—	—	54	350
81330	Frozen Dessert, sundae, hot fudge, A&W	1 ea	189	350	8	54	1	11	6.0	—	—	30	150
81311	Hamburger	1 ea	177	460	26	39	3	22	8.0	—	—	75	40
81314	Hot Dog, cheese, w/bun	1 ea	126	320	11	25	1	20	7.0	—	—	40	20
81315	Hot Dog, chili & cheese, w/bun	1 ea	154	350	13	27	2	21	8.0	—	—	45	40

Thia (mg)	Ribo (mg)	Niac (mg NE)	Vit B6 (mg)	Vit B12 (µg)	Fol (µg)	Vit C (mg)	Vit D (IU)	Vit E (mg AT)	Cal (mg)	Iron (mg)	Magn (mg)	Phos (mg)	Pota (mg)	Sodi (mg)	Zinc (mg)	Wat (%)	Alco (g)	Caff (mg)
—	—	—	—	—	—	0.0	—	—	0	0.36	—	—	—	90	—	65	0.00	0.00
—	—	—	—	—	—	0.0	—	—	0	0.36	—	—	—	240	—	—	0.00	0.00
0.14	0.03	1.51	0.07	0.17	7.9	2.0	—	0.3	13	1.19	13.7	56	112	48	0.4	65	0.03	0.00
0.10	0.07	0.74	0.28	0.00	14.6	3.2	—	0.3	40	0.81	33.2	63	448	73	0.4	77	0.00	0.00
0.05	0.09	0.37	0.10	0.00	35.4	44.4	—	—	40	0.69	21.6	50	179	320	—	—	0.00	0.00
—	—	—	—	—	—	32.4	—	—	31	0.70	15.1	42	191	439	—	—	0.00	0.00
—	—	—	—	0.00	—	5.6	—	—	33	0.27	—	—	—	281	—	—	0.00	0.00
—	—	—	—	0.00	—	9.1	—	—	3	0.10	—	—	—	9	—	—	0.00	0.00
—	—	—	—	0.00	—	21.0	—	—	20	0.00	—	—	—	510	—	—	0.00	0.00
—	—	—	—	0.00	—	0.0	—	—	3	0.27	—	—	—	12	—	86	0.00	0.00
0.02	0.03	0.07	0.03	0.00	3.1	14.6	—	0.3	41	0.07	7.1	20	112	14	0.0	95	0.00	0.00
0.17	0.11	1.74	0.00	0.00	27.5	0.0	—	0.0	15	1.08	6.4	26	26	183	0.2	29	0.00	0.00
0.56	0.43	8.34	0.27	2.06	91.2	2.7	—	2.0	169	4.71	36.5	349	390	921	4.1	47	0.00	0.00
0.47	0.56	11.17	0.28	2.52	74.0	0.0	22.2	—	91	5.46	38.9	422	644	1589	5.6	39	0.00	0.00
0.31	0.23	6.38	0.15	1.23	64.7	2.3	—	1.3	182	2.65	26.2	216	229	976	2.6	55	0.00	0.00
0.25	0.10	2.18	0.31	0.00	43.8	6.9	—	—	4	0.87	40.9	108	359	29	0.9	72	0.00	0.00
0.10	0.05	1.45	0.28	0.05	9.7	0.5	—	—	25	0.56	21.8	67	356	275	0.4	79	0.00	0.00
0.09	0.09	1.78	0.09	0.93	14.5	0.0	—	—	15	1.78	20.4	145	272	452	0.4	54	0.00	0.00
0.57	0.50	3.92	0.05	0.36	72.9	0.1	—	—	73	1.88	16.2	146	177	513	0.6	51	0.00	0.00
0.33	0.27	3.72	0.05	0.88	53.1	0.0	10.8	0.5	63	2.40	18.9	103	145	387	2.0	38	0.00	0.00
0.12	0.55	0.50	0.11	0.87	8.5	2.3	22.6	0.4	320	0.31	36.8	283	515	235	1.0	74	0.00	0.00
0.07	0.30	0.31	0.09	0.60	8.3	1.3	60.6	0.1	203	0.15	20.0	170	290	136	0.6	75	0.00	0.00
0.18	0.37	1.53	0.20	0.81	10.2	1.2	—	—	272	1.27	55.4	276	172	816	1.8	40	0.00	0.00
0.07	0.09	0.87	0.05	0.11	51.6	0.5	—	0.3	69	0.80	14.8	81	122	405	0.3	37	0.00	0.00
0.20	0.28	1.69	0.05	0.11	25.5	1.7	—	0.7	64	1.30	24.4	238	125	552	0.5	50	0.00	0.00
0.07	0.00	1.07	0.17	0.00	7.9	5.5	—	0.1	7	0.47	15.8	69	267	290	0.2	60	0.00	0.00
0.07	0.10	0.25	0.14	0.10	23.8	1.0	—	—	13	0.68	7.6	53	256	312	0.2	79	0.00	0.00
0.05	0.10	1.13	0.17	0.00	76.6	48.0	—	—	27	1.29	22.8	81	356	54	0.4	96	0.00	0.00
0.14	0.23	2.40	0.14	1.02	60.0	2.7	—	2.0	189	3.74	24.0	238	250	999	1.6	47	0.00	0.00
0.67	0.60	2.00	0.27	1.19	65.3	0.0	—	2.3	221	4.55	30.7	317	319	1382	2.2	55	0.00	0.00
0.30	0.49	2.15	0.10	0.62	57.1	0.1	—	3.3	82	2.90	19.0	388	238	891	1.0	50	0.00	0.00
0.18	0.37	1.50	0.10	0.76	47.0	0.1	—	—	244	2.20	21.6	348	174	551	1.8	45	0.00	0.00
0.34	0.34	2.19	0.11	0.86	45.1	2.2	—	—	151	2.19	23.2	276	201	889	1.9	44	0.00	0.00
0.69	0.25	4.13	0.15	0.68	66.7	1.3	—	1.3	168	2.25	24.1	186	215	1036	1.7	38	0.00	0.00
0.50	0.31	3.48	0.14	0.02	38.4	0.1	—	1.7	160	2.72	22.6	554	197	1433	1.6	28	0.00	0.00
—	—	—	—	—	—	2.4	—	—	150	4.50	—	—	—	870	—	—	0.00	0.00
—	—	—	—	—	—	6.0	—	—	200	5.40	—	—	—	1390	—	—	0.00	0.00
—	—	—	—	—	—	18.0	—	—	40	0.00	—	—	—	880	—	—	0.00	0.00
—	—	—	—	—	—	0.0	—	—	467	4.19	—	—	—	646	—	—	0.00	—
—	—	—	—	—	—	0.0	—	—	200	0.36	—	—	—	140	—	60	0.00	—
—	—	—	—	—	—	2.4	—	—	100	4.50	—	—	—	690	—	—	0.00	0.00
—	—	—	—	—	—	1.2	—	—	60	1.44	—	—	—	920	—	—	0.00	0.00
—	—	—	—	—	—	1.2	—	—	80	1.79	—	—	—	1080	—	—	0.00	0.00

Code	Food Name	Unit/ Amt	Wt (g)	Energy (kcal)	Prot (g)	Carb (g)	Fiber (g)	Fat (g)	Sat (g)	Mono (g)	Poly (g)	Chol (mg)	Vit A (RE)
81317	Hot Dog, w/bun	1 ea	90	280	11	22	1	17	6.0	—	—	35	20
81341	Ice Cream Float, root beer, med	1 ea	467	330	4	70	0	4	2.5	—	—	15	100
81348	Milk Shake, chocolate, med, A&W	1 ea	475	700	11	100	2	29	18.1	—	—	125	312
81358	Milk Shake, vanilla, med, A&W	1 ea	475	719	12	97	0	31	18.8	—	—	134	250
81343	Potatoes, french fries, sml svg	1 ea	113	313	4	45	4	13	3.3	—	—	0	0
81310	Sandwich, chicken, grilled	1 ea	262	430	37	37	4	15	3.5	—	—	90	40
Arby's													
42433	Biscuit, w/butter	1 ea	82	280	5	27	0	17	4.0	—	—	0	—
9008	Cheese, mozzarella sticks, 4.8 oz svg	1 ea	137	470	18	34	2	29	14.0	—	—	60	—
9011	Chicken, finger, 4 pack	1 ea	192	640	31	42	0	38	8.0	—	—	70	—
9009	Onion, petals	4 oz	113	410	4	43	2	24	3.5	—	—	0	—
8986	Potatoes, french fries, curly, med svg	1 ea	128	400	5	50	4	19	4.5	—	—	0	0
8997	Salad, caesar	1 ea	223	90	7	8	3	4	2.5	—	—	10	—
52074	Salad, garden	1 ea	349	70	4	14	6	1	0.0	—	—	0	518
8988	Sandwich, beef melt, w/cheddar	1 ea	150	320	16	36	2	14	6.0	—	—	45	—
69045	Sandwich, beef, Arby Q	1 ea	186	360	16	40	2	14	4.0	—	—	70	—
69055	Sandwich, beef, philly & swiss cheese, submarine	1 ea	311	670	36	46	4	40	16.0	—	—	75	—
56341	Sandwich, chicken, breast fillet	1 ea	208	550	24	47	2	30	5.0	—	—	90	—
69095	Sandwich, chicken, cordon bleu	1 ea	242	630	34	47	2	35	8.0	14.4	12.6	120	—
69046	Sandwich, chicken, grilled, deluxe	1 ea	252	450	29	37	2	22	4.0	—	—	110	88
69043	Sandwich, French dip, submarine	1 ea	285	410	28	43	2	16	9.0	—	—	45	—
56342	Sandwich, ham swiss, hot	1 ea	170	340	23	35	1	13	4.5	—	—	90	40
8992	Sandwich, roast beef swiss	1 ea	360	780	37	74	6	40	14.0	—	—	80	—
56336	Sandwich, roast beef, regular	1 ea	157	330	21	35	2	14	7.0	—	—	45	0
53256	Sauce, Arbys, pkt	1 ea	14	15	0	4	0	0	0.0	0.0	0.0	0	—
9025	Sauce, honey mustard, dipping	1 oz	28	130	0	5	0	12	1.5	—	—	10	—
Boston Market													
52109	Cole Slaw, svg	1 ea	430	310	7	29	10	22	3.0	—	—	20	—
57529	Dish, macaroni & cheese, svg	1 ea	192	280	13	33	1	11	6.0	—	—	30	—
7390	Dish, mashed potatoes, homestyle, svg	1 ea	173	210	4	30	2	9	5.0	—	—	25	—
57528	Dish, mashed potatoes, w/gravy, homestyle, svg	1 ea	201	230	4	32	3	9	5.0	—	—	25	—
57530	Dish, pot pie, chicken, original, svg	1 ea	425	750	26	57	2	46	14.0	—	—	110	—
53541	Gravy, chicken, 1 oz svg	1 ea	28	15	0	2	0	0	0.0	—	—	0	—
52104	Salad, caesar, svg	1 ea	269	470	14	17	3	40	9.0	—	—	35	—
1143	Sandwich, marinated grilled chicken	1 ea	284	670	42	45	2	36	6.0	—	—	105	—
50299	Soup, chicken noodle, hearty, svg	1 cup	190	100	6	8	0	4	1.5	—	—	30	—
7391	Spinach, creamed, svg	1 ea	181	260	9	11	2	20	13.0	—	—	55	—
Burger King													
56352	Cheeseburger	1 ea	136	370	20	31	2	18	9.0	—	—	55	60
57001	Cheeseburger, double	1 ea	197	570	35	32	2	34	17.0	—	—	110	100
56355	Cheeseburger, Whopper	1 ea	303	780	34	55	4	47	17.0	—	—	105	150
57000	Cheeseburger, Whopper Jr	1 ea	180	460	21	33	2	27	10.0	—	—	60	80
9087	Chicken, Tenders, 4 pce svg	1 ea	62	170	11	10	0	9	3.0	—	—	25	0
42429	French Toast, sticks, svg	1 ea	112	390	6	46	2	20	4.5	—	—	0	0
56351	Hamburger	1 ea	123	320	18	30	2	14	6.0	—	—	45	20
56354	Hamburger, Whopper	1 ea	278	680	29	53	4	39	12.0	—	—	80	100

Thia (mg)	Ribo (mg)	Niac (mg NE)	Vit B6 (mg)	Vit B12 (µg)	Fol (µg)	Vit C (mg)	Vit D (IU)	Vit E (mg AT)	Cal (mg)	Iron (mg)	Magn (mg)	Phos (mg)	Pota (mg)	Sodi (mg)	Zinc (mg)	Wat (%)	Alco (g)	Caff (mg)
—	—	—	—	—	—	0.0	—	—	40	1.44	—	—	—	710	—	—	0.00	0.00
—	—	—	—	—	—	0.0	—	—	150	0.36	—	—	—	120	—	—	0.00	0.00
—	—	—	—	—	—	0.0	—	—	281	1.69	—	—	—	200	—	—	0.00	—
—	—	—	—	—	—	0.0	—	—	438	1.69	—	—	—	212	—	—	0.00	0.00
—	—	—	—	—	—	19.6	—	—	0	0.00	—	—	—	465	—	—	0.00	0.00
—	—	—	—	—	—	6.0	—	—	100	3.59	—	—	—	1080	—	—	0.00	0.00
0.23	0.14	3.00	—	—	—	0.0	—	—	40	0.00	—	—	130	780	—	—	0.00	0.00
—	—	—	—	—	—	1.2	—	—	400	0.72	—	—	—	1330	—	—	0.00	0.00
—	—	—	—	—	—	0.0	—	—	20	2.70	—	—	—	1590	—	—	0.00	0.00
—	—	—	—	—	—	0.0	—	—	40	0.72	—	—	—	300	—	—	0.00	0.00
0.07	0.09	2.57	—	0.00	—	15.5	—	—	0	1.86	—	—	934	993	0.8	41	0.00	0.00
—	—	—	—	—	—	42.0	—	—	200	1.79	—	—	—	170	—	—	0.00	0.00
0.17	0.20	1.26	—	—	—	42.0	—	—	80	1.44	—	—	635	45	0.9	—	0.00	0.00
—	—	—	—	—	—	0.0	—	—	80	2.70	—	—	—	850	—	—	0.00	0.00
0.25	0.37	9.00	—	—	—	4.8	—	—	80	3.59	—	—	456	1530	—	—	0.00	0.00
0.44	0.72	13.89	—	—	—	9.0	—	—	300	2.70	—	—	646	1850	5.9	—	0.00	0.00
0.23	0.56	9.17	0.38	—	18.4	3.6	—	—	80	1.79	30.6	184	336	1160	0.2	—	0.00	0.00
0.44	0.68	10.97	—	—	—	1.2	—	—	200	0.89	—	—	499	1820	2.4	—	0.00	0.00
0.34	0.31	14.89	—	—	—	1.2	—	—	60	2.70	—	—	722	1050	—	—	0.00	0.00
0.36	0.87	15.55	—	—	—	1.2	—	—	80	4.50	—	—	679	1200	—	—	0.00	0.00
0.81	0.37	7.80	0.31	—	26.0	1.2	—	—	150	2.70	31.0	405	382	1450	0.9	—	0.00	0.00
—	—	—	—	—	—	2.4	—	—	200	2.70	—	—	—	1690	—	—	0.00	0.00
—	—	—	—	—	—	0.0	—	—	60	3.59	16.2	122	427	890	3.8	—	0.00	0.00
—	—	—	—	—	—	1.2	—	—	0	0.00	—	—	28	180	—	—	0.00	0.00
—	—	—	—	—	—	0.0	—	—	0	0.00	—	—	—	160	—	—	0.00	0.00
—	—	—	—	—	—	—	—	—	—	—	—	—	—	230	—	—	0.00	0.00
—	—	—	—	—	—	—	—	—	—	—	—	—	—	890	—	—	0.00	0.00
—	—	—	—	—	—	—	—	—	—	—	—	—	—	590	—	74	0.00	0.00
—	—	—	—	—	—	—	—	—	—	—	—	—	—	780	—	—	0.00	0.00
—	—	—	—	—	—	—	—	—	—	—	—	—	—	1530	—	—	0.00	0.00
—	—	—	—	—	—	—	—	—	—	—	—	—	—	180	—	89	0.00	0.00
—	—	—	—	—	—	—	—	—	—	—	—	—	—	1070	—	—	0.00	0.00
—	—	—	—	—	—	—	—	—	—	—	—	—	—	810	—	—	0.00	0.00
—	—	—	—	—	—	—	—	—	—	—	—	—	—	500	—	89	0.00	0.00
—	—	—	—	—	—	—	—	—	—	—	—	—	—	740	—	—	0.00	0.00
—	—	—	—	—	—	0.0	—	—	150	2.70	—	—	—	750	—	—	0.00	0.00
—	—	—	—	—	—	0.0	—	—	250	4.50	—	—	—	1020	—	—	0.00	0.00
—	—	—	—	—	—	9.0	—	—	250	5.40	—	—	—	1390	—	—	0.00	0.00
—	—	—	—	—	—	4.8	—	—	150	3.59	—	—	—	740	—	—	0.00	0.00
—	—	—	—	—	—	0.0	—	—	0	0.36	—	—	—	420	—	—	0.00	0.00
—	—	—	—	—	—	0.0	—	—	60	1.79	—	—	—	440	—	—	0.00	0.00
—	—	—	—	—	—	0.0	—	—	80	2.70	—	—	—	530	—	—	0.00	0.00
—	—	—	—	—	—	9.0	—	—	100	5.40	—	—	—	940	—	—	0.00	0.00

PAGE KEY: 2 Beverage and Beverage Mixes   4 Other Beverages   4 Beverages, Alcoholic   6 Candies and Confections, Gum   10 Cereals, Breakfast Type
14 Cheese and Cheese Substitutes   16 Dairy Products and Substitutes   18 Desserts   24 Dessert Toppings   24 Eggs, Substitutes, and Egg Dishes   26 Ethnic Foods
30 Fast Foods/Restaurants   44 Fats, Oils, Margarines, Shortenings, and Substitutes   44 Fish, Seafood, and Shellfish   46 Food Additives
46 Fruit, Vegetable, or Blended Juices   48 Grains, Flours, and Fractions   48 Grain Products, Prepared and Baked Goods

Code	Food Name	Unit/ Amt	Wt (g)	Energy (kcal)	Prot (g)	Carb (g)	Fiber (g)	Fat (g)	Sat (g)	Mono (g)	Poly (g)	Chol (mg)	Vit A (RE)
56999	Hamburger, Whopper Jr	1 ea	167	410	18	32	2	23	7.0	—	—	50	40
9041	Onion Rings, lrg	1 ea	137	480	7	60	5	23	6.0	—	—	0	0
56362	Sandwich, Big Fish	1 ea	263	710	24	67	4	38	14.0	—	—	50	20
56360	Sandwich, chicken	1 ea	224	660	25	53	3	39	8.0	—	—	70	20
9057	Sandwich, chicken tenders	1 ea	148	450	14	37	2	27	5.0	—	—	30	40
Carl's Junior													
91433	Burrito, breakfast	1 ea	185	480	27	26	2	30	13.0	—	—	465	150
91404	Cheeseburger, Western Bacon	1 ea	225	650	32	63	2	30	12.0	—	—	80	40
91419	Chicken, nuggets, Chicken Stars, svg	1 ea	90	280	12	15	0	19	4.5	—	—	40	0
91421	Dish, baked potato bacon cheese, Great Stuff	1 ea	411	630	20	76	6	29	7.0	—	—	35	150
91406	Hamburger, Jr	1 ea	134	330	18	34	1	13	5.0	—	—	45	0
91403	Hamburger, Super Star	1 ea	345	790	42	49	2	46	14.0	—	—	130	100
91414	Potatoes, french fries, svg	1 ea	92	290	5	37	3	14	3.0	—	—	0	0
91425	Salad, garden, Salad To Go	1 ea	137	50	3	4	2	2	1.5	—	—	10	600
91407	Sandwich, chicken, bbq, charbroiled	1 ea	199	280	25	37	2	3	1.0	—	—	60	60
91411	Sandwich, chicken, crispy, bacon swiss	1 ea	291	720	32	66	3	36	10.0	—	—	75	80
91413	Sandwich, fish, Carl's Catch	1 ea	201	510	18	50	1	27	7.0	—	—	80	60
Chick-Fil-A													
69188	Chicken, breast, fillet, brd	1 ea	105	230	23	10	0	11	2.5	—	—	60	40
52139	Salad, carrot raisin, sml	1 ea	91	130	1	22	2	5	1.0	—	—	0	1700
52135	Salad, Chick-N-Strips	1 ea	315	340	30	19	3	16	5.0	—	—	85	600
69152	Sandwich, chicken	1 ea	170	410	28	38	1	16	3.5	—	—	60	40
69183	Wrap, chicken caesar, Cool Wrap	1 ea	227	460	38	51	3	11	6.0	—	—	85	150
69182	Wrap, chicken, spicy	1 ea	225	390	31	51	3	7	3.5	—	—	70	40
Chili's Grill&Bar													
4822	Dinner, chicken, platter, Guiltless Grill	0.5 ea	326	282	19	42	2	4	1.5	—	—	29	368
4826	Salad, chicken, w/dressing	1 ea	445	272	29	27	6	5	1.0	—	—	47	416
4825	Sandwich, chicken, Guiltless Grill	1 ea	553	527	44	70	11	8	2.0	—	—	43	620
Dairy Queen													
56372	Cheeseburger, double, homestyle	1 ea	219	540	35	30	2	31	16.0	—	—	115	150
16287	Dinner, chicken, strip, basket, w/gravy	1 ea	415	1000	35	102	5	50	13.0	—	—	55	40
2131	Frozen Dessert, banana split, Royal Treats	1 ea	369	510	8	96	3	12	8.0	—	—	30	200
2352	Frozen Dessert, Misty Slush, med	1 ea	595	290	0	74	0	0	0.0	0.0	0.0	0	0
2368	Frozen Dessert, oreo, med, Dairy Queen Blizzard	1 ea	326	640	12	97	1	23	11.0	—	—	45	250
56368	Hamburger, homestyle	1 ea	138	290	17	29	2	12	5.0	—	—	45	40
56374	Hot Dog	1 ea	99	240	9	19	1	14	5.0	—	—	25	20
2222	Ice Cream Cone, chocolate, med	1 ea	198	340	8	53	0	11	7.0	—	—	30	150
2143	Ice Cream Cone, vanilla, med	1 ea	213	355	9	57	0	10	6.5	—	—	32	161
2134	Ice Cream Sandwich, Dairy Queen	1 ea	85	200	4	31	1	6	3.0	—	—	10	40
2348	Ice Cream, chocolate, soft serve, Dairy Queen	0.5 cup	94	150	4	22	0	5	3.5	—	—	15	100
2224	Milk Shake, chocolate, med, Dairy Queen	1 ea	539	770	17	130	0	20	13.0	—	—	70	400
56383	Onion Rings, svg	1 ea	113	320	5	39	3	16	4.0	—	—	0	0
71690	Sandwich, bbq beef	1 ea	142	300	16	37	2	9	3.5	—	—	35	40
Dennys													
1125	Biscuit, w/sausage gravy, svg	1 ea	198	398	8	45	0	21	6.0	—	—	12	0
25238	Breakfast, Country Slam	1 ea	510	1000	41	61	1	66	21.0	—	—	467	300
1077	Breakfast, sausage supreme skillet	1 ea	425	857	27	29	8	62	19.0	—	—	466	490

Thia (mg)	Ribo (mg)	Niac (mg NE)	Vit B6 (mg)	Vit B12 (μg)	Fol (μg)	Vit C (mg)	Vit D (IU)	Vit E (mg AT)	Cal (mg)	Iron (mg)	Magn (mg)	Phos (mg)	Pota (mg)	Sodi (mg)	Zinc (mg)	Wat (%)	Alco (g)	Caff (mg)
—	—	—	—	—	—	4.8	—	—	80	3.59	—	—	—	520	—	55	0.00	0.00
—	—	—	—	—	—	0.0	—	—	150	0.00	—	—	—	690	—	—	0.00	0.00
—	—	—	—	—	—	0.0	—	—	80	3.59	—	—	—	1200	—	—	0.00	0.00
—	—	—	—	—	—	0.0	—	—	80	2.70	—	—	—	1330	—	—	0.00	0.00
—	—	—	—	—	—	3.6	—	—	60	1.79	—	—	—	680	—	—	0.00	0.00
—	—	—	—	—	—	0.0	—	—	350	2.70	—	—	—	750	—	—	0.00	0.00
—	—	—	—	—	—	1.2	—	—	200	4.50	—	—	—	1430	—	—	0.00	0.00
—	—	—	—	—	—	0.0	—	—	20	1.08	—	—	—	330	—	47	0.00	0.00
—	—	—	—	—	—	36.0	—	—	150	4.50	—	—	—	1700	—	—	0.00	0.00
—	—	—	—	—	—	2.4	—	—	60	3.59	—	—	—	480	—	—	0.00	0.00
—	—	—	—	—	—	9.0	—	—	100	5.40	—	—	—	910	—	—	0.00	0.00
—	—	—	—	—	—	21.0	—	—	0	1.08	—	—	—	170	—	36	0.00	0.00
—	—	—	—	—	—	15.0	—	—	80	0.72	—	—	—	60	—	93	0.00	0.00
—	—	—	—	—	—	4.8	—	—	80	2.70	—	—	—	830	—	—	0.00	0.00
—	—	—	—	—	—	6.0	—	—	250	3.59	—	—	—	1610	—	—	0.00	0.00
—	—	—	—	—	—	2.4	—	—	150	1.79	—	—	—	1030	—	51	0.00	0.00
—	—	—	—	—	—	0.0	—	—	40	1.08	—	—	—	990	—	—	0.00	0.00
—	—	—	—	—	—	3.6	—	—	20	0.36	—	—	—	90	—	—	0.00	0.00
—	—	—	—	—	—	6.0	—	—	150	1.08	—	—	—	680	—	—	0.00	0.00
—	—	—	—	—	—	0.0	—	—	100	2.70	—	—	—	1300	—	—	0.00	0.00
—	—	—	—	—	—	0.0	—	—	400	3.59	—	—	—	1540	—	—	0.00	0.00
—	—	—	—	—	—	4.8	—	—	200	3.59	—	—	—	1150	—	—	0.00	0.00
—	—	—	—	—	—	16.5	—	—	86	4.00	—	—	—	1642	—	—	0.00	0.00
—	—	—	—	—	—	16.0	—	—	36	4.00	—	—	—	1475	—	—	0.00	0.00
—	—	—	—	—	—	26.0	—	—	306	9.00	—	—	—	2923	—	—	0.00	0.00
—	—	—	—	—	—	3.6	—	—	250	4.50	—	—	—	1130	—	—	0.00	0.00
—	—	—	—	—	—	9.0	—	—	60	4.50	—	—	—	2510	—	—	0.00	0.00
—	—	—	—	—	—	15.0	—	—	250	1.79	—	—	—	180	—	—	0.00	—
—	—	—	—	—	—	0.0	—	—	0	0.00	—	—	—	30	—	—	0.00	0.00
—	—	—	—	—	—	1.2	—	—	400	2.70	—	—	—	500	—	—	0.00	—
—	—	—	—	—	—	3.6	—	—	60	2.70	—	—	—	630	—	56	0.00	0.00
—	—	—	—	—	—	3.6	—	—	60	1.79	—	—	—	730	—	55	0.00	0.00
—	—	—	—	—	—	1.2	—	—	250	1.79	—	—	—	160	—	—	0.00	—
—	—	—	—	—	—	2.6	—	—	269	1.94	—	—	—	172	—	—	0.00	0.00
—	—	—	—	—	—	0.0	—	—	80	1.08	—	—	—	140	—	51	0.00	—
—	—	—	—	—	—	0.0	—	—	100	0.72	—	—	—	75	—	—	0.00	—
—	—	—	—	—	—	2.4	—	—	600	2.70	—	—	—	420	—	—	0.00	—
—	—	—	—	—	—	0.0	—	—	20	1.44	—	—	—	180	—	—	0.00	0.00
—	—	—	—	—	—	0.0	—	—	60	2.70	—	—	—	610	—	—	0.00	0.00
—	—	—	—	—	—	0.0	—	—	10	0.18	—	—	—	1267	—	—	0.00	0.00
—	—	—	—	—	—	0.0	—	—	70	4.13	—	—	—	2727	—	—	0.00	0.00
—	—	—	—	—	—	22.8	—	—	180	2.88	—	—	—	1700	—	—	0.00	0.00

36

PAGE KEY: 2 Beverage and Beverage Mixes   4 Other Beverages   4 Beverages, Alcoholic   6 Candies and Confections, Gum   10 Cereals, Breakfast Type   14 Cheese and Cheese Substitutes   16 Dairy Products and Substitutes   18 Desserts   24 Dessert Toppings   24 Eggs, Substitutes, and Egg Dishes   26 Ethnic Foods   30 Fast Foods/Restaurants   44 Fats, Oils, Margarines, Shortenings, and Substitutes   44 Fish, Seafood, and Shellfish   46 Food Additives   46 Fruit, Vegetable, or Blended Juices   48 Grains, Flours, and Fractions   48 Grain Products, Prepared and Baked Goods

Code	Food Name	Unit/ Amt	Wt (g)	Energy (kcal)	Prot (g)	Carb (g)	Fiber (g)	Fat (g)	Sat (g)	Mono (g)	Poly (g)	Chol (mg)	Vit A (RE)
17277	Chicken, breast, grilled, svg	1 ea	170	219	26	16	0	6	1.0	—	—	67	60
25249	Chicken, buffalo wings	1 ea	35	71	8	0	0	4	1.4	—	—	42	15
25248	Dish, appetizer sampler, w/chicken mozzarella onion & sauce	1 ea	482	1405	47	124	4	80	24.0	—	—	75	30
10432	Dish, fish & chips, w/tartar sauce, svg	1 ea	255	732	30	48	3	47	7.0	—	—	105	0
38655	French Toast, cinnamon swirl, w/o topping & margarine, svg	1 ea	341	1030	23	124	4	49	21.0	—	—	280	370
52144	Hamburger, classic	1 ea	312	673	37	42	3	40	15.0	—	—	106	200
12199	Hamburger, w/cheese, classic	1 ea	369	836	47	43	3	53	19.0	—	—	137	210
19548	Omelette, ham 'n cheddar, Dennys	1 ea	397	743	36	24	2	55	10.0	—	—	657	580
19547	Omelette, ultimate, Dennys	1 ea	482	780	31	29	4	62	14.0	—	—	639	540
38657	Onion Rings, basket	1 ea	255	824	11	83	1	50	12.0	—	—	14	30
25250	Quesadilla, chicken	1 ea	454	827	50	43	2	55	23.0	—	—	181	630
12195	Sandwich, club	1 ea	312	718	32	62	3	38	7.0	—	—	75	60
Dominos Pizza													
91365	Breadsticks	1 ea	37	116	3	18	1	4	0.8	—	—	0	4
91369	Chicken, buffalo wings	1 ea	25	50	6	2	0	2	0.6	—	—	26	8
56386	Pizza, cheese, hand tossed, 12"	2 pce	159	375	15	55	3	11	4.8	—	—	23	131
91360	Pizza, Hawaiian feast, hand tossed, 12"	2 pce	204	450	21	58	3	16	7.2	—	—	41	173
91361	Pizza, pepperoni feast, hand tossed, 12"	2 pce	196	534	24	56	3	25	10.9	—	—	57	175
91357	Pizza, veggie feast, hand tossed, 12"	2 pce	203	439	19	57	4	16	7.1	—	—	34	181
Dunkin' Donuts													
50720	Chowder, clam, New England, svg	1 ea	227	200	10	16	0	10	3.0	—	—	30	100
45742	Doughnut, Bismark	1 ea	80	310	4	42	1	14	4.0	—	—	0	0
45700	Doughnut, cake, chocolate	1 ea	59	210	3	19	1	14	3.0	—	—	0	0
45695	Doughnut, cake, old fash	1 ea	60	280	3	24	1	19	4.0	—	—	0	0
45708	Doughnut, raised, glazed	1 ea	46	160	3	23	1	7	2.0	—	—	0	0
42636	Fritter, apple	1 ea	95	300	5	41	2	13	3.0	—	—	0	0
69090	Sandwich, ham cheese, croissant	1 ea	192	710	33	29	0	32	13.0	—	—	85	100
50722	Soup, cream of broccoli, svg	1 ea	227	200	8	17	0	11	6.0	—	—	25	200
45749	Turnover, apple	1 ea	109	350	5	49	2	15	4.0	—	—	0	0
El Pollo Loco													
28110	Chicken, strips, svg	1 ea	213	558	41	48	0	25	5.0	—	—	76	0
49103	Frozen Dessert, banana split	1 ea	425	717	12	107	3	28	11.0	—	—	56	80
4012	Guacamole, 1.8 oz svg	1 ea	50	52	0	5	0	3	0.0	—	—	0	30
1655	Salad, garden, reg	1 ea	113	105	5	7	1	7	3.0	—	—	15	60
1656	Salad, tostada	1 ea	397	304	29	28	4	11	3.0	—	—	57	190
28104	Salsa, avocado	28.35 g	28	12	0	1	0	1	0.0	—	—	0	5
7204	Taco, chicken, soft	1 ea	128	238	17	15	0	12	4.0	—	—	74	120
49112	Tortilla, corn, 6"	1 ea	28	70	1	14	1	1	0.0	—	—	0	30
Hardees													
9280	Cheeseburger	1 ea	124	313	16	26	1	14	7.0	—	—	40	—
56412	Hamburger	1 ea	110	265	14	26	1	10	4.0	—	—	35	—
9286	Potatoes, french fries, Crispy Curls, reg svg	1 ea	96	340	5	41	0	18	4.0	—	—	0	—
6146	Potatoes, french fries, reg svg	1 ea	113	340	4	45	0	16	2.0	—	—	0	—
56418	Sandwich, roast beef, regular	1 ea	123	310	17	26	2	16	6.0	—	—	43	—

Thia (mg)	Ribo (mg)	Niac (mg NE)	Vit B6 (mg)	Vit B12 (µg)	Fol (µg)	Vit C (mg)	Vit D (IU)	Vit E (mg AT)	Cal (mg)	Iron (mg)	Magn (mg)	Phos (mg)	Pota (mg)	Sodi (mg)	Zinc (mg)	Wat (%)	Alco (g)	Caff (mg)
—	—	—	—	—	—	1.2	—	—	10	1.08	—	—	—	880	—	—	0.00	0.00
—	—	—	—	—	—	2.4	—	—	16	1.29	—	—	—	462	—	—	0.00	0.00
—	—	—	—	—	—	6.6	—	—	440	2.88	—	—	—	5305	—	—	0.00	0.00
—	—	—	—	—	—	0.0	—	—	0	1.44	—	—	—	1335	—	—	0.00	0.00
—	—	—	—	—	—	0.0	—	—	180	6.48	—	—	—	675	—	—	0.00	0.00
—	—	—	—	—	—	10.8	—	—	130	4.50	—	—	—	1142	—	—	0.00	0.00
—	—	—	—	—	—	10.8	—	—	340	4.50	—	—	—	1595	—	—	0.00	0.00
—	—	—	—	—	—	6.6	—	—	290	3.05	—	—	—	1518	—	—	0.00	0.00
—	—	—	—	—	—	37.8	—	—	90	3.59	—	—	—	1360	—	—	0.00	0.00
—	—	—	—	—	—	4.8	—	—	40	1.25	—	—	—	2173	—	—	0.00	0.00
—	—	—	—	—	—	54.0	—	—	640	1.79	—	—	—	1982	—	—	0.00	0.00
—	—	—	—	—	—	13.2	—	—	120	4.32	—	—	—	1666	—	—	0.00	0.00
—	—	—	—	—	—	0.1	—	—	6	0.87	—	—	—	152	—	—	0.00	0.00
—	—	—	—	—	—	0.1	—	—	6	0.31	—	—	—	175	—	—	0.00	0.00
—	—	—	—	—	—	0.0	—	—	187	2.99	—	—	—	776	—	—	0.00	0.00
—	—	—	—	—	—	1.9	—	—	274	3.29	—	—	—	1102	—	51	0.00	0.00
—	—	—	—	—	—	0.1	—	—	279	3.40	—	—	—	1349	—	44	0.00	0.00
—	—	—	—	—	—	1.3	—	—	279	3.44	—	—	—	987	—	53	0.00	0.00
—	—	—	—	—	—	3.6	—	—	150	2.70	—	—	—	1050	—	—	0.00	0.00
—	—	—	—	—	—	2.4	—	—	0	0.72	—	—	—	260	—	—	0.00	0.00
—	—	—	—	—	—	3.6	—	—	0	1.44	—	—	—	270	—	—	0.00	—
—	—	—	—	—	—	1.2	—	—	0	1.08	—	—	—	350	—	—	0.00	0.00
—	—	—	—	—	—	1.2	—	—	0	0.36	—	—	—	200	—	—	0.00	0.00
—	—	—	—	—	—	0.0	—	—	0	1.44	—	—	—	320	—	—	0.00	0.00
—	—	—	—	—	—	24.0	—	—	250	2.70	—	—	—	1840	—	—	0.00	0.00
—	—	—	—	—	—	18.0	—	—	250	0.36	—	—	—	1050	—	83	0.00	0.00
—	—	—	—	—	—	2.4	—	—	0	0.72	—	—	—	340	—	—	0.00	0.00
—	—	—	—	—	—	0.0	—	—	100	2.70	—	—	—	1876	—	—	0.00	0.00
—	—	—	—	—	—	22.2	—	—	270	1.98	—	—	—	310	—	—	0.00	0.00
—	—	—	—	—	—	4.2	—	—	40	0.73	—	—	—	282	—	—	0.00	0.00
—	—	—	—	—	—	6.6	—	—	110	0.36	—	—	—	99	—	—	0.00	0.00
—	—	—	—	—	—	22.8	—	—	180	3.24	—	—	—	1175	—	—	0.00	0.00
—	—	—	—	—	—	7.2	—	—	0	0.18	—	—	—	204	—	92	0.00	0.00
—	—	—	—	—	—	10.2	—	—	181	1.62	—	—	—	631	—	—	0.00	0.00
—	—	—	—	—	—	0.0	—	—	10	0.36	—	—	—	35	—	42	0.00	0.00
—	—	—	—	—	—	—	—	—	—	—	—	—	—	895	—	—	0.00	0.00
—	—	—	—	—	—	—	—	—	—	—	—	—	—	663	—	—	0.00	0.00
—	—	—	—	—	—	—	—	—	—	—	—	—	—	950	—	—	0.00	0.00
—	—	—	—	—	—	—	—	—	—	—	—	—	—	390	—	41	0.00	0.00
—	—	—	—	—	—	—	—	—	—	—	—	—	—	804	—	—	0.00	0.00

Code	Food Name	Unit/ Amt	Wt (g)	Energy (kcal)	Prot (g)	Carb (g)	Fiber (g)	Fat (g)	Sat (g)	Mono (g)	Poly (g)	Chol (mg)	Vit A (RE)
56404	Sandwich, sausage egg, w/biscuit	1 ea	156	617	19	44	—	41	12.9	—	—	224	—
56403	Sandwich, sausage, w/biscuit	1 ea	114	553	13	44	—	36	11.0	—	—	30	—
In-N-Out Burgers													
81119	Potatoes, french fries	1 ea	125	400	7	54	2	18	5.0	—	—	0	0
Jack in the Box													
56434	Cheeseburger	1 ea	116	300	14	31	2	13	6.0	—	—	40	40
15162	Chicken, strips, 5 pce svg	1 ea	150	360	27	24	1	17	3.0	—	—	80	40
62548	Dish, fish & chips	1 ea	281	780	19	86	6	39	9.0	—	—	45	20
56433	Hamburger	1 ea	104	250	12	30	2	9	3.5	—	—	30	0
2163	Milk Shake, chocolate, med, Jack in the Box	1 ea	332	630	11	85	1	27	16.0	—	—	85	150
2165	Milk Shake, vanilla, med, Jack in the Box	1 ea	332	610	12	73	0	31	18.0	—	—	95	150
56446	Onion Rings, svg	1 ea	120	450	7	50	3	25	5.0	—	—	0	40
56448	Salad, side	1 ea	86	50	2	3	1	3	1.5	—	—	10	75
69035	Sandwich, chicken	1 ea	164	400	15	38	3	21	3.0	—	—	40	40
56377	Taco	1 ea	90	170	7	12	2	10	3.5	—	—	15	60
Jamba Juice													
81280	Breadsticks, pizza, w/add prot, svg	1 ea	76	230	9	33	2	6	1.5	—	—	5	60
81227	Smoothie, Banana Berry, Jamba Juice	16 fl-oz	475	270	2	66	3	2	0.0	—	—	0	20
81245	Smoothie, Coldbuster, Jamba Juice	16 fl-oz	476	280	3	65	3	2	0.0	—	—	5	700
81266	Smoothie, Orange Dream Machine, Jamba Juice	16 fl-oz	504	410	15	84	1	2	1.0	—	—	5	80
81253	Smoothie, PowerBoost	16 fl-oz	519	280	4	67	6	1	0.0	—	—	0	600
81283	Smoothie, Razzmatazz, Jamba Juice	16 fl-oz	490	300	2	72	3	1	0.0	—	—	0	20
81362	Smoothie, strawberry banana	8 fl-oz	240	124	1	29	1	0	0.0	0.0	0.0	0	0
Kentucky Fried Chicken													
42331	Biscuit, buttermilk	1 ea	57	190	2	23	0	10	2.0	—	—	0	0
15163	Chicken, breast, original rec	1 ea	161	380	40	11	0	19	6.0	—	—	145	0
56451	Cole Slaw, svg	1 ea	130	190	1	22	3	11	2.0	—	—	5	250
6152	Corn, cob, large	1 ea	162	150	5	26	7	3	1.0	—	—	0	0
56453	Potatoes, mashed, w/gravy, svg	1 ea	136	130	2	18	1	4	1.0	—	—	0	20
6188	Potatoes, wedges, svg	1 ea	102	240	5	30	3	12	3.0	—	—	0	0
Long John Silvers													
91388	Cheese, cheesesticks, brd, fried, 0.5 oz ea	3 ea	45	140	4	12	1	8	2.0	—	—	10	40
56477	Cornbread, hush puppies, svg	1 ea	23	60	1	9	1	2	0.5	—	—	0	0
56461	Fish, batter dipped, reg, 3.3 oz	1 pce	92	230	11	16	0	13	4.0	—	—	30	0
69030	Sandwich, fish, batter dipped	1 ea	177	440	17	47	3	21	5.0	—	—	40	60
19108	Shrimp, battered	1 ea	14	45	2	3	0	3	1.0	—	—	15	0
McDonalds													
69009	Cheeseburger	1 ea	119	326	15	33	2	15	6.2	5.2	1.5	42	—
69010	Cheeseburger, Big Mac	1 ea	219	572	26	47	3	31	10.9	11.3	8.5	79	—
69012	Cheeseburger, Quarter Pounder	1 ea	199	535	30	39	2	29	13.8	12.1	2.6	96	—
15174	Chicken, nuggets, McNuggets, 4 pce svg	4 pce	72	190	10	13	1	11	2.5	—	—	35	0
47147	Cookie, McDonaldland, pkg	1 ea	57	230	3	38	1	8	2.0	—	—	0	0
19579	Eggs, scrambled, svg	1 ea	102	160	13	1	0	11	3.5	—	—	425	150
2171	Frozen Dessert, sundae, hot fudge, low fat	1 ea	179	340	8	52	1	12	9.0	—	—	30	100
69008	Hamburger	1 ea	105	270	13	32	2	10	3.6	4.1	1.3	27	—
69011	Hamburger, Quarter Pounder	1 ea	171	438	27	38	2	20	8.3	9.4	2.1	68	—
2169	Milk Shake, vanilla, sml, McDonalds	1 ea	293	360	11	59	0	9	6.0	—	—	40	60

Thia (mg)	Ribo (mg)	Niac (mg NE)	Vit B6 (mg)	Vit B12 (μg)	Fol (μg)	Vit C (mg)	Vit D (IU)	Vit E (mg AT)	Cal (mg)	Iron (mg)	Magn (mg)	Phos (mg)	Pota (mg)	Sodi (mg)	Zinc (mg)	Wat (%)	Alco (g)	Caff (mg)
—	—	—	—	—	—	—	—	—	—	—	—	—	—	1359	—	—	0.00	0.00
—	—	—	—	—	—	—	—	—	—	—	—	—	—	1305	—	—	0.00	0.00
—	—	—	—	—	—	0.0	—	—	20	1.79	—	—	—	245	—	—	0.00	0.00
—	—	—	—	—	—	0.0	—	—	150	3.59	—	—	180	840	—	—	0.00	0.00
—	—	—	—	—	—	1.2	—	—	0	1.79	—	—	430	970	—	—	0.00	0.00
—	—	—	—	—	—	15.0	—	—	20	2.70	—	—	1060	1740	—	—	0.00	0.00
—	—	—	—	—	—	0.0	—	—	100	3.59	—	—	155	610	—	—	0.00	0.00
—	—	—	—	—	—	0.0	—	—	350	0.36	—	—	720	330	—	—	0.00	—
—	—	—	—	—	—	0.0	—	—	400	0.00	—	—	730	320	—	64	0.00	0.00
—	—	—	—	—	—	18.0	—	—	40	2.70	—	—	150	780	—	30	0.00	0.00
—	—	—	—	—	—	0.0	—	—	80	0.72	—	—	160	75	—	—	0.00	0.00
—	—	—	—	—	—	4.8	—	—	100	2.70	—	—	200	770	—	—	0.00	0.00
—	—	—	—	—	—	0.2	—	—	100	1.08	40.4	168	235	390	1.4	66	0.00	0.00
0.37	0.25	3.00	0.03	0.00	80.0	4.8	0.0	0.8	80	2.70	8.0	20	130	450	0.3	—	0.00	0.00
0.05	0.10	0.80	0.60	0.11	16.0	9.0	0.0	0.4	80	0.72	24.0	40	540	35	0.3	—	0.00	0.00
0.23	0.14	2.00	0.30	0.00	100.0	684.0	0.0	10.1	60	0.72	40.0	60	800	15	7.5	—	0.00	0.00
0.23	0.25	0.80	0.11	0.47	60.0	78.0	100.0	0.0	400	0.72	32.0	300	540	230	0.6	—	0.00	0.00
2.70	2.89	34.00	3.59	4.80	360.0	198.0	240.0	12.1	600	1.44	240.0	80	810	30	7.5	—	0.00	0.00
0.05	0.17	4.00	0.69	0.11	100.0	36.0	0.0	0.0	80	1.08	24.0	60	570	45	0.3	—	0.00	0.00
—	—	—	—	—	—	60.0	—	—	0	0.89	—	—	475	10	—	—	0.00	0.00
—	—	—	—	—	—	0.0	—	—	0	0.72	—	—	—	580	—	36	0.00	0.00
—	—	—	—	—	—	0.0	—	—	0	1.79	—	—	—	1150	—	55	0.00	0.00
—	—	—	—	—	—	24.0	—	—	40	0.00	—	—	—	300	—	—	0.00	0.00
—	—	—	—	—	—	6.0	—	—	60	1.08	—	—	—	10	—	—	0.00	0.00
—	—	—	—	—	—	2.4	—	—	0	0.36	—	—	—	380	—	—	0.00	0.00
—	—	—	—	—	—	3.6	—	—	20	1.79	—	—	—	830	—	—	0.00	—
—	—	—	—	—	—	0.0	—	—	100	0.72	—	—	—	320	—	—	0.00	0.00
—	—	—	—	—	—	0.0	—	—	20	0.36	—	—	—	200	—	43	0.00	0.00
—	—	—	—	—	—	4.8	—	—	20	1.79	—	—	—	700	—	54	0.00	0.00
—	—	—	—	—	—	9.0	—	—	60	3.59	—	—	—	1120	—	—	0.00	0.00
—	—	—	—	—	—	1.2	—	—	0	0.00	—	—	—	125	—	43	0.00	0.00
0.34	0.18	4.82	0.09	1.57	30.9	0.4	—	0.1	219	1.75	29.8	179	234	739	2.4	45	0.00	0.00
0.40	0.43	7.94	0.37	2.77	59.1	0.7	—	0.1	278	3.06	54.8	298	399	1062	4.7	51	0.00	0.00
0.23	0.51	8.06	0.18	3.48	31.8	0.6	—	0.4	356	2.02	51.7	364	444	1176	5.6	48	0.00	0.00
—	—	4.92	0.20	—	—	0.0	—	0.9	9	0.70	16.4	191	202	360	0.7	51	0.00	0.00
—	—	2.03	—	—	—	0.0	—	1.0	20	1.79	11.3	71	63	250	0.4	13	0.00	0.00
0.07	0.50	0.05	0.11	1.11	44.0	0.0	—	0.9	40	1.08	10.0	172	126	170	1.1		0.00	0.00
—	—	—	—	—	—	1.2	—	—	250	0.72	—	—	—	170	—	59	0.00	—
0.31	0.07	4.55	0.10	1.17	29.4	0.3	—	0.1	130	1.77	25.2	112	204	502	2.0	45	0.00	0.00
0.27	0.34	7.94	0.25	2.83	37.6	0.5	—	0.1	149	2.96	41.0	207	385	640	5.2	49	0.00	0.00
—	—	—	—	—	—	1.2	—	—	350	0.36	—	327	534	250	—	—	0.00	0.00

Code	Food Name	Unit/ Amt	Wt (g)	Energy (kcal)	Prot (g)	Carb (g)	Fiber (g)	Fat (g)	Sat (g)	Mono (g)	Poly (g)	Chol (mg)	Vit A (RE)
56531	Pizza, Mexican	1 ea	216	550	21	46	7	31	11.0	—	—	45	150
57685	Quesadilla, cheese	1 ea	142	490	19	39	3	28	13.0	—	—	55	100
57689	Quesadilla, chicken	1 ea	184	540	28	40	3	30	13.0	—	—	80	150
56537	Salad, taco, w/salsa & shell	1 ea	533	790	31	73	13	42	15.0	—	—	65	300
53604	Sauce, border, mild, 1 oz svg	1 ea	28	5	0	1	0	0	0.0	0.0	0.0	0	60
56524	Taco	1 ea	78	170	8	13	3	10	4.0	—	—	25	60
56525	Taco, soft, beef	1 ea	90	191	9	19	2	9	4.1	—	—	23	55
56689	Taco, soft, chicken	1 ea	99	190	14	19	1	6	2.5	—	—	30	20
56528	Tostada	1 ea	170	250	11	29	7	10	4.0	—	—	15	100

Taco Johns

Code	Food Name	Unit/ Amt	Wt (g)	Energy (kcal)	Prot (g)	Carb (g)	Fiber (g)	Fat (g)	Sat (g)	Mono (g)	Poly (g)	Chol (mg)	Vit A (RE)
57576	Burrito, bean, w/cheese	1 ea	187	380	15	53	10	12	5.0	—	—	15	—
57577	Burrito, beefy	1 ea	187	430	22	41	8	20	9.0	—	—	55	—
49127	Dessert, churros	1 ea	55	230	2	31	1	11	2.0	—	—	10	—
57585	Dish, chimi platter, beef & bean	1 ea	422	760	27	88	9	34	11.0	—	—	50	—
57586	Enchilada, double	1 ea	422	720	37	54	11	40	18.0	—	—	105	—
57589	Mexi Rolls	1 ea	213	480	20	33	3	30	10.0	—	—	50	—
57593	Nachos, svg	1 ea	142	380	6	38	1	23	6.0	—	—	10	—
57596	Taco Burger, w/cheese	1 ea	142	280	14	28	3	12	5.0	—	—	35	—
57600	Taco, crispy	1 ea	94	180	9	13	3	10	4.0	—	—	25	—
57601	Taco, soft shell	1 ea	113	220	11	21	4	10	5.0	—	—	25	—

Taco Time

Code	Food Name	Unit/ Amt	Wt (g)	Energy (kcal)	Prot (g)	Carb (g)	Fiber (g)	Fat (g)	Sat (g)	Mono (g)	Poly (g)	Chol (mg)	Vit A (RE)
7141	Beans, refritos, svg	1 ea	201	326	18	44	13	10	5.0	—	—	22	44
56542	Burrito, bean, soft	1 ea	193	380	16	58	13	10	4.0	—	—	15	—
56621	Burrito, chicken, crisp	1 ea	150	422	17	32	2	25	8.0	—	—	54	—
56541	Burrito, meat, crispy	1 ea	163	552	34	39	7	30	10.0	—	—	58	—
56543	Burrito, meat, soft	1 ea	193	491	31	48	12	21	8.0	—	—	56	—
56620	Burrito, veggie	1 ea	321	491	21	70	10	16	6.0	—	—	24	—
56550	Cheeseburger, taco	1 ea	215	633	31	48	7	36	10.0	—	—	66	—
56551	Chimichanga, meat	1 ea	349	768	37	62	12	43	18.0	—	—	89	—
45586	Empanada, berry	1 ea	113	387	5	66	3	12	1.0	5.0	6.0	2	16
2488	Frozen Dessert, Choco Taco	1 ea	113	310	3	37	1	17	10.0	—	—	20	40
1696	Gordita, taco meat	1 ea	227	470	18	44	4	24	7.0	—	—	35	150
56554	Nachos, svg	1 ea	301	680	26	61	11	38	19.0	—	—	78	—
50979	Quesadilla, cheese	1 ea	93	205	11	17	1	11	6.0	—	—	30	—
56556	Salad, taco, w/o dressing, reg	1 ea	215	479	30	30	7	28	11.0	—	—	63	—
56545	Taco, crisp	1 ea	115	295	22	16	5	17	7.0	—	—	48	—
56674	Taco, fish	1 ea	231	470	19	32	2	29	8.0	—	—	60	—
56655	Taco, soft, value	1 ea	150	316	24	23	5	15	7.0	—	—	48	—
56856	Tostada, w/bean	1 ea	138	211	10	26	7	8	4.0	—	—	15	—
56548	Tostada, w/meat	1 ea	219	447	35	33	12	21	9.0	—	—	61	—
1705	Wrap, chicken, classic	1 ea	494	813	29	101	6	33	11.0	—	—	67	—

Wendy's

Code	Food Name	Unit/ Amt	Wt (g)	Energy (kcal)	Prot (g)	Carb (g)	Fiber (g)	Fat (g)	Sat (g)	Mono (g)	Poly (g)	Chol (mg)	Vit A (RE)
56570	Cheeseburger, jr	1 ea	129	310	17	34	2	12	6.0	—	—	45	60
56571	Cheeseburger, w/bacon, jr	1 ea	165	380	20	34	2	19	7.0	—	—	55	80
15176	Chicken, nuggets, 5 pce svg	1 ea	75	220	11	13	0	14	3.0	—	—	35	0
50311	Chili, sml svg	1 ea	227	200	17	21	5	6	2.5	—	—	35	150
56579	Dish, baked potato bacon cheese	1 ea	380	580	18	79	7	22	6.0	—	—	40	100

Thia (mg)	Ribo (mg)	Niac (mg NE)	Vit B6 (mg)	Vit B12 (μg)	Fol (μg)	Vit C (mg)	Vit D (IU)	Vit E (mg AT)	Cal (mg)	Iron (mg)	Magn (mg)	Phos (mg)	Pota (mg)	Sodi (mg)	Zinc (mg)	Wat (%)	Alco (g)	Caff (mg)
—	—	—	—	—	—	6.0	—	—	350	3.59	—	—	—	1030	—	—	0.00	0.00
—	—	—	—	—	—	0.0	—	—	500	1.44	—	—	—	1150	—	—	0.00	0.00
—	—	—	—	—	—	2.4	—	—	500	1.79	—	—	—	1380	—	—	0.00	0.00
—	—	—	—	—	—	21.0	—	—	400	6.30	—	—	—	1670	—	—	0.00	0.00
—	—	—	—	—	—	0.0	—	—	0	0.00	—	—	—	210	—	—	0.00	0.00
—	—	—	—	—	—	2.4	—	—	60	1.08	—	—	—	350	—	—	0.00	0.00
—	—	—	—	—	—	2.2	—	—	91	1.63	—	—	—	564	—	—	0.00	0.00
—	—	—	—	—	—	1.2	—	—	100	1.08	—	—	—	550	—	—	0.00	0.00
—	—	—	—	—	—	4.8	—	—	150	1.44	—	—	—	710	—	—	0.00	0.00
—	—	—	—	—	—	—	—	—	—	—	—	—	—	830	—	—	0.00	0.00
—	—	—	—	—	—	—	—	—	—	—	—	—	—	870	—	—	0.00	0.00
—	—	—	—	—	—	—	—	—	—	—	—	—	—	120	—	—	0.00	0.00
—	—	—	—	—	—	—	—	—	—	—	—	—	—	1930	—	—	0.00	0.00
—	—	—	—	—	—	—	—	—	—	—	—	—	—	2090	—	—	0.00	0.00
—	—	—	—	—	—	—	—	—	—	—	—	—	—	1270	—	—	0.00	0.00
—	—	—	—	—	—	—	—	—	—	—	—	—	—	970	—	—	0.00	0.00
—	—	—	—	—	—	—	—	—	—	—	—	—	—	600	—	—	0.00	0.00
—	—	—	—	—	—	—	—	—	—	—	—	—	—	270	—	—	0.00	0.00
—	—	—	—	—	—	—	—	—	—	—	—	—	—	470	—	—	0.00	0.00
0.23	0.15	1.00	0.37	0.00	13.2	3.0	—	—	218	3.03	—	256	340	525	2.0	—	0.00	0.00
—	—	—	—	—	—	—	—	—	—	—	—	—	—	—	—	—	0.00	0.00
—	—	—	—	—	—	—	—	—	—	—	—	—	—	795	—	—	0.00	0.00
—	—	—	—	—	—	—	—	—	—	—	—	—	—	—	—	—	0.00	0.00
—	—	—	—	—	—	—	—	—	—	—	—	—	—	—	—	—	0.00	0.00
—	—	—	—	—	—	—	—	—	—	—	—	—	—	643	—	—	0.00	0.00
—	—	—	—	—	—	—	—	—	—	—	—	—	—	—	—	—	0.00	0.00
—	—	—	—	—	—	—	—	—	—	—	—	—	—	—	—	—	0.00	0.00
0.15	0.20	2.00	0.05	—	20.0	10.0	—	—	84	3.00	—	56	170	1	0.0	—	0.00	0.00
—	—	—	—	—	—	0.0	—	—	60	0.72	—	—	—	100	—	—	0.00	—
—	—	—	—	—	—	12.0	—	—	150	3.59	—	—	—	940	—	—	0.00	0.00
—	—	—	—	—	—	—	—	—	—	—	—	—	—	—	—	—	0.00	0.00
—	—	—	—	—	—	—	—	—	—	—	—	—	—	255	—	—	0.00	0.00
—	—	—	—	—	—	—	—	—	—	—	—	—	—	—	—	—	0.00	0.00
—	—	—	—	—	—	—	—	—	—	—	—	—	—	—	—	—	0.00	0.00
—	—	—	—	—	—	—	—	—	—	—	—	—	—	660	—	—	0.00	0.00
—	—	—	—	—	—	—	—	—	—	—	—	—	—	599	—	—	0.00	0.00
—	—	—	—	—	—	—	—	—	—	—	—	—	—	215	—	—	0.00	0.00
—	—	—	—	—	—	—	—	—	—	—	—	—	—	—	—	—	0.00	0.00
—	—	—	—	—	—	—	—	—	—	—	—	—	—	1688	—	—	0.00	0.00
—	—	—	—	—	—	3.6	—	—	150	3.59	—	—	230	820	—	49	0.00	0.00
—	—	—	—	—	—	9.0	—	—	150	3.59	—	—	320	890	—	—	0.00	0.00
—	—	—	—	—	—	1.2	—	—	20	0.72	—	—	190	480	—	48	0.00	0.00
—	—	—	—	—	—	2.4	—	—	80	1.79	—	—	470	870	—	—	0.00	0.00
—	—	—	—	—	—	42.0	—	—	200	3.59	—	—	1410	950	—	—	0.00	0.00

Code	Food Name	Unit/ Amt	Wt (g)	Energy (kcal)	Prot (g)	Carb (g)	Fiber (g)	Fat (g)	Sat (g)	Mono (g)	Poly (g)	Chol (mg)	Vit A (RE)
56580	Dish, baked potato broccoli cheese	1 ea	411	480	9	81	9	14	3.0	—	—	5	350
71834	Frozen Dessert, Frosty, dairy, jr	1 ea	113	170	4	28	0	4	2.5	—	—	20	80
2177	Frozen Dessert, Frosty, dairy, med	1 ea	298	440	11	73	0	11	7.0	—	—	50	200
56574	Hamburger, Big Bacon Classic	1 ea	282	570	34	46	3	29	12.0	—	—	100	150
71831	Potatoes, french fries, med, svg	1 ea	142	390	4	56	6	17	3.0	—	—	0	0
52080	Salad, caesar, w/o dressing, side	1 ea	99	70	7	2	1	4	2.0	—	—	15	450
56588	Salad, taco, supremo, w/o chips	1 ea	495	360	27	29	8	17	9.0	—	—	65	500
69059	Sandwich, chicken, grilled	1 ea	188	300	24	36	2	7	1.5	—	—	55	40

FATS, OILS, MARGARINES, SHORTENINGS, AND SUBSTITUTES

Fat Substitutes

Fats and Oils, Animal

Code	Food Name	Unit/ Amt	Wt (g)	Energy (kcal)	Prot (g)	Carb (g)	Fiber (g)	Fat (g)	Sat (g)	Mono (g)	Poly (g)	Chol (mg)	Vit A (RE)
8000	Butter, salted	1 Tbs	14	100	0	0	0	11	7.2	2.9	0.4	30	98
8003	Fat, bacon grease	1 tsp	4	39	0	0	0	4	1.7	1.9	0.5	4	0
8107	Fat, lard	1 Tbs	13	115	0	0	0	13	5.0	5.8	1.4	12	0

Fats and Oils, Vegetable

Code	Food Name	Unit/ Amt	Wt (g)	Energy (kcal)	Prot (g)	Carb (g)	Fiber (g)	Fat (g)	Sat (g)	Mono (g)	Poly (g)	Chol (mg)	Vit A (RE)
8084	Oil, canola	1 Tbs	14	124	0	0	0	14	1.0	8.2	4.1	0	0
8009	Oil, corn, salad or cooking	1 Tbs	14	120	0	0	0	14	1.8	3.8	7.4	0	0
8008	Oil, olive, salad or cooking	1 Tbs	14	119	0	0	0	14	1.8	10.0	1.4	0	0
90965	Oil, veg, pure	1 Tbs	14	120	0	0	0	14	1.5	6.0	6.0	0	0

Margarines and Spreads

Code	Food Name	Unit/ Amt	Wt (g)	Energy (kcal)	Prot (g)	Carb (g)	Fiber (g)	Fat (g)	Sat (g)	Mono (g)	Poly (g)	Chol (mg)	Vit A (RE)
8490	Margarine, soft, safflower oil	1 Tbs	14	100	0	0	0	11	1.0	8.0	2.0	0	100

Shortenings

Code	Food Name	Unit/ Amt	Wt (g)	Energy (kcal)	Prot (g)	Carb (g)	Fiber (g)	Fat (g)	Sat (g)	Mono (g)	Poly (g)	Chol (mg)	Vit A (RE)
8007	Shortening, household, hydrog soybean & cttnsd oil	1 Tbs	13	113	0	0	0	13	3.2	5.7	3.3	0	0

FISH, SEAFOOD, AND SHELLFISH

Code	Food Name	Unit/ Amt	Wt (g)	Energy (kcal)	Prot (g)	Carb (g)	Fiber (g)	Fat (g)	Sat (g)	Mono (g)	Poly (g)	Chol (mg)	Vit A (RE)
19049	Clams, bkd/brld, sml	15 ea	150	210	23	5	0	11	1.9	4.4	2.9	60	223
19151	Crab, imit	3 oz	85	99	11	11	0	1	0.1	0.1	0.3	42	6
17002	Fish Sticks, heated f/fzn, 4" x 1" x 1/2"	1 ea	28	76	4	7	0	3	0.9	1.4	0.9	31	9
17179	Fish, catfish, channel, fillet, bkd/brld, farmed	3 oz	85	129	16	0	0	7	1.5	3.5	1.2	54	13
17090	Fish, haddock, fillet, bkd/brld	3 oz	85	95	21	0	0	1	0.1	0.1	0.3	63	16
70260	Fish, halibut, battered, fzn	3 ea	113	330	13	22	0	21	3.0	8.0	1.5	20	—
17049	Fish, mackerel, Atlantic, fillet, bkd/brld	3 oz	85	223	20	0	0	15	3.6	6.0	3.7	64	46
17121	Fish, orange roughy, fillet, bkd/brld	3 oz	85	76	16	0	0	1	0.0	0.5	0.0	22	20
17093	Fish, perch, ocean, Atlantic, fillet, bkd/brld	3 oz	85	103	20	0	0	2	0.3	0.7	0.5	46	12
17171	Fish, salmon, pink, fillet, bkd/brld	3 oz	85	127	22	0	0	4	0.6	1.0	1.5	57	35
17068	Fish, sole, fillet, bkd/brld	3 oz	85	100	21	0	0	1	0.3	0.2	0.5	58	11
71139	Fish, sturgeon, filled, bkd/brld mixed species 4.5" x 2" 1/8" x 7/8"	3 oz	85	115	18	0	0	4	1.0	2.1	0.8	65	224
17101	Fish, tuna, bluefin, fillet, bkd/brld	3 oz	85	156	25	0	0	5	1.4	1.7	1.6	42	644
19056	Lobster, bkd/brld	1 ea	125	146	25	2	0	4	2.0	1.1	0.2	96	60
19061	Scallops, bkd/brld	4 ea	100	134	20	3	0	4	0.7	1.5	1.2	40	46
19065	Shrimp, bkd/brld, w/margarine & salt, med	2 ea	10	16	2	0	0	1	0.1	0.2	0.2	18	9
19401	Shrimp, cocktail	1 cup	230	218	28	21	5	3	0.5	0.4	1.0	196	72
70702	Shrimp, popcorn, breaded, fzn	20 ea	112	270	11	28	1	13	2.0	5.0	2.0	35	0

Thia (mg)	Ribo (mg)	Niac (mg NE)	Vit B6 (mg)	Vit B12 (µg)	Fol (µg)	Vit C (mg)	Vit D (IU)	Vit E (mg AT)	Cal (mg)	Iron (mg)	Magn (mg)	Phos (mg)	Pota (mg)	Sodi (mg)	Zinc (mg)	Wat (%)	Alco (g)	Caff (mg)
—	—	—	—	—	—	72.0	—	—	200	4.50	—	—	1400	510	—	—	0.00	0.00
—	—	—	—	—	—	0.0	—	—	150	0.72	—	—	290	100	—	—	0.00	—
—	—	—	—	—	—	0.0	—	—	400	1.44	—	—	770	260	—	—	0.00	—
—	—	—	—	—	—	15.0	—	—	200	5.40	—	—	580	1460	—	—	0.00	0.00
—	—	—	—	—	—	3.6	—	—	20	1.44	—	—	770	340	—	—	0.00	0.00
—	—	—	—	—	—	21.0	—	—	150	1.08	—	—	280	250	—	—	0.00	0.00
—	—	—	—	—	—	27.0	—	—	350	3.59	—	—	950	1090	—	—	0.00	0.00
—	—	—	—	—	—	9.0	—	—	80	2.70	—	—	430	740	—	—	0.00	0.00
0.00	0.00	0.00	0.00	0.01	0.4	0.0	7.8	0.3	3	0.00	0.3	3	3	81	0.0	16	0.00	0.00
0.00	0.00	0.00	0.00	0.00	0.0	0.0	—	0.0	0	0.00	0.0	0	0	6	0.0	0	0.00	0.00
0.00	0.00	0.00	0.00	0.00	0.0	0.0	—	0.1	0	0.00	0.0	0	0	0	0.0	0	0.00	0.00
0.00	0.00	0.00	0.00	0.00	0.0	0.0	—	2.4	0	0.00	0.0	0	0	0	0.0	0	0.00	0.00
0.00	0.00	0.00	0.00	0.00	0.0	0.0	—	1.9	0	0.00	0.0	0	0	0	0.0	0	0.00	0.00
0.00	0.00	0.00	0.00	0.00	0.0	0.0	—	1.9	0	0.09	0.0	0	0	0	0.0	0	0.00	0.00
—	—	—	—	—	—	0.0	—	3.0	0	0.00	—	—	—	0	—	0	0.00	0.00
—	—	—	—	—	—	0.0	—	—	0	0.00	—	—	—	90	—	19	0.00	0.00
0.00	0.00	0.00	0.00	0.00	0.0	0.0	—	0.1	0	0.00	0.0	0	0	0	0.0	0	0.00	0.00
0.12	0.30	2.96	0.10	82.93	26.9	21.8	6.0	3.1	84	24.69	16.2	301	559	202	2.4	72	0.00	0.00
0.02	0.10	1.91	0.15	1.77	1.7	0.0	—	0.1	36	0.33	39.8	131	209	52	0.3	72	0.00	0.00
0.03	0.05	0.60	0.01	0.50	12.0	0.0	1.9	0.1	6	0.20	7.0	51	73	163	0.2	46	0.00	0.00
0.36	0.05	2.14	0.14	2.38	6.0	0.7	—	1.1	8	0.69	22.1	208	273	68	0.9	72	0.00	0.00
0.02	0.03	3.94	0.28	1.17	11.1	0.0	—	0.4	36	1.14	42.5	205	339	74	0.4	74	0.00	0.00
																48	0.00	0.00
0.14	0.34	5.82	0.38	16.15	1.7	0.3	—	1.6	13	1.34	82.5	236	341	71	0.8	53	0.00	0.00
0.10	0.15	3.10	0.28	1.96	6.8	0.0	—	0.5	32	0.20	32.3	218	327	69	0.8	69	0.00	0.00
0.10	0.10	2.06	0.23	0.98	8.5	0.7	—	1.4	117	1.00	33.2	236	298	82	0.5	73	0.00	0.00
0.17	0.05	7.25	0.20	2.94	4.3	0.0	—	1.1	14	0.83	28.1	251	352	73	0.6	70	0.00	0.00
0.07	0.10	1.85	0.20	2.13	7.7	72.0	—	0.6	15	0.28	49.3	246	293	89	0.5	73	0.00	0.00
0.07	0.07	8.59	0.20	2.13	14.5	0.0	—	0.5	14	0.76	38.3	230	310	59	0.5	70	0.00	0.00
0.23	0.25	8.96	0.44	9.25	1.7	0.0	—	1.1	9	1.11	54.4	277	275	43	0.7	59	0.00	0.00
0.00	0.07	1.29	0.09	3.77	13.6	0.0	7.0	1.3	75	0.47	42.5	225	428	492	3.5	74	0.00	0.00
0.00	0.05	1.33	0.17	1.75	18.5	3.5	4.0	1.7	30	0.34	68.0	266	392	231	1.2	71	0.00	0.00
0.00	0.00	0.28	0.00	0.12	0.3	0.2	14.0	0.1	6	0.28	4.5	25	23	21	0.1	68	0.00	0.00
0.10	0.10	4.30	0.25	1.26	47.7	25.7	147.2	3.5	91	3.76	59.4	307	576	1129	1.6	75	0.00	0.00
—	—	—	—	—	—	0.0	—	—	40	1.44	—	—	—	610	—	—	0.00	0.00

Code	Food Name	Unit/ Amt	Wt (g)	Energy (kcal)	Prot (g)	Carb (g)	Fiber (g)	Fat (g)	Sat (g)	Mono (g)	Poly (g)	Chol (mg)	Vit A (RE)
FOOD ADDITIVES													
ALGINATES													
Bases and Preps													
54032	Prep, consomme, chicken style, w/o msg, vgtrn, dry mix	1 cup	246	522	21	76	—	15	2.0	—	—	1	—
Chemicals													
Colors, Flavors, and Aromas													
26624	Flavor, vanilla extract	1 tsp	4	12	0	1	0	0	0.0	0.0	0.0	0	0
Gums, Fibers, Starches, Pectins, Emulsifiers													
30000	Cornstarch	1 Tbs	8	30	0	7	0	0	0.0	0.0	0.0	0	0
Ingredient Sweeteners													
Nutraceuticals													
Nutritional Additives													
JUICE—100% FRUIT, VEGETABLE, OR BLENDED													
3008	Juice, apple, unswtnd, cnd/btld	1 cup	248	117	0	29	0	0	0.0	0.0	0.1	0	0
3455	Juice, grapefruit, pink, fresh	1 cup	247	96	1	23	0	0	0.0	0.0	0.1	0	109
3090	Juice, orange, fresh	1 cup	248	112	2	26	0	0	0.1	0.1	0.1	0	50
3561	Juice, orange, fzn, conc	2.2 oz	63	110	1	27	0	0	0.0	0.0	0.0	0	0
Fruits													
3001	Apples, fresh, lrg, 3 1/4"	1 ea	212	110	1	29	5	0	0.1	0.0	0.1	0	13
3147	Applesauce, swtnd, unsalted, cnd	1 cup	255	194	0	51	3	0	0.1	0.0	0.1	0	5
3157	Apricots, fresh, whole	1 ea	35	17	0	4	1	0	0.0	0.1	0.0	0	67
3016	Avocado, avg, fresh	1 ea	201	322	4	17	13	29	4.3	19.7	3.7	0	28
3020	Banana, fresh, med, 7" to 7 7/8" long	1 ea	118	105	1	27	3	0	0.1	0.0	0.1	0	7
3029	Blueberries, fresh	0.5 cup	68	39	1	10	2	0	0.0	0.0	0.1	0	4
3026	Boysenberries, fresh	0.5 cup	72	31	1	7	4	0	0.0	0.0	0.2	0	16
3036	Cherries, sweet, fresh	1 ea	7	4	0	1	0	0	0.0	0.0	0.0	0	0
3191	Currants, red, fresh	1 cup	112	63	2	15	5	0	0.0	0.0	0.1	0	4
3676	Figs, fresh, lrg, 2 1/2"	1 ea	64	47	0	12	2	0	0.0	0.0	0.1	0	9
3203	Gooseberries, fresh	0.5 cup	75	33	1	8	3	0	0.0	0.0	0.2	0	22
3818	Grapefruit, pink, fresh, 3 3/4"	0.5 ea	123	52	1	13	2	0	0.0	0.0	0.0	0	143
3820	Grapefruit, red, fresh, 3 3/4"	0.5 ea	123	52	1	13	2	0	0.0	0.0	0.0	0	143
3638	Kiwi, fresh	1 cup	177	108	2	26	5	1	0.1	0.1	0.5	0	14
3067	Lemon Peel, fresh	1 Tbs	6	3	0	1	1	0	0.0	0.0	0.0	0	0
3071	Limes, peeled, fresh, 2"	1 ea	67	20	0	7	2	0	0.0	0.0	0.0	0	3
71769	Mandarin Oranges, fresh, med, 2 3/8"	1 ea	84	45	1	11	2	0	0.0	0.1	0.1	0	57
71774	Mandarin Oranges, w/light syrup, cnd	1 cup	252	154	1	41	2	0	0.0	0.0	0.1	0	212
3221	Mango, fresh, whole	0.5 ea	104	67	1	18	2	0	0.1	0.1	0.1	0	79
3076	Melon, cantaloupe, fresh, med, 5"	1 ea	552	188	5	45	5	1	0.3	0.0	0.4	0	1866
71102	Melon, honeydew, fresh, 5 1/4"	1 ea	1000	360	5	91	8	1	0.4	0.0	0.6	0	60
3309	Mulberries, fresh	10 ea	15	6	0	1	0	0	0.0	0.0	0.0	0	0
3215	Nectarines, fresh, 2 1/2"	1 ea	136	60	1	14	2	0	0.0	0.1	0.2	0	46
3082	Oranges, fresh, med, 2 5/8"	1 ea	131	62	1	15	3	0	0.0	0.0	0.0	0	29
3720	Papaya, fresh, lrg, 5 3/4"–x 3 1/"4	1 ea	380	148	2	37	7	1	0.2	0.1	0.1	0	418
3096	Peaches, fresh, med, w/o skin, 2 1/2"	1 ea	98	38	1	9	1	0	0.0	0.1	0.1	0	31
3103	Pears, fresh, bartlett, med	1 ea	166	96	1	26	5	0	0.0	0.0	0.0	0	3
71114	Pineapple, chunks, w/juice, cnd, not drained	0.5 cup	124	75	1	20	1	0	0.0	0.0	0.0	0	5

Thia (mg)	Ribo (mg)	Niac (mg NE)	Vit B6 (mg)	Vit B12 (µg)	Fol (µg)	Vit C (mg)	Vit D (IU)	Vit E (mg AT)	Cal (mg)	Iron (mg)	Magn (mg)	Phos (mg)	Pota (mg)	Sodi (mg)	Zinc (mg)	Wat (%)	Alco (g)	Caff (mg)
—	—	—	—	—	—	—	—	—	—	—	—	—	492	46494	—	—	0.00	0.00
0.00	0.00	0.01	0.00	0.00	0.0	0.0	—	0.0	0	0.00	0.5	0	6	0	0.0	53	1.49	0.00
0.00	0.00	0.00	0.00	0.00	0.0	0.0	—	0.0	0	0.03	0.2	1	0	1	0.0	8	0.00	0.00
0.05	0.03	0.25	0.07	0.00	0.0	2.2	—	0.0	17	0.92	7.4	17	295	7	0.1	88	0.00	0.00
0.10	0.05	0.49	0.10	0.00	24.7	93.9	0.0	0.1	22	0.49	29.6	37	400	2	0.1	90	0.00	0.00
0.21	0.07	0.99	0.10	0.00	74.4	124.0	—	0.1	27	0.50	27.3	42	496	2	0.1	88	0.00	0.00
0.00	—	0.00	0.00	—	10.0	78.0	—	0.0	20	0.00	—		430	5	—	53	0.00	0.00
0.03	0.05	0.18	0.09	0.00	6.4	9.8	—	0.4	13	0.25	10.6	23	227	2	0.1	86	0.00	0.00
0.02	0.07	0.47	0.07	0.00	2.5	4.3	—	0.5	10	0.88	7.6	18	156	8	0.1	80	0.00	0.00
0.00	0.00	0.20	0.01	0.00	3.1	3.5	—	0.3	5	0.14	3.5	8	91	0	0.1	86	0.00	0.00
0.12	0.25	3.49	0.51	0.00	162.8	20.1	—	4.2	24	1.11	58.3	105	975	14	1.3	73	0.00	0.00
0.03	0.09	0.77	0.43	0.00	23.6	10.3	—	0.1	6	0.31	31.9	26	422	1	0.2	75	0.00	0.00
0.02	0.02	0.28	0.03	0.00	4.1	6.6	—	0.4	4	0.18	4.1	8	52	1	0.1	84	0.00	0.00
0.00	0.01	0.46	0.01	0.00	18.0	15.1	—	0.8	21	0.44	14.4	16	117	1	0.4	88	0.00	0.00
0.00	0.00	0.00	0.00	0.00	0.3	0.5	—	0.0	1	0.01	0.7	1	15	0	0.0	82	0.00	0.00
0.03	0.05	0.10	0.07	0.00	9.0	45.9	—	0.1	37	1.12	14.6	49	308	1	0.3	84	0.00	0.00
0.03	0.02	0.25	0.07	0.00	3.8	1.3	—	0.1	22	0.23	10.9	9	148	1	0.1	79	0.00	0.00
0.02	0.01	0.23	0.05	0.00	4.5	20.8	—	0.3	19	0.23	7.5	20	148	1	0.1	88	0.00	0.00
0.05	0.03	0.25	0.07	0.00	16.0	38.4	—	0.2	27	0.10	11.1	22	166	0	0.1	88	0.00	0.00
0.05	0.03	0.25	0.07	0.00	16.0	38.4	—	0.2	27	0.10	11.1	22	166	0	0.1	88	0.00	0.00
0.05	0.03	0.60	0.10	0.00	44.2	164.1	—	2.6	60	0.55	30.1	60	552	5	0.2	83	0.00	0.00
0.00	0.00	0.01	0.00	0.00	0.8	7.7	—	0.0	8	0.05	0.9	1	10	0	0.0	82	0.00	0.00
0.01	0.00	0.12	0.02	0.00	5.4	19.5	—	0.1	22	0.40	4.0	12	68	1	0.1	88	0.00	0.00
0.05	0.02	0.31	0.07	0.00	13.4	22.4	—	0.2	31	0.12	10.1	17	139	2	0.1	85	0.00	0.00
0.12	0.10	1.12	0.10	0.00	12.6	49.9	—	0.3	18	0.93	20.2	25	197	15	0.6	83	0.00	0.00
0.05	0.05	0.60	0.14	0.00	14.5	28.7	—	1.2	10	0.12	9.3	11	161	2	0.0	82	0.00	0.00
0.23	0.10	4.05	0.40	0.00	115.9	202.6	—	0.3	50	1.15	66.2	83	1474	88	1.0	90	0.00	0.00
0.37	0.11	4.17	0.87	0.00	190.0	180.0	—	0.2	60	1.70	100.0	110	2280	180	0.9	90	0.00	0.00
0.00	0.01	0.09	0.00	0.00	0.9	5.5	0.0	0.1	6	0.28	2.7	6	29	2	0.0	88	0.00	0.00
0.05	0.03	1.52	0.02	0.00	6.8	7.3	—	1.0	8	0.37	12.2	35	273	0	0.2	88	0.00	0.00
0.10	0.05	0.37	0.07	0.00	39.3	69.7	—	0.2	52	0.12	13.1	18	237	0	0.1	87	0.00	0.00
0.10	0.11	1.27	0.07	0.00	144.4	234.8	—	2.8	91	0.37	38.0	19	977	11	0.3	89	0.00	0.00
0.01	0.02	0.79	0.01	0.00	3.9	6.5	—	0.7	6	0.25	8.8	20	186	0	0.2	89	0.00	0.00
0.01	0.03	0.25	0.05	0.00	11.6	7.0	—	0.2	15	0.28	11.6	18	198	2	0.2	84	0.00	0.00
0.11	0.01	0.34	0.09	0.00	6.2	11.8	—	0.0	17	0.34	17.4	7	152	1	0.1	84	0.00	0.00

48

PAGE KEY: 2 Beverage and Beverage Mixes 4 Other Beverages 4 Beverages, Alcoholic 6 Candies and Confections, Gum 10 Cereals, Breakfast Type
14 Cheese and Cheese Substitutes 16 Dairy Products and Substitutes 18 Desserts 24 Dessert Toppings 24 Eggs, Substitutes, and Egg Dishes 26 Ethnic Foods
30 Fast Foods/Restaurants 44 Fats, Oils, Margarines, Shortenings, and Substitutes 44 Fish, Seafood, and Shellfish 46 Food Additives
46 Fruit, Vegetable, or Blended Juices 48 Grains, Flours, and Fractions 48 Grain Products, Prepared and Baked Goods

Code	Food Name	Unit/ Amt	Wt (g)	Energy (kcal)	Prot (g)	Carb (g)	Fiber (g)	Fat (g)	Sat (g)	Mono (g)	Poly (g)	Chol (mg)	Vit A (RE)
3112	Pineapple, fresh	1 ea	472	227	3	60	7	1	0.0	0.1	0.2	0	28
3121	Plums, fresh, 2 1/8"	1 ea	66	30	0	8	1	0	0.0	0.1	0.0	0	22
3197	Pomegranate, fresh, 3 3/8"	1 ea	154	105	1	26	1	0	0.1	0.1	0.1	0	15
3202	Raisins, golden, seedless, packed cup	0.25 cup	41	125	1	33	2	0	0.1	0.0	0.1	0	0
3209	Rhubarb, fresh, diced	0.5 cup	61	13	1	3	1	0	0.0	0.0	0.1	0	6
3134	Strawberries, fresh, whole	1 cup	144	46	1	11	3	0	0.0	0.1	0.2	0	3
3087	Tangelo, fresh, 2 3/8"	1 ea	96	45	1	11	2	0	0.0	0.0	0.0	0	21
3717	Tangerines, fresh, lrg, 2 1/2"	1 ea	98	52	1	13	2	0	0.0	0.1	0.1	0	67
3143	Watermelon, fresh, slice, 1/16 melon	1 pce	286	86	2	22	1	0	0.0	0.1	0.1	0	160

GRAINS, FLOURS, AND FRACTIONS

Code	Food Name	Unit/ Amt	Wt (g)	Energy (kcal)	Prot (g)	Carb (g)	Fiber (g)	Fat (g)	Sat (g)	Mono (g)	Poly (g)	Chol (mg)	Vit A (RE)
38650	Dish, wheat pilaf, dry mix	2 oz	57	184	6	42	5	1	0.2	0.1	0.4	0	7
28018	Flour, all purpose, self-rising, bleached, enrich	0.25 cup	30	100	3	22	0	0	0.0	0.0	0.0	0	0
38030	Flour, all purpose, white, bleached, enrich	0.25 cup	31	114	3	24	1	0	0.0	0.0	0.1	0	0
46086	Flour, cake, white, enrich, unsifted	0.25 cup	34	124	3	27	1	0	0.0	0.0	0.1	0	0
38032	Flour, whole wheat	0.25 cup	30	102	4	22	4	1	0.1	0.1	0.2	0	0
38017	Oats, old fash, dry	0.5 cup	40	148	5	27	4	3	0.4	0.8	0.9	0	0
38575	Oats, steel cut, Irish style, dry	0.25 cup	40	148	5	27	4	3	0.4	0.8	0.9	0	0
2730	Tapioca, dry	1.5 tsp	6	20	0	5	0	0	0.0	0.0	0.0	0	0
38027	Wheat, bulgur, dry	0.25 cup	35	120	4	27	6	0	0.1	0.1	0.2	0	0
38026	Wheat, germ, tstd	1 cup	113	432	33	56	17	12	2.1	1.7	7.5	0	11
38068	Wheat, sprouted	1 cup	108	214	8	46	1	1	0.2	0.2	0.6	0	0

GRAIN PRODUCTS, PREPARED AND BAKED GOODS
Bagels

Code	Food Name	Unit/ Amt	Wt (g)	Energy (kcal)	Prot (g)	Carb (g)	Fiber (g)	Fat (g)	Sat (g)	Mono (g)	Poly (g)	Chol (mg)	Vit A (RE)
71165	Bagel, egg, 3"	1 ea	57	158	6	30	1	1	0.2	0.2	0.4	14	19
8846	Bagel, plain, classic, 4 oz svg	1 ea	112	296	11	60	3	2	—	—	—	0	0

Biscuits

Code	Food Name	Unit/ Amt	Wt (g)	Energy (kcal)	Prot (g)	Carb (g)	Fiber (g)	Fat (g)	Sat (g)	Mono (g)	Poly (g)	Chol (mg)	Vit A (RE)
42001	Biscuit, buttermilk, prep f/recipe, 2 1/2"	1 ea	60	212	4	27	1	10	2.6	4.2	2.5	2	14
71195	Biscuit, plain, prep f/recipe, 2 1/2"	1 ea	60	212	4	27	1	10	2.6	4.2	2.5	2	14
42205	Biscuit, whole wheat	1 ea	63	199	6	30	5	7	1.7	3.0	2.2	2	14

Breads and Rolls

Code	Food Name	Unit/ Amt	Wt (g)	Energy (kcal)	Prot (g)	Carb (g)	Fiber (g)	Fat (g)	Sat (g)	Mono (g)	Poly (g)	Chol (mg)	Vit A (RE)
71024	Bread Crumbs, white, soft, enrich	1 cup	45	120	3	23	1	1	0.3	0.3	0.6	0	0
71021	Bread, 7 grain, slice	1 pce	26	65	3	12	2	1	0.2	0.4	0.2	0	0
42052	Bread, Boston brown, cnd, slice	1 pce	45	88	2	19	2	1	0.1	0.1	0.3	0	11
42042	Bread, cracked wheat, slice, reg	1 pce	25	65	2	12	1	1	0.2	0.5	0.2	0	0
71207	Bread, French, slice, lrg	1 pce	96	263	8	50	3	3	0.6	1.2	0.7	0	0
42049	Bread, oatmeal, slice	1 pce	27	73	2	13	1	1	0.2	0.4	0.5	0	1
42007	Bread, pita, white, enrich, lrg, 6 1/2"	1 ea	60	165	5	33	1	1	0.1	0.1	0.3	0	0
42051	Bread, raisin, enrich, slice	1 pce	26	71	2	14	1	1	0.3	0.6	0.2	0	0
57235	Bread, rye, mild	1 pce	32	70	3	13	4	0	0.0	—	—	0	0
42003	Bread, sourdough starter	1 cup	250	359	17	70	5	2	0.2	—	—	1	38
42012	Bread, wheat, slice	1 pce	25	65	2	12	1	1	0.2	0.4	0.2	0	0
42138	Bread, white, prep w/2% milk f/recipe, slice	1 pce	42	120	3	21	1	2	0.5	0.5	1.2	1	10
71020	Bread, whole grain, slice	1 pce	26	65	3	12	2	1	0.2	0.4	0.2	0	0
71939	Bread, wraps, thin thin	1 ea	35	110	4	21	0	1	0.0	—	—	0	0
42036	Breadsticks, plain, 7 5/8" x 5/8"	1 ea	10	41	1	7	0	1	0.1	0.4	0.4	0	0

Thia (mg)	Ribo (mg)	Niac (mg NE)	Vit B6 (mg)	Vit B12 (µg)	Fol (µg)	Vit C (mg)	Vit D (IU)	Vit E (mg AT)	Cal (mg)	Iron (mg)	Magn (mg)	Phos (mg)	Pota (mg)	Sodi (mg)	Zinc (mg)	Wat (%)	Alco (g)	Caff (mg)
0.37	0.15	2.30	0.51	0.00	70.8	170.9	—	0.1	61	1.32	56.6	38	543	5	0.5	86	0.00	0.00
0.01	0.01	0.28	0.01	0.00	3.3	6.3	—	0.2	4	0.10	4.6	11	104	0	0.1	87	0.00	0.00
0.05	0.05	0.46	0.15	0.00	9.2	9.4	—	0.9	5	0.46	4.6	12	399	5	0.2	81	0.00	0.00
0.00	0.07	0.46	0.12	0.00	1.2	1.3	—	0.0	22	0.74	14.4	47	308	5	0.1	15	0.00	0.00
0.00	0.01	0.18	0.00	0.00	4.3	4.9	—	0.2	52	0.12	7.3	9	176	2	0.1	94	0.00	0.00
0.02	0.02	0.56	0.07	0.00	34.6	84.7	—	0.4	23	0.60	18.7	35	220	1	0.2	91	0.00	0.00
0.07	0.03	0.27	0.05	0.00	28.8	51.1	—	0.2	38	0.10	9.6	13	174	0	0.1	87	0.00	0.00
0.05	0.03	0.37	0.07	0.00	15.7	26.2	—	0.2	36	0.15	11.8	20	163	2	0.1	85	0.00	0.00
0.09	0.05	0.50	0.12	0.00	8.6	23.2	—	0.1	20	0.68	28.6	31	320	3	0.3	91	0.00	0.00
0.17	0.10	2.47	0.11	0.00	12.1	1.2	0.0	0.3	23	1.10	10.8	49	213	645	0.6	9	0.00	0.00
0.15	0.10	1.60	—	—	40.0	0.0	—	—	60	1.44	—	—	35	400	—	16	0.00	0.00
0.25	0.15	1.84	0.00	0.00	57.2	0.0	—	0.0	5	1.45	6.9	34	33	1	0.2	12	0.00	0.00
0.31	0.15	2.32	0.00	0.00	63.7	0.0	—	0.0	5	2.50	5.5	29	36	1	0.2	13	0.00	0.00
0.12	0.05	1.90	0.10	0.00	13.2	0.0	—	0.2	10	1.15	41.4	104	122	2	0.9	10	0.00	0.00
0.21	0.05	0.33	0.03	0.00	19.5	0.0	0.0	0.3	19	1.86	107.9	183	143	1	1.3	9	0.00	0.00
0.21	0.05	0.33	0.03	0.00	19.5	0.0	0.0	0.3	19	1.86	107.9	183	143	1	1.3	9	0.00	0.00
—	—	—	—	—	—	0.0	—	—	0	0.00	—	0	0	0	—	—	0.00	0.00
0.07	0.03	1.78	0.11	0.00	9.4	0.0	—	0.0	12	0.86	57.4	105	144	6	0.7	9	0.00	0.00
1.88	0.93	6.32	1.11	0.00	397.8	6.8	0.0	18.1	51	10.27	361.6	1295	1070	5	18.8	6	0.00	0.00
0.23	0.17	3.32	0.28	0.00	41.0	2.8	—	0.1	30	2.30	88.6	216	183	17	1.8	48	0.00	0.00
0.31	0.12	1.96	0.05	0.09	50.2	0.3	—	0.1	7	2.26	14.2	48	39	288	0.4	33	0.00	0.00
0.47	0.31	3.96	0.00	0.00	0.1	0.1	0.0	0.0	14	3.32	0.4	71	80	510	0.0	34	0.00	0.00
0.20	0.18	1.76	0.01	0.05	36.6	0.1	—	0.8	141	1.74	10.8	98	73	348	0.3	29	0.00	0.00
0.20	0.18	1.76	0.01	0.05	36.6	0.1	—	0.8	141	1.74	10.8	98	73	348	0.3	29	0.00	0.00
0.15	0.11	2.20	0.12	0.07	13.0	0.2	10.1	1.3	155	1.69	56.9	199	200	210	1.2	28	0.00	0.00
0.20	0.15	1.97	0.03	0.00	49.9	0.0	—	0.1	68	1.67	10.3	45	45	306	0.3	36	0.00	0.00
0.10	0.09	1.12	0.09	0.01	30.7	0.1	—	0.1	24	0.89	13.8	46	53	127	0.3	38	0.00	0.00
0.00	0.05	0.50	0.03	0.00	4.9	0.0	—	0.1	32	0.93	28.3	50	143	284	0.2	47	0.00	0.00
0.09	0.05	0.92	0.07	0.00	15.2	0.0	—	0.1	11	0.69	13.0	38	44	134	0.3	36	0.00	0.00
0.50	0.31	4.55	0.03	0.00	142.1	0.0	—	0.3	72	2.43	25.9	101	108	585	0.8	34	0.00	0.00
0.10	0.05	0.85	0.01	0.00	16.7	0.0	—	0.1	18	0.73	10.0	34	38	162	0.3	37	0.00	0.00
0.36	0.20	2.77	0.01	0.00	64.2	0.0	—	0.2	52	1.57	15.6	58	72	322	0.5	32	0.00	0.00
0.09	0.10	0.89	0.01	0.00	27.6	0.0	—	0.1	17	0.75	6.8	28	59	101	0.2	34	0.00	0.00
0.15	0.14	3.00	0.30	0.89	80.0	0.0	—	—	100	1.79	60.0	—	—	70	2.2	47	0.00	0.00
1.00	1.35	10.68	0.30	0.31	508.7	0.5	35.2	0.1	123	6.17	42.9	358	522	57	1.9	64	0.00	0.00
0.10	0.07	1.02	0.01	0.00	22.8	0.0	—	0.1	26	0.82	11.5	38	50	132	0.3	37	0.00	0.00
0.17	0.15	1.50	0.01	0.02	38.2	0.1	—	0.4	24	1.25	8.0	48	61	151	0.3	35	0.00	0.00
0.10	0.09	1.12	0.09	0.01	30.7	0.1	—	0.1	24	0.89	13.8	46	53	127	0.3	38	0.00	0.00
—	—	—	—	—	—	0.0	—	—	40	1.44	—	—	—	190	—	—	0.00	0.00
0.05	0.05	0.52	0.00	0.00	16.2	0.0	—	0.1	2	0.43	3.2	12	12	66	0.1	6	0.00	0.00

50

PAGE KEY: 2 Beverage and Beverage Mixes 4 Other Beverages 4 Beverages, Alcoholic 6 Candies and Confections, Gum 10 Cereals, Breakfast Type
14 Cheese and Cheese Substitutes 16 Dairy Products and Substitutes 18 Desserts 24 Dessert Toppings 24 Eggs, Substitutes, and Egg Dishes 26 Ethnic Foods
30 Fast Foods/Restaurants 44 Fats, Oils, Margarines, Shortenings, and Substitutes 44 Fish, Seafood, and Shellfish 46 Food Additives
46 Fruit, Vegetable, or Blended Juices 48 Grains, Flours, and Fractions 48 Grain Products, Prepared and Baked Goods

Code	Food Name	Unit/Amt	Wt (g)	Energy (kcal)	Prot (g)	Carb (g)	Fiber (g)	Fat (g)	Sat (g)	Mono (g)	Poly (g)	Chol (mg)	Vit A (RE)
42020	Buns, hamburger	1 ea	43	120	4	21	1	2	0.5	0.5	0.8	0	0
42021	Buns, hot dog/frankfurter	1 ea	43	120	4	21	1	2	0.5	0.5	0.8	0	0
42649	Cornbread, homestyle, prep f/dry mix, 2" x 3" pce	1 pce	52	150	3	26	1	4	1.0	1.5	1.0	5	0
42015	Croissant, butter, med	1 ea	57	231	5	26	1	12	6.6	3.1	0.6	38	120
45520	Dumpling, plain	1 ea	32	40	1	7	0	1	0.3	0.4	0.3	1	4
43512	Matzoh Balls	3 ea	42	58	2	7	0	2	0.5	0.8	0.5	44	20
71886	Pretzels, soft, garlic	1 ea	120	320	9	66	2	1	0.0	—	—	0	0
42018	Rolls, dinner, brown & serve, browned	1 ea	28	84	2	14	1	2	0.5	1.0	0.3	0	0
42158	Rolls, dinner, prep f/recipe w/2% milk, 2 1/2"	1 ea	35	111	3	19	1	3	0.6	1.0	0.7	12	32
42022	Rolls, hard, 3 1/2"	1 ea	57	167	6	30	1	2	0.3	0.6	1.0	0	0
71358	Rolls, hoagie, whole wheat, med	1 ea	94	250	8	48	7	4	0.8	1.1	2.0	0	0
71359	Rolls, submarine, whole wheat, med	1 ea	94	250	8	48	7	4	0.8	1.1	2.0	0	0

Bread Crumbs, Croutons, Breading Mixes & Batters

Code	Food Name	Unit/Amt	Wt (g)	Energy (kcal)	Prot (g)	Carb (g)	Fiber (g)	Fat (g)	Sat (g)	Mono (g)	Poly (g)	Chol (mg)	Vit A (RE)
42004	Bread Crumbs, plain, grated, dry	1 Tbs	7	27	1	5	0	0	0.1	0.1	0.1	0	0
42016	Croutons, plain, dry	0.25 cup	8	31	1	6	0	0	0.1	0.2	0.1	0	0

Crackers

43503	Cracker Crumbs, graham, plain	1 cup	84	355	6	65	2	8	1.3	3.4	3.2	0	0
71273	Crackers, cheese, 1" square	30 ea	30	151	3	17	1	8	2.8	3.6	0.7	4	9
11712	Crackers, club style	1 ea	7	32	1	5	0	1	0.3	—	—	0	0
11745	Crackers, ea, Town House	5 ea	16	83	1	9	0	5	0.9	—	—	0	1
47253	Crackers, graham, honey	3 ea	21	92	2	16	1	3	0.7	—	—	0	0
43535	Crackers, matzoh, egg, svg	1 oz	28	111	3	22	1	1	0.2	0.2	0.1	24	4
43509	Crackers, melba toast, plain, pce, 3 3/4" x 1 3/4" x 1/8"	1 pce	5	20	1	4	0	0	0.0	0.0	0.1	0	0
70963	Crackers, original, svg	5 ea	16	79	1	10	0	4	0.6	2.8	0.3	0	0
43506	Crackers, saltines	4 ea	12	51	1	9	0	1	0.2	0.8	0.1	0	0
43581	Crackers, wheat, original	16 ea	29	136	2	20	1	6	0.9	2.0	0.4	0	0

Muffins

44585	English Muffin, traditional	1 ea	57	130	5	26	2	0	0.0	—	—	0	0
44515	Muffin, plain, prep f/recipe w/2% milk	1 ea	57	169	4	24	2	6	1.2	1.6	3.3	22	23
42295	Popover, unenrich, dry mix, 6 oz pkg	1 ea	170	631	18	121	—	7	1.7	3.4	1.4	0	0

Pancakes, French Toast, and Waffles

45033	Crepe, suzette	1 ea	66	159	4	16	0	9	3.8	3.2	1.3	83	81
42156	French Toast, prep f/recipe w/2% milk	1 pce	65	149	5	16	1	7	1.8	2.9	1.7	75	84
45192	Pancakes, buttermilk	1 ea	43	99	3	16	0	3	0.6	1.3	0.9	5	73
45152	Waffles, buttermilk egg, 7" prep f/dry mix	1 ea	81	230	6	37	2	7	1.0	3.5	2.5	10	0

Pasta

57411	Dish, ravioli, beef, square, preckd	9 pce	146	300	14	40	1	8	3.8	—	—	77	—
92216	Dish, tortellini, cheese filled	1 cup	108	332	15	51	2	8	3.9	2.2	0.5	45	42
91205	Pasta, acini di pepe, enrich, dry, all brands	3.6 oz	100	364	14	74	3	1	0.4	—	—	0	0
38365	Pasta, egg noodles	0.75 cup	68	200	8	33	1	4	1.0	—	—	40	0
38580	Pasta, elbow twist, semolina, dry	0.75 cup	56	201	7	41	2	1	0.3	0.2	0.8	0	0
91211	Pasta, lasagna noodles, enrich, dry, all brands	3.6 oz	100	364	14	74	3	1	0.4	—	—	0	0
38102	Pasta, macaroni noodles, enrich, ckd	1 cup	140	197	7	40	2	1	0.1	0.1	0.4	0	0
38551	Pasta, rice noodle, ckd	0.5 cup	88	96	1	22	1	0	0.0	0.0	0.0	0	0
38105	Pasta, shells, sml, enrich, ckd	0.5 cup	58	81	3	16	1	0	0.1	0.0	0.2	0	0
38118	Pasta, spaghetti noodles, enrich, ckd	0.5 cup	70	99	3	20	1	0	0.1	0.1	0.2	0	0

Thia (mg)	Ribo (mg)	Niac (mg NE)	Vit B6 (mg)	Vit B12 (µg)	Fol (µg)	Vit C (mg)	Vit D (IU)	Vit E (mg AT)	Cal (mg)	Iron (mg)	Magn (mg)	Phos (mg)	Pota (mg)	Sodi (mg)	Zinc (mg)	Wat (%)	Alco (g)	Caff (mg)
0.17	0.14	1.78	0.02	0.09	47.7	0.0	—	0.0	59	1.42	9.0	27	40	206	0.3	35	0.00	0.00
0.17	0.14	1.78	0.02	0.09	47.7	0.0	—	0.0	59	1.42	9.0	27	40	206	0.3	35	0.00	0.00
—	—	—	—	—	—	0.0	—	—	9	0.49	—	90	40	280	—	35	0.00	0.00
0.21	0.14	1.25	0.02	0.09	50.2	0.1	—	0.5	21	1.15	9.1	60	67	424	0.4	23	0.00	0.00
0.05	0.05	0.41	0.00	0.01	1.8	0.1	—	0.1	45	0.43	3.0	28	20	66	0.1	72	0.00	0.00
0.02	0.07	0.31	0.01	0.09	4.5	0.0	—	0.3	6	0.43	3.3	26	22	13	0.2	72	0.00	0.00
—	—	—	—	—	—	0.0	—	—	20	2.16	—	—	—	830	—	—	0.00	0.00
0.14	0.09	1.12	0.01	0.01	27.4	0.0	—	0.1	33	0.87	6.4	32	37	146	0.2	32	0.00	0.00
0.14	0.14	1.21	0.01	0.05	31.5	0.1	—	0.3	21	1.03	6.7	44	53	145	0.2	29	0.00	0.00
0.27	0.18	2.42	0.01	0.00	54.1	0.0	—	0.2	54	1.87	15.4	57	62	310	0.5	31	0.00	0.00
0.23	0.14	3.46	0.18	0.00	28.2	0.0	—	0.8	100	2.26	79.9	211	256	449	1.9	33	0.00	0.00
0.23	0.14	3.46	0.18	0.00	28.2	0.0	—	0.8	100	2.26	79.9	211	256	449	1.9	33	0.00	0.00
0.07	0.02	0.44	0.00	0.01	7.2	0.0	—	0.0	12	0.33	2.9	11	13	49	0.1	7	0.00	0.00
0.05	0.01	0.40	0.00	0.00	9.9	0.0	—	0.0	6	0.31	2.3	9	9	52	0.1	6	0.00	0.00
0.18	0.25	3.46	0.05	0.00	38.6	0.0	—	0.3	20	3.13	25.2	87	113	508	0.7	4	0.00	0.00
0.17	0.12	1.39	0.17	0.14	45.6	0.0	—	0.0	45	1.42	10.8	65	44	298	0.3	3	0.00	0.00
—	—	—	—	—	—	0.0	—	—	2	0.15	—	—	—	70	—	7	0.00	0.00
—	—	—	—	—	—	0.2	—	—	4	0.47	—	—	—	155	—	—	0.00	0.00
—	—	—	—	—	—	0.0	—	—	17	0.73	—	—	—	114	—	3	0.00	0.00
0.21	0.18	1.44	0.01	0.05	6.8	0.0	—	0.3	11	0.76	6.8	42	43	6	0.2	6	0.00	0.00
0.01	0.00	0.20	0.00	0.00	6.2	0.0	—	0.0	5	0.18	3.0	10	10	41	0.1	5	0.00	0.00
0.03	0.05	0.61	0.00	0.00	9.6	0.0	—	—	24	0.64	3.2	48	15	124	0.2	3	0.00	0.00
0.00	0.05	0.62	0.00	0.00	16.7	0.0	—	0.1	8	0.68	2.6	12	18	129	0.1	5	0.00	0.00
0.09	0.09	1.15	0.02	—	12.2	0.0	—	—	23	1.07	15.1	60	56	168	—	2	0.00	0.00
—	—	—	—	—	—	0.0	—	—	80	1.08	—	—	—	250	—	43	0.00	0.00
0.15	0.17	1.32	0.01	0.09	29.1	0.2	—	1.0	114	1.36	9.7	87	69	266	0.3	38	0.00	0.00
0.17	0.03	1.76	0.07	0.14	42.5	0.2	—	1.8	54	1.38	42.5	170	170	1541	1.5	12	0.00	0.00
0.07	0.17	0.60	0.03	0.23	10.7	3.0	21.1	0.6	45	0.75	8.3	69	86	74	0.4	56	0.00	0.00
0.12	0.20	1.05	0.05	0.20	27.9	0.2	—	0.7	65	1.09	11.0	76	87	311	0.4	55	0.00	0.00
0.10	0.11	1.47	0.15	0.43	22.1	0.6	—	0.0	15	1.32	7.7	145	44	225	0.3	47	0.00	0.00
—	—	—	—	—	—	0.0	—	—	43	1.50	—	450	130	900	—	—	0.00	0.00
—	—	—	—	—	—	—	—	—	119	2.10	—	—	—	400	—	—	0.00	0.00
0.34	0.33	2.91	0.05	0.17	79.9	0.0	—	0.2	164	1.62	22.7	229	96	372	1.1	30	0.00	0.00
0.80	0.44	5.36	—	—	214.0	0.0	—	—	18	3.21	53.7	141	144	5	1.2	10	0.00	0.00
—	—	—	—	—	—	0.0	—	—	0	1.79	—	—	—	140	—	—	0.00	0.00
0.49	0.20	3.33	0.07	0.00	10.3	0.0	—	0.1	12	1.61	—	105	—	3	0.7	11	0.00	0.00
0.80	0.44	5.36	—	—	214.0	0.0	—	—	18	3.21	53.7	141	144	5	1.2	10	0.00	0.00
0.28	0.14	2.33	0.05	0.00	107.8	0.0	—	0.1	10	1.96	25.2	76	43	1	0.7	66	0.00	0.00
0.01	0.00	0.05	0.00	0.00	2.6	0.0	—	—	4	0.11	2.6	18	4	17	0.2	74	0.00	0.00
0.11	0.05	0.95	0.01	0.00	44.3	0.0	—	0.0	4	0.80	10.3	31	18	1	0.3	66	0.00	0.00
0.14	0.07	1.16	0.01	0.00	53.9	0.0	—	0.0	5	0.98	12.6	38	22	1	0.4	66	0.00	0.00

Code	Food Name	Unit/ Amt	Wt (g)	Energy (kcal)	Prot (g)	Carb (g)	Fiber (g)	Fat (g)	Sat (g)	Mono (g)	Poly (g)	Chol (mg)	Vit A (RE)
Rice													
38013	Rice, white, long grain, ckd	1 cup	158	205	4	45	1	0	0.1	0.1	0.1	0	0
Stuffing and Mixes													
38491	Baking Mix, dry, Bisquick	0.33 cup	40	162	3	24	1	6	1.6	2.5	0.5	0	0
42037	Stuffing, bread, prep f/dry mix	0.5 cup	100	178	3	22	3	9	1.7	3.8	2.6	0	125
Tortillas and Taco/Tostada Shells													
42359	Taco Shells	2 ea	27	130	2	18	2	6	1.0	3.8	1.2	0	0
Granola Bars, Cereal Bars, Diet Bars, Scones, and Tarts													
53227	Bar, cereal, mixed berry	1 ea	37	137	2	27	1	3	0.6	1.9	0.4	0	150
23100	Bar, granola, almond, hard	1 ea	24	117	2	15	1	6	3.0	1.8	0.9	0	1
47591	Bar, granola, cinnamon	2 ea	42	180	4	29	2	6	0.5	—	—	0	0
63342	Bar, granola, fruit & nut	3.6 oz	100	397	8	77	5	6	0.7	0.2	4.8	0	28
47592	Bar, granola, oats 'n honey	2 ea	42	180	4	29	2	6	0.5	—	—	0	0
23059	Bar, granola, plain, hard	1 ea	24	115	2	16	1	5	0.6	1.1	3.0	0	4
42071	Scones	1 ea	42	150	4	19	1	6	2.0	2.6	1.3	49	69
MEALS AND DISHES													
Canned Meals and Dishes													
92620	Dish, ravioli, beef, w/meat sauce, cnd	1 cup	212	260	11	39	5	7	3.0	—	—	10	100
FROZEN OR REFRIGERATED MEALS AND DISHES													
Frozen/Refrigerated Breakfasts													
70830	Eggs, scrambled, low fat	1 ea	170	240	12	18	2	13	3.0	—	—	40	225
70826	Sandwich, breakfast, sausage egg cheese, w/biscuit	1 ea	156	460	16	37	3	28	11.0	—	—	115	0
Frozen/Refrigerated Children's Meals													
Frozen/Refrigerated Dinners													
70023	Dinner, beef noodles, w/veg, fzn	1 ea	298	407	14	59	3	14	4.8	5.6	2.4	31	312
11118	Dinner, beef, pot roast, fzn, Healthy Choice	1 ea	312	300	20	41	8	6	2.0	—	—	40	250
15957	Dinner, chicken & noodles, homestyle, ckd f/fzn	1 cup	340	390	12	44	7	19	7.0	—	—	50	700

Thia (mg)	Ribo (mg)	Niac (mg NE)	Vit B6 (mg)	Vit B12 (μg)	Fol (μg)	Vit C (mg)	Vit D (IU)	Vit E (mg AT)	Cal (mg)	Iron (mg)	Magn (mg)	Phos (mg)	Pota (mg)	Sodi (mg)	Zinc (mg)	Wat (%)	Alco (g)	Caff (mg)
0.25	0.01	2.32	0.15	0.00	91.6	0.0	—	0.1	16	1.89	19.0	68	55	2	0.8	68	0.00	0.00
0.20	0.15	1.67	—	—	—	0.0	—	—	60	1.39	—	—	50	499	—	—	0.00	0.00
0.14	0.10	1.48	0.03	0.00	39.0	0.0	—	1.4	32	1.09	12.0	42	74	543	0.3	65	0.00	0.00
—	—	—	—	—	—	0.0	—	—	40	0.72	—	—	63	190	—	2	0.00	0.00
0.37	0.40	4.98	0.51	0.00	40.0	0.0	—	0.0	14	1.80	9.6	36	70	110	1.5	14	0.00	0.00
0.07	0.01	0.14	0.00	0.00	2.8	0.0	—	0.4	8	0.58	19.1	54	64	60	0.4	3	0.00	0.00
—	—	—	—	—	—	0.0	—	—	0	1.08	—	—	—	160	—	—	0.00	0.00
0.49	0.43	5.11	0.80	0.00	160.0	0.0	—	1.1	36	5.30	85.0	243	238	251	1.9	7	0.00	0.00
—	—	—	—	—	—	0.0	—	—	0	1.08	—	—	—	160	—	—	0.00	0.00
0.05	0.02	0.38	0.01	0.00	5.6	0.2	—	0.3	15	0.72	23.8	68	82	72	0.5	4	0.00	0.00
0.15	0.15	1.21	0.02	0.10	7.9	0.1	6.7	0.7	80	1.32	7.1	74	49	171	0.3	27	0.00	0.00
0.15	0.17	4.00	—	—	60.0	0.0	—	—	40	1.79	—	—	—	1070	—	—	0.00	0.00
—	—	—	—	—	—	4.8	—	—	40	0.72	—	—	—	620	—	73	0.00	0.00
—	—	—	—	—	—	0.0	—	—	150	1.79	—	—	—	1060	—	46	0.00	0.00
0.25	0.25	3.44	0.20	0.87	38.0	16.5	—	1.3	116	2.02	43.5	210	466	2756	2.3	68	0.00	0.00
—	—	—	—	—	—	18.0	—	—	20	1.79	—	—	—	600	—	—	0.00	0.00
0.27	0.28	5.69	—	—	—	0.0	—	—	60	1.79	—	—	374	1080	—	—	0.00	0.00

54

PAGE KEY: 2 Beverage and Beverage Mixes   4 Other Beverages   4 Beverages, Alcoholic   6 Candies and Confections, Gum   10 Cereals, Breakfast Type   14 Cheese and Cheese Substitutes   16 Dairy Products and Substitutes   18 Desserts   24 Dessert Toppings   24 Eggs, Substitutes, and Egg Dishes   26 Ethnic Foods   30 Fast Foods/Restaurants   44 Fats, Oils, Margarines, Shortenings, and Substitutes   44 Fish, Seafood, and Shellfish   46 Food Additives   46 Fruit, Vegetable, or Blended Juices   48 Grains, Flours, and Fractions   48 Grain Products, Prepared and Baked Goods

Code	Food Name	Unit/ Amt	Wt (g)	Energy (kcal)	Prot (g)	Carb (g)	Fiber (g)	Fat (g)	Sat (g)	Mono (g)	Poly (g)	Chol (mg)	Vit A (RE)
446	Dinner, egg roll, w/fried rice & chicken, ckd f/fzn	1 ea	241	330	12	51	5	9	3.0	—	—	60	200
70151	Dinner, enchilada, cheese, w/beans & rice, fzn	1 ea	340	515	19	71	14	18	7.8	6.7	2.3	32	121
1756	Dinner, fish, sticks, ckd f/fzn	1 ea	187	290	11	33	4	13	4.5	—	—	30	100
70766	Dinner, meatloaf, Swanson	1 ea	468	640	24	65	6	31	14.0	—	—	45	60
11071	Dinner, steak, salisbury, Swanson	1 ea	461	610	34	46	10	33	17.0	—	—	80	150
57293	Dinner, stir fry, teriyaki veg, fzn	1 cup	108	92	4	17	1	1	0.3	—	—	1	175
16912	Dinner, turkey, breast, traditional, fzn, Healthy Choice	1 ea	298	290	22	40	5	4	2.0	—	—	45	80
Frozen/Refrigerated Dishes													
56668	Corn Dog	1 ea	175	460	17	56	—	19	5.2	9.1	3.5	79	61
16167	Dish, chicken & noodles, casserole, Swanson	1 ea	284	300	18	36	2	9	3.0	—	—	50	20
70749	Dish, fish & chips, Swanson	1 ea	156	350	16	38	4	15	4.5	—	—	30	40
16163	Dish, pot pie, chicken, Swanson	1 ea	198	410	10	43	2	22	9.0	—	—	25	200
16915	Dish, pot pie, turkey, Swanson	1 ea	198	400	10	42	3	21	8.0	—	—	25	100
57845	Dish, rice bowl, chicken & veg	1 ea	340	360	21	56	3	5	1.5	—	—	25	—
52165	Dish, rice bowl, chicken, sweet & sour	1 ea	340	360	17	65	2	3	0.5	—	—	30	—
83063	Dish, rice bowl, fried	1 ea	340	450	18	77	6	8	0.5	—	—	0	700
57140	Dish, tortellini, three cheese, fzn	2.9 oz	81	250	11	37	2	7	3.5	—	—	35	0
Frozen/Refrigerated Dinners/Dishes—Vegetarian													
8869	Corn Dog, vegetarian	1 ea	71	159	8	22	1	4	0.5	1.2	2.5	0	0
Prepared Generic or Homemade Meals and Dishes													
7037	Beans, baked, prep f/recipe	1 cup	253	382	14	54	14	13	4.9	5.4	1.9	13	0
56258	Chicken, liver, chopped, w/egg & onion	1 cup	208	472	27	6	1	37	11.2	15.2	7.2	753	4581
11013	Dish, beef curry	1 cup	236	436	27	13	3	31	7.0	14.5	7.4	69	367
56195	Dish, chicken & noodles, w/cream sauce	1 cup	224	320	22	32	1	11	3.2	4.3	2.5	81	100
56200	Dish, chicken & noodles, w/tomato sauce	1 cup	224	291	20	31	2	9	2.1	3.8	2.5	74	143
15904	Dish, chicken cacciatore	1 cup	244	459	42	13	2	26	6.3	9.7	7.2	128	132
56213	Dish, chicken dumplings	1 cup	244	372	26	22	1	19	5.1	7.8	4.6	89	52
56287	Dish, egg foo young, chicken	1 ea	86	121	8	4	1	8	1.9	2.8	2.3	167	87
56110	Dish, egg roll, w/o meat	1 ea	64	101	3	10	1	6	1.2	2.9	1.3	30	16
11000	Dish, goulash, beef	1 cup	249	270	33	7	1	12	3.2	4.3	2.5	84	31
56239	Dish, jambalaya, shrimp	1 cup	243	310	27	28	1	9	1.8	3.8	2.8	181	133
56140	Dish, meatballs, Swedish, w/cream sauce	1 cup	246	406	31	17	1	23	9.5	9.0	1.3	163	94
56180	Dish, pork & potatoes, w/gravy	1 cup	252	255	21	21	2	10	3.2	4.3	1.1	57	1
56100	Dish, spaghetti w/meatballs, prep f/recipe	1 cup	248	362	18	28	3	18	4.8	—	—	65	164
57523	Dish, spring roll, fresh	1 ea	64	113	5	9	1	6	1.4	3.0	1.3	37	16
11008	Dish, stroganoff, beef	1 cup	256	408	26	16	1	27	10.6	7.9	6.3	85	99
56130	Dish, tortellini, meat	1 cup	190	373	25	33	1	15	5.4	5.7	2.1	240	134
56215	Dish, turkey & stuffing	1 cup	200	273	35	19	2	5	1.4	1.7	1.3	105	19
56242	Gumbo, w/rice, New Orleans style	1 cup	244	193	14	17	2	8	1.6	2.6	2.7	40	63
56150	Hash, beef	1 cup	190	312	21	21	2	16	4.9	5.7	3.3	57	0
56231	Pie, shepherds, w/beef	1 cup	243	278	17	32	3	9	2.6	4.0	1.7	37	78
Pizza													
56995	Pizza, bagel, cheese & pepperoni, fzn	2 pce	22	52	3	6	1	2	0.8	—	—	4	20
56993	Pizza, bagel, cheese, extra, fzn	4 pce	88	190	11	24	3	6	2.0	—	—	10	80
81030	Pizza, Canadian bacon, fzn	1 ea	195	440	17	50	2	19	3.5	—	—	15	0

PAGE KEY: 52 Granola Bars, Cereal Bars, Diet Bars, Scones, and Tarts   52 Meals and Dishes   56 Meats   62 Nuts, Seeds, and Products   64 Poultry   66 Salad Dressings, Dips, and Mayonnaise   66 Salads   68 Sandwiches   70 Sauces and Gravies   70 Snack Foods—Chips, Pretzels, Popcorn   72 Soups, Stews, and Chilis   74 Spices, Flavors, and Seasonings   76 Sports Bars and Drinks   76 Supplemental Foods and Formulas   78 Sweeteners and Sweet Substitutes   78 Vegetables and Legumes   92 Weight Loss Bars and Drinks   94 Miscellaneous

Thia (mg)	Ribo (mg)	Niac (mg NE)	Vit B6 (mg)	Vit B12 (µg)	Fol (µg)	Vit C (mg)	Vit D (IU)	Vit E (mg AT)	Cal (mg)	Iron (mg)	Magn (mg)	Phos (mg)	Pota (mg)	Sodi (mg)	Zinc (mg)	Wat (%)	Alco (g)	Caff (mg)
—	—	—	—	—	—	0.0	—	—	40	1.08	—	—	—	1270	—	—	0.00	0.00
0.31	0.27	2.21	0.33	0.18	112.4	6.0	—	1.8	289	4.36	99.1	414	645	1967	2.7	66	0.00	0.00
—	—	—	—	—	—	3.6	—	—	60	1.79	—	—	—	820	—	—	0.00	0.00
—	—	—	—	—	—	18.0	—	—	150	5.40	—	—	—	1870	—	73	0.00	0.00
—	—	—	—	—	—	4.8	—	—	200	5.40	—	—	—	1620	—	74	0.00	0.00
—	—	—	—	—	—	10.2	—	—	73	0.58	—	—	—	717	—	—	0.00	0.00
0.44	0.25	6.00	—	—	—	36.0	—	—	20	1.44	—	270	540	460	—	—	0.00	0.00
0.28	0.69	4.15	0.09	0.43	103.2	0.0	—	0.7	102	6.17	17.5	166	262	973	1.3	47	0.00	0.00
—	—	—	—	—	—	0.0	—	—	200	3.59	—	—	—	940	—	76	0.00	0.00
—	—	—	—	—	—	1.2	—	—	150	1.44	—	—	—	930	—	54	0.00	0.00
—	—	—	—	—	—	1.2	—	—	20	1.79	—	—	—	780	—	—	0.00	0.00
—	—	—	—	—	—	2.4	—	—	20	1.79	—	—	—	700	—	62	0.00	0.00
—	—	—	—	—	—	—	—	—	—	—	—	—	—	1020	—	—	0.00	0.00
—	—	—	—	—	—	—	—	—	—	—	—	—	—	620	—	—	0.00	0.00
—	—	—	—	—	—	3.6	—	—	150	6.30	—	—	—	1090	—	—	0.00	0.00
—	—	—	—	—	—	0.0	—	—	0	0.00	—	—	—	300	—	30	0.00	0.00
0.10	0.05	0.00	—	—	—	0.0	—	—	12	0.64	—	113	66	527	0.2	49	0.00	0.00
0.34	0.11	1.02	0.23	0.00	121.4	2.8	—	1.3	154	5.03	108.8	276	906	1068	1.8	65	0.00	0.00
0.18	1.79	4.19	0.63	18.23	734.3	17.9	—	2.5	41	8.32	28.1	365	256	92	4.5	66	0.00	0.00
0.18	0.34	5.42	0.47	3.04	20.3	24.6	—	5.9	44	4.23	59.0	292	978	802	6.1	68	0.00	0.00
0.25	0.34	4.94	0.20	0.37	14.6	0.8	—	0.9	132	2.36	42.0	237	276	139	2.0	71	0.00	0.00
0.27	0.23	5.73	0.31	0.20	16.5	11.8	—	2.1	34	2.90	47.2	177	478	658	1.9	72	0.00	0.00
0.18	0.31	13.98	0.72	0.43	16.5	14.8	29.3	3.0	61	3.02	56.1	305	690	247	3.1	66	0.44	0.00
0.23	0.31	9.32	0.30	0.31	11.0	1.9	—	0.9	128	2.50	34.5	261	297	244	1.9	72	0.00	0.00
0.05	0.23	0.88	0.11	0.34	22.3	3.1	—	1.1	27	0.81	11.4	96	136	132	0.8	76	0.00	0.00
0.07	0.10	0.80	0.05	0.05	13.4	2.9	—	0.9	14	0.81	9.1	38	97	274	0.3	70	0.00	0.00
0.15	0.31	5.73	0.46	3.25	21.3	8.7	14.9	1.8	18	3.57	45.6	336	698	225	5.3	78	0.00	0.00
0.28	0.10	4.76	0.21	1.17	12.2	16.9	—	2.3	104	4.38	63.6	300	439	370	1.7	72	0.00	0.00
0.30	0.52	6.57	0.31	2.41	20.2	2.7	—	0.3	124	3.19	43.4	326	573	407	5.5	70	0.00	0.00
0.56	0.25	5.90	0.50	0.52	16.4	14.9	—	0.3	22	1.73	40.6	262	821	651	2.4	78	0.00	0.00
0.25	0.30	4.38	0.28	0.94	67.7	16.3	16.9	2.5	92	3.32	43.7	173	479	1133	3.4	71	0.00	0.00
0.15	0.12	1.27	0.09	0.11	9.9	2.1	—	0.8	15	0.82	10.0	57	124	274	0.5	66	0.00	0.00
0.18	0.38	4.51	0.28	2.60	20.2	1.8	—	2.4	92	3.64	40.4	308	556	677	4.9	72	0.00	0.00
0.46	0.56	4.48	0.21	0.89	29.1	0.0	—	1.1	178	3.11	28.1	290	231	437	2.2	61	0.00	0.00
0.23	0.31	13.10	0.44	0.36	28.7	2.9	—	0.6	43	2.27	47.5	293	403	511	2.5	70	0.00	0.00
0.20	0.15	4.51	0.20	2.41	45.6	13.5	—	1.4	71	2.60	40.1	152	446	542	15.2	83	0.00	0.00
0.15	0.20	3.74	0.49	1.79	16.5	7.1	—	1.2	19	2.46	36.4	204	587	470	5.0	69	0.00	0.00
0.20	0.18	3.90	0.58	1.25	21.1	16.4	—	1.3	40	2.18	46.9	193	764	312	3.9	75	0.00	0.00
—	—	—	—	—	—	2.2	—	—	25	0.36	—	—	38	162	—	—	0.00	0.00
—	—	—	—	—	—	9.0	—	—	150	0.72	—	—	150	490	—	—	0.00	0.00
—	—	—	—	—	—	0.0	—	—	150	3.59	—	—	—	1160	—	—	0.00	0.00

Code	Food Name	Unit/ Amt	Wt (g)	Energy (kcal)	Prot (g)	Carb (g)	Fiber (g)	Fat (g)	Sat (g)	Mono (g)	Poly (g)	Chol (mg)	Vit A (RE)
56782	Pizza, cheese, for one, fzn	1 ea	184	497	21	48	4	24	—	—	—	40	—
56781	Pizza, deluxe, for one, fzn	1 ea	234	582	23	51	4	32	10.0	9.0	3.0	20	245
56779	Pizza, pepperoni, for one, fzn	1 ea	191	546	20	50	4	30	9.0	7.0	2.0	20	263
70898	Pizza, pepperoni, fzn, svg	1 ea	146	432	16	42	3	22	7.0	10.0	3.4	22	61
56778	Pizza, sausage, for one, fzn	1 ea	213	571	23	49	4	32	10.0	7.0	3.0	20	272
57178	Pizza, supreme, fzn, 1/5 of 12"	1 pce	130	300	14	30	3	14	6.0	—	—	30	60

MEATS
Beef

Code	Food Name	Unit/ Amt	Wt (g)	Energy (kcal)	Prot (g)	Carb (g)	Fiber (g)	Fat (g)	Sat (g)	Mono (g)	Poly (g)	Chol (mg)	Vit A (RE)
10820	Beef, average of all cuts, ckd, 1/8" trim	3 oz	85	247	22	0	0	17	6.6	7.2	0.6	74	0
10095	Beef, average of all cuts, ckd, choice, 1/4" trim	3 oz	85	274	22	0	0	20	8.0	8.6	0.7	75	0
10099	Beef, average of all cuts, ckd, prime, 1/4" trim	3 oz	85	274	22	0	0	20	8.1	8.6	0.7	71	0
10097	Beef, average of all cuts, ckd, select, 1/4" trim	3 oz	85	247	22	0	0	17	6.7	7.2	0.6	73	0
10705	Beef, average of all cuts, lean, ckd, 1/4" trim	3 oz	85	184	25	0	0	8	3.2	3.5	0.3	73	0
47441	Beef, chuck, ground, extra lean, raw	4 oz	113	130	22	0	0	5	2.0	2.0	0.5	60	0
10740	Beef, cubed patty	1 ea	91	251	15	2	0	20	8.1	—	—	64	11
58115	Beef, ground, hamburger, bkd, 10% fat	3 oz	85	182	23	0	0	9	3.7	4.0	0.3	73	0
58120	Beef, ground, hamburger, bkd, 15% fat	3 oz	85	204	22	0	0	12	4.6	5.3	0.4	77	0
58125	Beef, ground, hamburger, bkd, 20% fat	3 oz	85	216	21	0	0	14	5.9	6.1	0.4	77	0
58110	Beef, ground, hamburger, bkd, 5% fat	3 oz	85	148	23	0	0	5	2.5	2.4	0.3	62	0
10051	Beef, jerky, lrg pce	1 ea	20	81	7	2	0	5	2.1	2.2	0.2	10	0
53688	Beef, meat stick, spicy	0.63 oz	18	100	4	1	1	8	3.0	—	—	25	0
11019	Beef, meatballs	4 ea	112	240	19	7	0	14	5.1	6.3	0.7	93	21
11020	Beef, patty, brd, 3.6 oz	1 ea	101	216	17	6	0	13	4.6	5.7	0.7	84	19
11487	Beef, porterhouse steak, brld, 1/8"– trim	3 oz	85	253	20	0	0	19	7.2	8.2	0.7	60	0
11407	Beef, prime rib, brld, 1/8" trim	3 oz	85	301	21	0	0	24	9.8	10.3	0.8	71	0
11386	Beef, rib pot roast, brld, 1/8" trim	3 oz	85	287	18	0	0	23	9.4	9.8	0.9	68	0
11015	Beef, ribs, w/bbq sauce	3 oz	85	148	18	2	0	7	2.6	2.9	0.3	52	16
11815	Beef, roast, Italian style, deli meat	2 oz	57	60	11	1	0	1	0.5	—	—	20	0
11681	Beef, roast, lean, rstd	3 oz	85	169	24	0	0	7	2.8	3.0	0.2	66	0
11680	Beef, roast, rstd	3 oz	85	227	22	0	0	15	5.8	6.3	0.5	68	0
10737	Beef, salisbury steak, patty, ckd, 3 oz	1 ea	85	280	12	5	0	23	10.7	—	—	59	7
11678	Beef, steak, brld/bkd	3.6 oz	100	255	28	0	0	15	5.9	6.3	0.5	83	0
11679	Beef, steak, lean, brld/bkd	3.6 oz	100	199	30	0	0	8	3.1	3.3	0.3	81	0
10049	Beef, stew meat, ckd	0.75 cup	105	322	29	0	0	22	8.5	9.4	0.8	106	0
10050	Beef, stew meat, lean, ckd	0.75 cup	105	248	33	0	0	12	4.5	5.2	0.4	107	0
10806	Beef, T-bone steak, brld, 0" trim	3 oz	85	210	21	0	0	14	5.2	6.1	0.5	51	0
10805	Beef, T-bone steak, brld, 1/4" trim	3 oz	85	260	20	0	0	19	7.6	8.6	0.7	55	0
11491	Beef, T-bone steak, brld, 1/8" trim	3 oz	85	238	21	0	0	17	6.4	7.3	0.6	53	0
10933	Beef, tenderloin, filet mignon, rstd, 1/8" trim	3 oz	85	276	20	0	0	21	8.3	8.7	0.9	72	0
10908	Beef, top round steak, brsd, 1/8" trim	3 oz	85	202	29	0	0	9	3.2	3.5	0.4	77	0
10943	Beef, top sirloin steak, raw, 1/8" trim	4 oz	113	228	23	0	0	14	5.8	6.2	0.5	53	0
11014	Beef, w/bbq sauce	1 cup	263	457	56	8	1	21	7.9	9.0	1.1	160	49
11016	Beef, w/sweet & sour	1 cup	252	336	16	28	2	18	6.1	7.2	2.6	54	33
10846	Beef, whole rib, brld, 1/8" trim	3 oz	85	287	19	0	0	23	9.2	9.7	0.8	70	0

PAGE KEY: 52 Granola Bars, Cereal Bars, Diet Bars, Scones, and Tarts   52 Meals and Dishes   56 Meats   62 Nuts, Seeds, and Products   64 Poultry   66 Salad Dressings, Dips, and Mayonnaise   66 Salads   68 Sandwiches   70 Sauces and Gravies   70 Snack Foods—Chips, Pretzels, Popcorn   72 Soups, Stews, and Chilis   74 Spices, Flavors, and Seasonings   76 Sports Bars and Drinks   76 Supplemental Foods and Formulas   78 Sweeteners and Sweet Substitutes   78 Vegetables and Legumes   92 Weight Loss Bars and Drinks   94 Miscellaneous

Thia (mg)	Ribo (mg)	Niac (mg NE)	Vit B6 (mg)	Vit B12 (µg)	Fol (µg)	Vit C (mg)	Vit D (IU)	Vit E (mg AT)	Cal (mg)	Iron (mg)	Magn (mg)	Phos (mg)	Pota (mg)	Sodi (mg)	Zinc (mg)	Wat (%)	Alco (g)	Caff (mg)
—	—	—	—	—	—	—	—	2.0	—	—	48.0	386	342	—	4.0	46	0.00	0.00
0.30	0.81	3.52	0.25	2.00	80.0	0.0	—	2.0	332	2.56	61.0	480	498	1367	5.0	53	0.00	0.00
0.25	0.70	2.57	0.20	2.00	97.0	0.0	—	4.0	336	2.03	53.0	443	416	1353	4.0	45	0.00	0.00
0.33	0.34	3.60	0.14	0.82	68.6	2.8	—	1.6	220	3.51	35.0	302	289	902	2.2	42	0.00	0.00
0.30	0.76	2.84	0.23	2.00	109.0	0.0	—	4.0	371	2.27	60.0	505	456	1363	0.0	48	0.00	0.00
—	—	—	—	—	—	0.0	—	—	150	1.44	—	—	—	690	—	—	0.00	0.00
0.07	0.18	3.16	0.28	2.09	6.0	0.0	—	0.2	8	2.27	19.6	177	271	54	5.1	53	0.00	0.00
0.07	0.18	3.03	0.27	2.04	6.0	0.0	10.2	0.1	9	2.19	18.7	169	260	52	4.9	50	0.00	0.00
0.07	0.18	3.64	0.31	2.07	6.8	0.0	—	0.2	8	2.07	20.4	168	295	53	4.6	51	0.00	0.00
0.07	0.18	3.11	0.28	2.07	6.0	0.0	—	0.1	9	2.25	19.6	174	269	53	5.1	52	0.00	0.00
0.09	0.20	3.50	0.31	2.25	6.8	0.0	—	0.1	8	2.53	22.1	198	306	57	5.9	59	0.00	0.00
—	—	5.00	—	2.40	—	0.0	—	—	0	1.79	—	—	—	65	4.5	—	0.00	0.00
0.10	—	—	—	—	—	8.0	—	—	17	1.89	—	—	—	53	—	58	0.00	0.00
0.02	0.15	4.44	0.30	2.13	5.1	0.0	—	0.3	11	2.46	17.9	164	255	52	5.7	61	0.00	0.00
0.02	0.15	4.19	0.28	2.11	5.1	0.0	—	0.4	15	2.32	17.0	158	243	54	5.5	59	0.00	0.00
0.03	0.14	3.94	0.28	2.10	6.0	0.0	—	0.4	20	2.19	16.2	152	230	57	5.3	58	0.00	0.00
0.02	0.15	4.69	0.30	2.13	5.1	0.0	—	0.3	7	2.58	18.7	169	268	49	5.8	65	0.00	0.00
0.02	0.02	0.34	0.03	0.20	26.5	0.0	—	0.1	4	1.07	10.1	81	118	438	1.6	23	0.00	0.00
—	—	—	—	—	—	0.0	—	—	0	0.72	—	—	—	350	—	23	0.00	0.00
0.07	0.28	4.17	0.15	1.72	12.4	0.6	—	0.1	45	2.10	23.3	167	306	138	3.8	62	0.00	0.00
0.07	0.25	3.75	0.12	1.54	11.2	0.6	—	0.1	40	1.89	21.0	151	276	124	3.4	62	0.00	0.00
0.09	0.18	3.46	0.30	1.83	6.0	0.0	—	0.2	7	2.32	19.6	159	273	54	3.9	53	0.00	0.00
0.07	0.15	3.46	0.28	2.50	6.0	0.0	—	0.2	11	1.89	18.7	151	282	54	4.9	47	0.00	0.00
0.05	0.14	2.35	0.20	2.46	5.1	0.0	—	0.2	9	1.86	16.2	155	263	54	4.3	49	0.00	0.00
0.05	0.12	2.61	0.20	2.19	5.8	1.3	—	0.3	12	2.08	19.9	150	295	204	4.1	66	0.00	0.00
—	—	—	—	—	—	0.0	—	—	0	1.08	—	—	—	360	—	73	0.00	0.00
0.07	0.18	3.42	0.28	2.17	6.9	0.0	10.2	0.1	5	2.19	22.3	191	321	57	5.5	62	0.00	0.00
0.07	0.17	3.06	0.27	2.03	6.1	0.0	10.2	0.2	6	1.98	19.6	173	290	53	4.8	56	0.00	0.00
0.07	—	—	—	—	—	4.0	—	—	51	1.20	—	—	—	621	—	—	0.00	0.00
0.09	0.21	4.57	0.38	2.45	8.3	0.0	12.0	0.1	9	2.61	25.4	209	365	61	5.2	55	0.00	0.00
0.10	0.23	5.26	0.46	2.53	9.3	0.0	12.0	0.1	9	2.75	28.8	228	411	66	5.9	60	0.00	0.00
0.07	0.25	3.10	0.30	2.58	7.3	0.0	12.6	0.2	11	3.27	21.6	231	265	66	7.9	50	0.00	0.00
0.07	0.28	3.35	0.31	2.76	8.2	0.0	12.6	0.1	11	3.73	24.6	259	291	70	9.3	56	0.00	0.00
0.09	0.20	3.63	0.31	1.86	6.0	0.0	—	0.2	4	2.84	20.4	169	257	57	4.0	58	0.00	0.00
0.07	0.18	3.36	0.28	1.80	6.0	0.0	—	0.2	6	2.63	18.7	157	240	57	3.7	52	0.00	0.00
0.09	0.18	3.51	0.30	1.85	6.0	0.0	—	0.2	7	2.41	20.4	164	286	56	4.0	55	0.00	0.00
0.07	0.21	2.54	0.20	2.08	6.8	0.0	—	0.2	8	2.65	18.7	173	282	48	3.4	48	0.00	0.00
0.05	0.20	3.09	0.23	2.23	7.7	0.0	—	0.1	4	2.69	20.4	183	271	38	3.7	55	0.00	0.00
0.07	0.10	6.78	0.62	1.19	12.5	0.0	—	0.4	27	1.67	23.8	212	357	59	4.0	66	0.00	0.00
0.15	0.40	8.10	0.61	6.76	17.9	4.0	—	0.9	36	6.44	61.6	463	913	632	12.7	66	0.00	0.00
0.11	0.18	2.61	0.31	1.59	12.7	21.6	—	1.2	27	2.69	33.7	151	336	930	3.9	74	0.00	0.00
0.07	0.14	2.77	0.23	2.46	5.1	0.0	—	0.2	9	1.86	17.0	152	268	54	4.5	48	0.00	0.00

Code	Food Name	Unit/ Amt	Wt (g)	Energy (kcal)	Prot (g)	Carb (g)	Fiber (g)	Fat (g)	Sat (g)	Mono (g)	Poly (g)	Chol (mg)	Vit A (RE)
Game Meats													
40559	Bison, ground, raw	4 oz	113	253	21	0	0	18	7.7	7.1	0.8	79	0
14009	Bison, rstd	3 oz	85	122	24	0	0	2	0.8	0.8	0.2	70	0
40565	Deer, ground, raw	4 oz	113	178	25	0	0	8	3.8	1.5	0.4	91	0
40551	Deer, rstd	3 oz	85	134	26	0	0	3	1.1	0.7	0.5	95	0
40560	Elk, ground, raw	4 oz	113	195	25	0	0	10	3.9	2.8	0.5	75	0
14014	Elk, rstd	3 oz	85	124	26	0	0	2	0.6	0.4	0.3	62	0
14068	Rabbit, brd, ckd	3.6 oz	100	245	28	6	0	11	2.9	4.0	2.8	86	0
14013	Venison, rstd	3 oz	85	134	26	0	0	3	1.1	0.7	0.5	95	0
Goat													
Lamb													
40354	Lamb, Austl, average of all cuts, ckd, 1/8" trim	3 oz	85	218	21	0	0	14	6.8	5.7	0.6	74	—
13628	Lamb, average of all cuts, ckd, choice, 1/8" trim	3 oz	85	230	22	0	0	15	6.3	6.5	1.1	82	0
13669	Lamb, ground, ckd	3.6 oz	100	283	25	0	0	20	8.1	8.3	1.4	97	0
Lunchmeats and Sausages													
13250	Frank, beef, fat free	1 ea	50	39	7	3	0	0	0.1	0.1	0.0	15	0
57967	Frank, beef, rducd fat	1 ea	49	120	6	0	0	10	4.5	—	—	25	0
13283	Frankfurter, beef	3.6 oz	100	326	13	2	0	29	12.3	14.0	1.4	64	0
13284	Frankfurter, beef & pork	3.6 oz	100	331	12	3	0	30	10.9	14.1	2.9	52	0
58290	Frankfurter, beef, low fat	1 cup	151	352	18	2	0	29	12.2	14.8	0.9	60	0
13318	Frankfurter, beef, low fat	1 ea	50	80	6	7	0	2	1.0	—	—	15	0
13260	Frankfurter, chicken	1 ea	45	116	6	3	0	9	2.5	3.8	1.8	45	18
13274	Frankfurter, low sod	1 ea	57	180	7	1	0	16	6.9	7.8	0.8	35	0
13012	Frankfurter, turkey	1 ea	45	102	6	1	0	8	2.7	2.5	2.2	48	0
13325	Hot Dog, fat free	1 ea	50	36	6	2	0	0	0.1	0.1	0.1	14	0
13000	Lunchmeat, beef, thin slice	1 oz	28	42	5	0	0	2	0.8	0.9	0.1	20	0
13177	Lunchmeat, bologna, beef	1 oz	28	90	3	1	0	8	3.6	4.3	0.3	18	0
58284	Lunchmeat, bologna, beef, low fat	1 cup	138	282	16	7	0	20	7.5	8.9	0.7	61	0
10439	Lunchmeat, bologna, beef, slice	1 pce	38	100	5	1	0	8	3.5	—	—	20	0
11829	Lunchmeat, bologna, chicken, slice	1 pce	38	100	4	1	0	9	2.5	—	—	45	20
13251	Lunchmeat, bologna, fat free, 1 oz svg	1 pce	28	22	4	2	0	0.1	0.1	0.0	7	0
13245	Lunchmeat, chicken breast, honey glazed, slice	1 oz	28	31	6	1	0	0	0.1	0.2	0.1	15	0
13257	Lunchmeat, chicken breast, oven rstd, fat free, slice	1 oz	28	24	5	0	0	0	0.0	0.0	0.0	12	0
58149	Lunchmeat, chicken breast, oven rstd, 1 oz slice	1 pce	28	20	5	0	0	0	0.0	0.0	0.0	10	—
58167	Lunchmeat, ham, brown sugar, deli, 0.8 oz slice	2 pce	45	60	8	4	0	1	0.0	—	—	10	0
13262	Lunchmeat, ham, extra lean, 5% fat, sliced	1 cup	135	148	23	4	0	4	1.2	1.7	0.5	65	0
11819	Lunchmeat, ham, smkd, deli meat	2 oz	57	60	9	2	0	2	0.5	—	—	30	0
58199	Lunchmeat, roast beef, choice, deli, 0.8 oz slice	2 pce	45	50	9	0	0	2	0.5	—	—	25	0
13114	Lunchmeat, turkey breast, oven rstd, fat free, slice	1 oz	28	24	4	1	0	0	0.1	0.1	0.0	9	0
13255	Lunchmeat, turkey breast, smkd, fat free, slice	1 oz	28	23	4	1	0	0	0.1	0.0	0.0	9	0
13020	Pastrami, turkey, slices	1 oz	28	35	5	1	0	1	0.3	0.4	0.3	19	1
13201	Salami, hard, slice	1 oz	28	104	7	0	0	8	3.1	4.2	0.8	27	2
58014	Salami, Italian, pork	3 oz	85	361	18	1	0	31	11.1	15.5	3.1	68	0
13025	Salami, turkey, ckd, 1 oz slice	2 pce	57	86	9	0	0	5	1.6	1.8	1.4	43	1
13182	Sausage, beef, smokies	1 ea	43	127	5	1	0	11	4.8	5.5	0.4	27	0

Thia (mg)	Ribo (mg)	Niac (mg NE)	Vit B6 (mg)	Vit B12 (µg)	Fol (µg)	Vit C (mg)	Vit D (IU)	Vit E (mg AT)	Cal (mg)	Iron (mg)	Magn (mg)	Phos (mg)	Pota (mg)	Sodi (mg)	Zinc (mg)	Wat (%)	Alco (g)	Caff (mg)
0.15	0.25	5.57	0.40	2.02	12.5	0.0	—	0.3	12	2.95	21.5	205	348	75	4.9	64	0.00	0.00
0.09	0.23	3.16	0.34	2.43	6.8	0.0	—	0.3	7	2.91	22.1	178	307	48	3.1	67	0.00	0.00
0.62	0.33	6.46	0.52	2.11	4.5	0.0	—	0.5	12	3.30	23.8	228	374	85	4.8	71	0.00	0.00
0.15	0.50	5.71	0.31	2.70	4.0	0.0	—	0.2	6	3.79	20.4	192	285	46	2.3	65	0.00	0.00
0.14	0.28	5.55	0.37	2.42	7.9	0.0	—	0.3	14	3.11	24.9	221	365	90	6.1	69	0.00	0.00
—	—	—	—	5.53	7.7	0.0	—	0.0	4	3.08	20.4	153	279	52	2.7	66	0.00	0.00
0.10	0.15	6.55	0.30	5.65	9.5	0.0	12.0	1.4	35	3.26	24.3	212	291	103	2.2	52	0.00	0.00
0.15	0.50	5.71	0.31	2.70	4.0	0.0	—	0.2	6	3.79	20.4	192	285	46	2.3	65	0.00	0.00
0.10	0.28	4.63	0.31	2.44	—	—	—	—	14	1.63	18.7	166	256	65	4.0	59	0.00	0.00
0.09	0.21	5.57	0.11	2.19	16.2	0.0	—	0.1	14	1.63	20.4	164	270	61	4.0	56	0.00	0.00
0.10	0.25	6.69	0.14	2.60	19.0	0.0	—	0.2	22	1.78	24.0	201	339	81	4.7	55	0.00	0.00
—	—	—	—	—	—	0.0	—	—	10	0.98	9.5	64	234	464	1.2	78	0.00	0.00
—	—	—	—	—	—	0.0	—	—	0	0.72	—	—	—	360	—	64	0.00	0.00
0.05	0.10	2.30	0.10	1.38	3.6	0.0	—	0.2	21	1.51	3.0	88	168	1037	2.3	53	0.00	0.00
0.18	0.11	2.51	0.10	1.17	3.6	0.0	—	0.2	12	1.22	10.1	87	169	1132	2.0	52	0.00	0.00
0.07	0.15	3.47	0.15	2.10	6.0	1.5	—	0.3	12	1.74	16.6	288	195	1572	3.0	64	0.00	0.00
—	—	—	—	—	—	2.4	—	—	0	0.36	—	—	—	400	—	66	0.00	0.00
0.02	0.05	1.38	0.14	0.10	1.8	0.0	0.0	0.1	43	0.89	4.5	48	38	616	0.5	58	0.00	0.00
0.02	0.05	1.37	0.07	0.87	2.3	0.0	—	0.1	11	0.81	1.7	50	95	177	1.2	57	0.00	0.00
0.01	0.07	1.86	0.10	0.12	3.6	0.0	—	0.3	48	0.82	6.3	60	81	642	1.4	63	0.00	0.00
—	—	—	—	—	—	0.0	—	—	8	0.46	10.5	81	236	487	0.6	79	0.00	0.00
0.01	0.05	1.21	0.10	0.73	3.1	0.0	—	0.1	3	0.58	5.4	48	122	401	1.1	69	0.00	0.00
0.00	0.02	0.68	0.05	0.40	3.7	0.0	9.1	—	3	0.38	4.0	31	48	334	0.6	54	0.00	0.00
0.07	0.14	3.45	0.20	1.92	6.9	1.4	—	0.3	12	1.37	16.6	246	203	1628	2.5	65	0.00	0.00
—	—	—	—	—	—	0.0	—	—	0	0.36	—	—	—	340	—	60	0.00	0.00
—	—	—	—	—	—	1.2	—	—	40	0.72	—	—	—	350	—	60	0.00	0.00
—	—	—	—	—	—	0.0	—	—	4	0.25	6.2	43	44	274	0.3	78	0.00	0.00
—	—	—	—	—	1.1	0.0	—	—	3	0.31	10.2	82	93	408	0.2	70	0.00	0.00
—	—	—	—	—	—	0.0	—	—	3	0.37	10.2	73	90	352	0.2	76	0.00	0.00
—	—	—	—	—	—	—	—	—	—	—	—	—	—	240	—	77	0.00	0.00
—	—	—	—	—	—	0.0	—	—	0	0.36	—	—	—	490	—	—	0.00	0.00
1.25	0.30	6.75	0.62	1.00	5.4	0.0	—	0.4	12	1.08	23.0	294	472	1493	2.6	74	0.00	0.00
—	—	—	—	—	—	0.0	—	—	0	0.36	—	—	—	430	—	74	0.00	0.00
—	—	—	—	—	—	0.0	—	—	0	1.08	—	—	—	250	—	—	0.00	0.00
—	—	—	—	—	—	0.0	—	—	3	0.31	7.7	66	58	338	0.2	76	0.00	0.00
—	—	—	—	—	—	0.0	—	—	3	0.21	8.5	69	62	310	0.2	78	0.00	0.00
0.01	0.07	1.00	0.07	0.07	1.4	4.6	—	0.1	3	1.19	4.0	57	98	278	0.6	72	0.00	0.00
0.15	0.07	1.42	0.11	0.52	0.9	0.0	17.6	—	3	0.51	6.0	51	101	560	0.9	38	0.00	0.00
0.79	0.28	4.76	0.46	2.38	1.7	0.0	—	0.2	9	1.28	18.7	195	289	1607	3.6	35	0.00	0.00
0.23	0.17	2.25	0.23	0.56	5.7	0.0	13.3	0.1	23	0.70	12.5	151	122	569	1.3	72	0.00	0.00
—	—	—	—	—	4.7	0.0	—	—	5	0.75	6.5	99	74	416	1.3	56	0.00	0.00

60

PAGE KEY: 2 Beverage and Beverage Mixes 4 Other Beverages 4 Beverages, Alcoholic 6 Candies and Confections, Gum 10 Cereals, Breakfast Type
14 Cheese and Cheese Substitutes 16 Dairy Products and Substitutes 18 Desserts 24 Dessert Toppings 24 Eggs, Substitutes, and Egg Dishes 26 Ethnic Foods
30 Fast Foods/Restaurants 44 Fats, Oils, Margarines, Shortenings, and Substitutes 44 Fish, Seafood, and Shellfish 46 Food Additives
46 Fruit, Vegetable, or Blended Juices 48 Grains, Flours, and Fractions 48 Grain Products, Prepared and Baked Goods

Code	Food Name	Unit/ Amt	Wt (g)	Energy (kcal)	Prot (g)	Carb (g)	Fiber (g)	Fat (g)	Sat (g)	Mono (g)	Poly (g)	Chol (mg)	Vit A (RE)
58242	Sausage, chicken & beef, smkd, pieces	1 cup	138	408	26	0	0	33	9.9	14.1	6.5	97	43
13021	Sausage, pepperoni, beef & pork, slice, 1 3/8" x 1/8"	1 pce	6	26	1	0	0	2	0.9	1.0	0.1	6	0
58353	Sausage, pork, link, USDA, ckd f/fzn	3.6 oz	100	267	20	0	0	20	5.5	8.7	2.3	98	15
13184	Sausage, smokies, links	1 ea	43	130	5	1	0	12	4.0	5.7	1.2	27	0
58232	Sausage, turkey, ckd	3.6 oz	100	196	24	0	0	10	2.3	3.0	2.7	92	15

Pork and Ham

Code	Food Name	Unit/ Amt	Wt (g)	Energy (kcal)	Prot (g)	Carb (g)	Fiber (g)	Fat (g)	Sat (g)	Mono (g)	Poly (g)	Chol (mg)	Vit A (RE)
27096	Bacon Bits	1 Tbs	7	24	3	0	0	1	0.5	0.7	0.2	5	0
92207	Bacon, cured, microwv	1 pce	8	38	3	0	0	3	0.9	1.2	0.3	9	1
92208	Bacon, cured, pan fried	1 pce	8	42	3	0	0	3	1.0	1.4	0.4	9	1
28143	Canadian Bacon, 2 oz svg	1 ea	56	68	9	1	—	3	1.0	1.4	0.3	27	0
12118	Pork, avg of retail cuts, leg shoulder & loin, lean, ckd	3 oz	85	180	25	0	0	8	2.9	3.7	0.6	73	2
12309	Pork, avg of retail cuts, leg shoulder loin & sparerib, ckd	3 oz	85	232	23	0	0	15	5.3	6.5	1.2	77	2
12240	Pork, avg of retail cuts, loin & shoulder blade, ckd	3 oz	85	214	24	0	0	13	4.5	5.6	1.0	73	2
12311	Pork, avg of retail cuts, loin & shoulder blade, lean, ckd	3 oz	85	179	25	0	0	8	2.8	3.6	0.6	72	2
12184	Pork, chop, blade loin, brld	3 oz	85	272	19	0	0	21	7.9	9.1	1.9	73	2
12081	Pork, chop, breaded, brld/bkd, 3.6 oz svg	1 ea	100	259	25	6	0	14	5.1	6.2	1.5	72	2
12192	Pork, chop, center loin, brld	3 oz	85	204	24	0	0	11	4.1	5.0	0.8	70	3
12126	Pork, chop, w/bbq sauce	1 ea	116	209	23	3	0	11	3.7	4.9	1.2	65	23
12243	Pork, cured ham, dinner 3 oz slice, add wtr	1 ea	84	83	14	0	0	3	1.0	1.5	0.3	41	0
12307	Pork, cured ham, lean, 8% fat, rstd	1 cup	140	231	31	1	0	11	3.7	5.2	1.5	80	0
12099	Pork, ground, ckd	3 oz	85	253	22	0	0	18	6.6	7.9	1.6	80	2
12010	Pork, ribs, spareribs, brsd	3 oz	85	338	25	0	0	26	9.5	11.5	2.3	103	3
12060	Pork, roast, top loin, rstd	3 oz	85	192	25	0	0	10	3.5	4.5	0.7	66	2
92798	Pork, shred, w/original bbq sauce, ckd	0.25 cup	56	90	6	11	0	2	0.5	—	—	15	40
12900	Pork, sweet & sour	3 oz	85	87	6	9	1	3	0.8	1.2	0.9	14	12
12237	Pork, tenderloin, chop, brld	3 oz	85	171	25	0	0	7	2.5	2.8	0.6	80	2

Veal

Code	Food Name	Unit/ Amt	Wt (g)	Energy (kcal)	Prot (g)	Carb (g)	Fiber (g)	Fat (g)	Sat (g)	Mono (g)	Poly (g)	Chol (mg)	Vit A (RE)
11531	Veal, avg of all cuts, ckd	3 oz	85	196	26	0	0	10	3.6	3.7	0.7	97	0

Variety Meats and By-Products

Code	Food Name	Unit/ Amt	Wt (g)	Energy (kcal)	Prot (g)	Carb (g)	Fiber (g)	Fat (g)	Sat (g)	Mono (g)	Poly (g)	Chol (mg)	Vit A (RE)
10472	Beef, liver, brsd	3 oz	85	162	25	4	0	4	1.4	0.6	0.5	337	8042

Meat Substitutes, Soy Tofu and Vegetable

Code	Food Name	Unit/ Amt	Wt (g)	Energy (kcal)	Prot (g)	Carb (g)	Fiber (g)	Fat (g)	Sat (g)	Mono (g)	Poly (g)	Chol (mg)	Vit A (RE)
27044	Bacon Bits, meatless	1 Tbs	7	33	2	2	1	2	0.3	0.4	0.9	0	0
7509	Bacon Substitute, vegetarian, strips	3 ea	15	46	2	1	0	4	0.7	1.1	2.3	0	1
7732	Beef Substitute, vegetarian, burger	0.25 cup	55	60	9	2	1	2	0.3	0.5	1.1	0	0
7558	Beef Substitute, vegetarian, fillet	1 ea	85	246	20	8	5	15	2.4	3.7	7.9	0	0
7561	Beef Substitute, vegetarian, patty	1 ea	56	110	12	4	3	5	0.8	1.2	2.6	0	0
7547	Chicken Substitute, vegetarian	1 cup	168	376	40	6	6	21	3.1	4.6	12.2	0	0
7549	Fish Sticks Substitute, vegetarian	1 ea	28	81	6	3	2	5	0.8	1.2	2.6	0	0
92148	Hot Dog Substitute	1 ea	70	163	14	5	3	10	1.4	2.7	5.5	0	0
7550	Hot Dog Substitute, vegetarian	1 ea	51	102	10	4	2	5	0.8	1.2	2.6	0	0
7551	Lunchmeat Substitute, vegetarian, 0.5 oz slice	1 pce	14	26	2	1	0	2	0.2	0.3	0.6	0	0
90626	Sausage Substitute, vegetarian, breakfast slices, 1 oz	1 ea	28	72	5	3	1	5	0.8	1.3	2.6	0	0
7564	Tempeh	0.5 cup	83	160	15	8	—	9	1.8	2.5	3.2	0	0
7519	Tofu, dried, fzn, 0.6 oz svg	1 pce	17	82	8	2	1	5	0.7	1.1	2.9	0	9
7522	Tofu, fermented & salted, block	3 oz	85	99	7	4	0	7	1.0	1.5	3.8	0	14
90040	Tofu, fermented & salted, w/calc sulfate, block, 0.4 oz	1 ea	11	13	1	1	0	1	0.1	0.2	0.5	0	2

PAGE KEY: 52 Granola Bars, Cereal Bars, Diet Bars, Scones, and Tarts   52 Meals and Dishes   56 Meats   62 Nuts, Seeds, and Products   64 Poultry
66 Salad Dressings, Dips, and Mayonnaise   66 Salads   68 Sandwiches   70 Sauces and Gravies   70 Snack Foods—Chips, Pretzels, Popcorn
72 Soups, Stews, and Chilis   74 Spices, Flavors, and Seasonings   76 Sports Bars and Drinks   76 Supplemental Foods and Formulas
78 Sweeteners and Sweet Substitutes   78 Vegetables and Legumes   92 Weight Loss Bars and Drinks   94 Miscellaneous

Thia (mg)	Ribo (mg)	Niac (mg NE)	Vit B6 (mg)	Vit B12 (µg)	Fol (µg)	Vit C (mg)	Vit D (IU)	Vit E (mg AT)	Cal (mg)	Iron (mg)	Magn (mg)	Phos (mg)	Pota (mg)	Sodi (mg)	Zinc (mg)	Wat (%)	Alco (g)	Caff (mg)
0.05	0.17	5.59	0.23	0.51	5.5	0.0	—	0.7	15	1.49	19.3	153	192	1408	2.4	56	0.00	0.00
0.02	0.00	0.30	0.01	0.09	0.3	0.0	0.5	0.0	1	0.07	1.0	10	17	98	0.2	31	0.00	0.00
0.73	0.23	2.79	0.28	0.88	1.0	0.0	—	0.7	9	1.14	19.0	190	239	540	2.8	59	0.00	0.00
—	—	—	—	—	—	0.0	—	—	4	0.50	7.3	103	77	433	0.9	56	0.00	0.00
0.07	0.25	5.71	0.31	1.23	6.0	0.7	—	0.2	22	1.49	21.0	202	298	665	3.9	65	0.00	0.00
—	—	—	—	—	—	0.0	—	—	2	0.20	4.6	43	39	224	0.3	35	0.00	0.00
0.03	0.01	0.75	0.02	0.11	0.2	0.0	—	0.0	1	0.10	2.3	36	37	155	0.3	16	0.00	0.00
0.03	0.01	0.91	0.02	0.10	0.2	0.0	—	0.0	1	0.10	2.8	44	47	192	0.3	12	0.00	0.00
—	—	—	—	—	—	0.8	—	—	3	0.50	10.6	—	156	569	1.0	73	0.00	0.00
0.72	0.28	4.40	0.37	0.63	0.9	0.3	—	0.2	18	0.93	22.1	202	319	50	2.5	60	0.00	0.00
0.64	0.28	4.19	0.34	0.64	5.1	0.3	—	0.2	21	0.93	20.4	197	301	53	2.5	55	0.00	0.00
0.72	0.28	4.21	0.34	0.62	5.1	0.3	10.2	0.2	20	0.83	20.4	193	308	48	2.2	57	0.00	0.00
0.74	0.28	4.46	0.37	0.63	5.1	0.3	—	0.4	19	0.91	22.1	199	321	48	2.4	60	0.00	0.00
0.55	0.25	3.49	0.31	0.70	3.4	0.6	—	0.3	25	0.79	18.7	180	293	60	2.9	52	0.00	0.00
0.81	0.30	4.75	0.41	0.62	5.8	0.5	12.0	0.4	24	1.00	26.8	240	400	415	2.2	52	0.00	0.00
0.91	0.23	4.46	0.36	0.62	5.1	0.3	—	0.3	28	0.68	21.3	197	304	49	1.9	58	0.00	0.00
0.73	0.28	4.90	0.36	0.64	5.0	1.9	—	0.5	19	1.30	24.1	221	373	860	2.4	65	0.00	0.00
0.60	0.18	3.93	0.31	0.40	—	0.0	—	—	4	1.01	16.9	203	221	1018	1.7	75	0.00	0.00
1.02	0.38	7.44	0.49	0.94	4.2	0.0	—	0.4	11	1.96	26.6	347	507	1939	3.7	66	0.00	0.00
0.60	0.18	3.57	0.33	0.46	5.1	0.6	10.2	0.2	19	1.10	20.4	192	308	62	2.7	53	0.00	0.00
0.34	0.31	4.65	0.30	0.92	3.4	0.0	—	0.3	40	1.57	20.4	222	272	79	3.9	40	0.00	0.00
0.51	0.25	4.36	0.31	0.46	6.8	0.3	—	0.3	4	0.68	19.6	183	291	37	1.9	59	0.00	0.00
—	—	—	—	—	—	0.0	—	—	0	0.72	—	—	—	380	—	—	0.00	0.00
0.20	0.07	1.37	0.15	0.12	3.9	7.4	10.2	0.4	11	0.54	12.9	56	145	316	0.6	77	0.00	0.00
0.81	0.31	4.30	0.43	0.82	5.1	0.9	—	0.3	4	1.17	29.8	247	378	54	2.5	61	0.00	0.00
0.05	0.27	6.78	0.25	1.34	12.8	0.0	—	0.3	19	0.98	22.1	203	276	74	4.0	57	0.00	0.00
0.15	2.91	14.90	0.86	60.02	215.2	1.6	—	0.4	5	5.55	17.9	423	299	67	4.5	59	0.00	0.00
0.03	0.00	0.10	0.00	0.07	8.9	0.1	—	0.5	7	0.05	6.7	15	10	124	0.1	8	0.00	0.00
0.66	0.07	1.12	0.07	0.00	6.3	0.0	—	1.0	3	0.36	2.9	10	26	220	0.1	49	0.00	0.00
0.12	0.10	1.96	0.23	1.13	—	0.0	—	—	4	1.73	—	56	25	269	0.4	71	0.00	0.00
0.93	0.75	10.19	1.27	3.56	86.7	0.0	—	2.9	81	1.70	19.6	382	510	416	1.2	45	0.00	0.00
0.50	0.34	5.59	0.67	1.34	43.7	0.0	—	1.0	16	1.17	10.1	193	101	308	1.0	58	0.00	0.00
1.14	0.40	2.44	1.17	3.66	127.7	0.0	—	4.5	59	5.48	28.6	563	91	1191	1.2	59	0.00	0.00
0.31	0.25	3.35	0.41	1.17	28.6	0.0	—	1.1	27	0.56	6.4	126	168	137	0.4	45	0.00	0.00
0.31	0.57	2.20	0.05	1.63	54.6	0.0	—	1.3	23	0.99	12.6	241	69	330	0.8	58	0.00	0.00
0.56	0.61	8.15	0.50	1.22	39.8	0.0	—	1.0	17	0.92	9.2	175	76	219	0.6	58	0.00	0.00
0.56	0.03	1.55	0.11	0.56	14.0	0.0	—	0.4	6	0.25	3.2	62	28	100	0.2	65	0.00	0.00
0.66	0.10	3.13	0.23	0.00	7.3	0.0	—	0.6	18	1.03	10.1	63	65	249	0.4	50	0.00	0.00
0.05	0.30	2.19	0.18	0.07	19.9	0.0	—	0.0	92	2.24	67.2	221	342	7	0.9	60	0.00	0.00
0.07	0.05	0.20	0.05	0.00	15.6	0.1	—	0.0	62	1.64	10.0	82	3	1	0.8	6	0.00	0.00
0.12	0.09	0.31	0.07	0.00	24.7	0.2	—	0.0	39	1.67	44.2	62	64	2443	1.3	70	0.00	0.00
0.01	0.00	0.03	0.00	0.00	3.2	0.0	—	0.0	135	0.21	6.4	8	8	316	0.2	70	0.00	0.00

Code	Food Name	Unit/ Amt	Wt (g)	Energy (kcal)	Prot (g)	Carb (g)	Fiber (g)	Fat (g)	Sat (g)	Mono (g)	Poly (g)	Chol (mg)	Vit A (RE)
NUTS, SEEDS, AND PRODUCTS													
4572	Almond Butter	1 cup	250	1582	38	53	9	148	14.0	95.9	31.0	0	0
4507	Coconut, fresh, shredded	1 cup	80	283	3	12	7	27	23.8	1.1	0.3	0	0
4559	Coconut, milk, cnd	2 Tbs	28	56	1	1	0	6	5.3	0.3	0.1	0	0
4575	Coconut, tstd f/dried	2 Tbs	9	55	0	4	1	4	3.9	0.2	0.0	0	0
4571	Nuts, almonds, dry rstd, salted, whole	22 ea	28	169	6	5	3	15	1.1	9.5	3.6	0	0
4549	Nuts, almonds, dry rstd, unsalted, whole	1 cup	138	824	30	27	16	73	5.6	46.4	17.5	0	0
4620	Nuts, almonds, oil rstd, salted	22 ea	28	172	6	5	3	16	1.2	9.9	3.8	0	0
4505	Nuts, almonds, oil rstd, unsalted	22 ea	28	172	6	5	3	16	1.2	9.9	3.8	0	0
4642	Nuts, beechnuts, dried	2 oz	57	327	4	19	2	28	3.2	12.4	11.4	0	0
4536	Nuts, Brazil, dried, lrg	6 ea	28	186	4	3	2	19	4.3	7.0	5.8	0	0
4750	Nuts, Brazil, dried, unblanched, shelled	1 cup	140	918	20	17	10	93	21.2	34.4	28.8	0	0
4519	Nuts, cashews, dry rstd, salted	0.25 cup	34	197	5	11	1	16	3.1	9.4	2.7	0	0
4621	Nuts, cashews, dry rstd, unsalted	0.25 cup	34	197	5	11	1	16	3.1	9.4	2.7	0	0
4596	Nuts, cashews, oil rstd, salted	0.25 cup	32	189	5	10	1	16	2.8	8.4	2.8	0	0
4622	Nuts, cashews, oil rstd, unsalted	0.25 cup	32	188	5	10	1	16	2.8	8.4	2.8	0	0
63431	Nuts, filberts, whole	1 cup	135	848	20	23	13	82	6.0	61.6	10.7	0	3
4513	Nuts, hazelnuts, whole	1 cup	135	848	20	23	13	82	6.0	61.6	10.7	0	3
4516	Nuts, macadamia, dried	11 ea	28	204	2	4	2	21	3.4	16.7	0.4	0	0
4595	Nuts, mixed, w/o peanuts, oil rstd, salted	0.25 cup	36	221	6	8	2	20	3.3	11.9	4.1	0	0
4594	Nuts, mixed, w/o peanuts, oil rstd, unsalted	0.25 cup	36	221	6	8	2	20	3.3	11.9	4.1	0	1
4592	Nuts, mixed, w/peanuts, dry rstd, salted	0.25 cup	34	203	6	9	3	18	2.4	10.8	3.7	0	0
4591	Nuts, mixed, w/peanuts, dry rstd, unsalted	0.25 cup	34	203	6	9	3	18	2.4	10.8	3.7	0	1
4593	Nuts, mixed, w/peanuts, oil rstd, salted	0.25 cup	36	219	6	8	3	20	3.1	11.3	4.7	0	0
4533	Nuts, mixed, w/peanuts, oil rstd, unsalted	0.25 cup	36	219	6	8	4	20	3.1	11.3	4.7	0	1
4541	Nuts, peanuts, dry rstd, salted	30 ea	30	176	7	6	2	15	2.1	7.4	4.7	0	0
4756	Nuts, peanuts, dry rstd, unsalted	30 ea	30	176	7	6	2	15	2.1	7.4	4.7	0	0
4763	Nuts, peanuts, oil rstd, salted	30 ea	27	162	8	4	3	14	2.3	7.0	4.1	0	0
4755	Nuts, peanuts, oil rstd, unsalted	32 ea	28	163	7	5	2	14	1.9	6.8	4.4	0	0
4542	Nuts, peanuts, oil rstd, unsalted, chpd	1 cup	133	773	35	25	9	66	9.1	32.5	20.7	0	0
4699	Nuts, peanuts, Spanish, oil rstd, salted	0.5 cup	74	426	21	13	7	36	5.6	16.2	12.5	0	0
4665	Nuts, peanuts, Spanish, oil rstd, unsalted	1 cup	147	851	41	26	13	72	11.1	32.4	25.0	0	0
4517	Nuts, peanuts, Spanish, raw	0.25 cup	36	208	10	6	3	18	2.8	8.1	6.3	0	0
4578	Nuts, pecans, halves	1 cup	108	746	10	15	10	78	6.7	44.1	23.3	0	6
4624	Nuts, pine	10 ea	1	7	0	0	0	1	0.1	0.2	0.3	0	0
4525	Nuts, walnuts, black, dried, chpd	1 cup	125	772	30	12	8	74	4.2	18.8	43.8	0	5
4626	Peanut Butter, chunky	2 Tbs	32	188	8	7	3	16	2.6	7.9	4.7	0	0
4576	Peanut Butter, chunky, unsalted	2 Tbs	32	188	8	7	3	16	2.6	7.9	4.7	0	0
4627	Peanut Butter, creamy	2 Tbs	32	188	8	6	2	16	3.3	7.6	4.4	0	0
63338	Peanut Butter, creamy, rducd fat	3.6 oz	100	520	26	36	5	34	7.4	16.2	10.3	0	0
4636	Peanut Butter, creamy, unsalted	2 Tbs	32	188	8	6	2	16	3.3	7.6	4.4	0	0
62939	Peanut Butter, crunchy, rducd fat	2 Tbs	36	190	8	15	2	12	2.5	—	—	0	0
4747	Peanut Butter, rducd fat	1 Tbs	16	81	4	5	1	5	1.0	2.8	1.6	0	—
62949	Peanut Butter, w/grape jelly, Goober	3 Tbs	53	230	7	24	2	13	2.0	—	—	0	0
4777	Seeds, flax/linseed	1 cup	155	763	30	53	43	53	5.0	10.6	34.8	0	0
4545	Seeds, sunflower, kernels, dried	1 cup	144	821	33	27	15	71	7.5	13.6	47.1	0	9

Thia (mg)	Ribo (mg)	Niac (mg NE)	Vit B6 (mg)	Vit B12 (µg)	Fol (µg)	Vit C (mg)	Vit D (IU)	Vit E (mg AT)	Cal (mg)	Iron (mg)	Magn (mg)	Phos (mg)	Pota (mg)	Sodi (mg)	Zinc (mg)	Wat (%)	Alco (g)	Caff (mg)
0.33	1.52	7.19	0.18	0.00	162.5	1.8	—	65.0	675	9.25	757.5	1308	1895	1125	7.6	1	0.00	0.00
0.05	0.01	0.43	0.03	0.00	20.8	2.6	—	0.2	11	1.94	25.6	90	285	16	0.9	47	0.00	0.00
0.00	0.00	0.18	0.00	0.00	4.0	0.3	—	0.2	5	0.93	13.0	27	62	4	0.2	73	0.00	0.00
0.00	0.00	0.05	0.02	0.00	0.8	0.1	—	0.1	2	0.31	8.5	20	51	3	0.2	1	0.00	0.00
0.01	0.23	1.09	0.03	0.00	9.4	0.0	—	7.4	75	1.27	81.1	139	211	96	1.0	3	0.00	0.00
0.10	1.19	5.30	0.17	0.00	45.5	0.0	—	35.9	367	6.21	394.7	675	1029	1	4.9	3	0.00	0.00
0.02	0.21	1.03	0.02	0.00	7.7	0.0	—	7.4	82	1.03	77.7	132	198	96	0.9	3	0.00	0.00
0.02	0.21	1.03	0.02	0.00	7.7	0.0	—	7.4	82	1.03	77.7	132	198	0	0.9	3	0.00	0.00
0.17	0.20	0.50	0.38	0.00	64.1	8.8	—	—	1	1.38	0.0	0	577	22	0.2	7	0.00	0.00
0.17	0.00	0.07	0.02	0.00	6.2	0.2	—	1.6	45	0.68	106.6	206	187	1	1.2	3	0.00	0.00
0.86	0.05	0.40	0.14	0.00	30.8	1.0	—	8.0	224	3.40	526.4	1015	923	4	5.7	3	0.00	0.00
0.07	0.07	0.47	0.09	0.00	23.6	0.0	—	0.3	15	2.05	89.1	168	194	219	1.9	2	0.00	0.00
0.07	0.07	0.47	0.09	0.00	23.6	0.0	—	0.3	15	2.05	89.1	168	194	5	1.9	2	0.00	0.00
0.11	0.07	0.56	0.10	0.00	8.1	0.1	—	0.3	14	1.97	88.7	173	205	100	1.7	2	0.00	0.00
0.11	0.07	0.56	0.10	0.00	8.1	0.1	—	0.3	14	1.97	88.7	173	205	4	1.7	3	0.00	0.00
0.87	0.15	2.43	0.75	0.00	152.6	8.5	—	20.3	154	6.34	220.1	392	918	0	3.3	5	0.00	0.00
0.87	0.15	2.43	0.75	0.00	152.6	8.5	—	20.3	154	6.34	220.1	392	918	0	3.3	5	0.00	0.00
0.34	0.05	0.69	0.07	0.00	3.1	0.3	—	0.2	24	1.04	36.9	53	104	1	0.4	1	0.00	0.00
0.18	0.17	0.70	0.05	0.00	20.2	0.2	—	3.0	38	0.93	90.4	162	196	110	1.7	2	0.00	0.00
0.18	0.17	0.70	0.05	0.00	20.2	0.2	—	2.2	38	0.93	90.4	162	196	4	1.7	3	0.00	0.00
0.07	0.07	1.61	0.10	0.00	17.1	0.1	—	3.7	24	1.26	77.1	149	204	229	1.3	2	0.00	0.00
0.07	0.07	1.61	0.10	0.00	17.1	0.1	—	2.1	24	1.26	77.1	149	204	4	1.3	2	0.00	0.00
0.18	0.07	1.79	0.09	0.00	29.5	0.2	—	2.6	38	1.13	83.4	165	206	149	1.8	2	0.00	0.00
0.18	0.07	1.79	0.09	0.00	29.5	0.2	—	2.1	38	1.13	83.4	165	206	4	1.8	2	0.00	0.00
0.12	0.02	4.05	0.07	0.00	43.5	0.0	—	2.3	16	0.68	52.8	107	197	244	1.0	2	0.00	0.00
0.12	0.02	4.05	0.07	0.00	43.5	0.0	—	2.1	16	0.68	52.8	107	197	2	1.0	2	0.00	0.00
0.01	0.01	3.73	0.11	0.00	32.4	0.2	—	1.9	16	0.40	47.5	107	196	86	0.9	1	0.00	0.00
0.07	0.02	4.00	0.07	0.00	35.3	0.0	—	1.9	25	0.50	51.8	145	191	2	1.9	2	0.00	0.00
0.34	0.14	18.98	0.34	0.00	167.6	0.0	—	9.2	117	2.43	246.1	688	907	8	8.8	2	0.00	0.00
0.23	0.05	10.97	0.18	0.00	92.6	0.0	0.0	5.4	74	1.67	123.5	284	570	318	1.5	2	0.00	0.00
0.46	0.11	21.95	0.37	0.00	185.2	0.0	—	10.9	147	3.34	247.0	569	1141	9	2.9	2	0.00	0.00
0.25	0.05	5.80	0.12	0.00	87.6	0.0	—	2.7	39	1.42	68.6	142	272	8	0.8	6	0.00	0.00
0.70	0.14	1.25	0.23	0.00	23.8	1.2	—	1.5	76	2.73	130.7	299	443	0	4.9	4	0.00	0.00
—	—	—	—	0.00	—	0.0	—	—	0	0.05	—	—	—	0	—	2	0.00	0.00
0.07	0.15	0.58	0.73	0.00	38.8	2.1	—	2.2	76	3.90	251.2	641	654	2	4.2	5	0.00	0.00
0.02	0.03	4.38	0.12	0.00	29.4	0.0	0.0	2.0	14	0.61	51.2	102	238	156	0.9	1	0.00	0.00
0.02	0.03	4.38	0.12	0.00	29.4	0.0	—	2.0	14	0.61	51.2	102	238	5	0.9	1	0.00	0.00
0.01	0.02	4.28	0.17	0.00	23.7	0.0	—	2.9	14	0.60	49.3	115	208	147	0.9	2	0.00	0.00
0.27	0.05	14.60	0.31	0.00	60.0	0.0	—	6.7	35	1.89	170.0	369	669	540	2.8	1	0.00	0.00
0.01	0.02	4.28	0.17	0.00	23.7	0.0	—	2.9	14	0.60	49.3	115	208	5	0.9	2	0.00	0.00
—	—	5.00	0.11	0.00	24.0	0.0	—	—	0	0.72	60.0	—	—	220	0.9	—	0.00	0.00
—	—	2.07	—	0.00	—	—	—	—	6	0.31	—	59	115	89	—	3	0.00	0.00
—	—	—	—	0.00	—	0.0	—	—	0	0.36	—	—	—	160	—	—	0.00	0.00
0.25	0.25	2.17	1.44	0.00	430.9	2.0	—	0.5	308	9.64	561.1	772	1056	53	6.5	9	0.00	0.00
3.29	0.36	6.48	1.11	0.00	326.9	2.0	—	49.7	167	9.75	509.8	1015	992	4	7.3	5	0.00	0.00

64

Code	Food Name	Unit/ Amt	Wt (g)	Energy (kcal)	Prot (g)	Carb (g)	Fiber (g)	Fat (g)	Sat (g)	Mono (g)	Poly (g)	Chol (mg)	Vit A (RE)
4597	Seeds, sunflower, kernels, dry rstd, salted	0.25 cup	32	186	6	8	3	16	1.7	3.0	10.5	0	0
4551	Seeds, sunflower, kernels, dry rstd, unsalted	0.25 cup	32	186	6	8	4	16	1.7	3.0	10.5	0	0
4546	Seeds, sunflower, kernels, oil rstd, unsalted	1 cup	135	799	27	31	14	69	9.5	10.9	46.3	0	1
4552	Seeds, sunflower, oil rstd, salted	0.25 cup	34	200	7	8	4	17	2.4	2.7	11.6	0	0
63261	Soy Nuts, wheat free	1.8 oz	50	241	20	14	6	11	1.7	—	—	1	4

POULTRY

Chicken—BBQ, Breaded, Fried, Glazed, Grilled, Raw

Code	Food Name	Unit/ Amt	Wt (g)	Energy (kcal)	Prot (g)	Carb (g)	Fiber (g)	Fat (g)	Sat (g)	Mono (g)	Poly (g)	Chol (mg)	Vit A (RE)
15064	Chicken, breast & wing, white meat, brd, fried	3 oz	85	258	19	10	1	15	4.1	6.4	3.5	77	30
81202	Chicken, breast, fillet, grilled	1 ea	85	100	20	1	0	2	—	—	—	45	0
81186	Chicken, breast, oven rstd, fat free, 0.75 oz slice	2 pce	42	33	7	1	0	0	0.1	0.1	0.0	15	0
15921	Chicken, breast, sweet & sour	1 ea	131	118	8	15	1	3	0.5	0.9	1.4	23	22
15915	Chicken, breast, teriyaki	3 oz	85	118	18	4	0	2	0.6	0.7	0.6	55	11
15057	Chicken, broiler/fryer, breast, w/o skin, fried	3 oz	85	159	28	0	0	4	1.1	1.5	0.9	77	6
15004	Chicken, broiler/fryer, breast, w/o skin, rstd	3 oz	85	140	26	0	0	3	0.9	1.1	0.7	72	5
15039	Chicken, broiler/fryer, breast, w/o skin, stwd	3 oz	85	128	25	0	0	3	0.7	0.9	0.6	65	5
15013	Chicken, broiler/fryer, breast, w/skin, batter fried	3 oz	85	221	21	8	0	11	3.0	4.6	2.6	72	17
15003	Chicken, broiler/fryer, breast, w/skin, flour fried	3 oz	85	189	27	1	0	8	2.1	3.0	1.7	76	13
15001	Chicken, broiler/fryer, breast, w/skin, rstd	3 oz	85	168	25	0	0	7	1.9	2.6	1.4	71	23
15113	Chicken, broiler/fryer, dark meat, w/skin, batter fried	3 oz	85	253	19	8	0	16	4.2	6.4	3.8	76	26
15079	Chicken, broiler/fryer, dark meat, w/skin, flour fried	3 oz	85	242	23	3	0	14	3.9	5.7	3.3	78	26
15080	Chicken, broiler/fryer, dark meat, w/skin, rstd	3 oz	85	215	22	0	0	13	3.7	5.3	3.0	77	51
15903	Chicken, buffalo wings, w/bone, spicy	1 pce	16	49	4	0	0	3	0.9	1.3	0.9	13	9
15063	Chicken, drumstick & thigh, dark meat, brd, fried	3 oz	85	247	17	9	1	15	4.1	6.3	3.6	95	38
81198	Chicken, ground, raw	4 oz	113	150	18	0	0	9	2.5	—	—	75	0
15243	Chicken, nuggets	4 pce	73	207	12	11	0	13	4.0	6.2	1.6	44	22
15902	Chicken, patty, brd, ckd	1 ea	75	213	12	11	0	13	4.1	6.4	1.7	45	22
15136	Chicken, roasting, dark meat, w/o skin, raw	4 oz	113	128	21	0	0	4	1.1	1.3	1.0	82	20
15134	Chicken, roasting, light meat, w/o skin, raw	4 oz	113	124	25	0	0	2	0.4	0.5	0.5	65	9
49158	Chicken, tenders, breast meat, fat free, bkd	3 ea	85	120	13	16	2	0	0.0	0.0	0.0	30	0
49171	Chicken, tenders, breast, ckd f/fzn	3 ea	85	240	11	16	1	14	4.0	—	—	25	0

Turkey

Code	Food Name	Unit/ Amt	Wt (g)	Energy (kcal)	Prot (g)	Carb (g)	Fiber (g)	Fat (g)	Sat (g)	Mono (g)	Poly (g)	Chol (mg)	Vit A (RE)
16086	Turkey, avg, breast, w/skin, rstd	3 oz	85	161	24	0	0	6	1.8	2.1	1.5	63	0
51101	Turkey, avg, dark meat, w/o skin, rstd	3 oz	85	159	24	0	0	6	2.1	1.4	1.8	72	0
16028	Turkey, avg, dark meat, w/skin, rstd	3 oz	85	188	23	0	0	10	3.0	3.1	2.6	76	0
16158	Turkey, avg, light meat, w/o skin, rstd	3 oz	85	134	25	0	0	3	0.9	0.5	0.7	59	0
16027	Turkey, avg, light meat, w/skin, rstd	3 oz	85	168	24	0	0	7	2.0	2.4	1.7	65	0
16071	Turkey, avg, skin, rstd	1 ea	496	2192	98	0	0	197	51.3	83.8	45.0	560	0
16000	Turkey, avg, w/o skin, rstd	3 oz	85	145	25	0	0	4	1.4	0.9	1.2	65	0
16204	Turkey, ground, 10% fat, raw	3 oz	85	137	16	0	0	8	2.6	3.1	2.5	73	0
51133	Turkey, ground, 99% fat free, raw	4 oz	113	120	28	0	0	2	—	—	—	45	0
16351	Turkey, jerky, original, Original California	1 oz	28	80	14	3	0	1	0.0	—	—	30	60

Duck, Emu, Ostrich and Other

Code	Food Name	Unit/ Amt	Wt (g)	Energy (kcal)	Prot (g)	Carb (g)	Fiber (g)	Fat (g)	Sat (g)	Mono (g)	Poly (g)	Chol (mg)	Vit A (RE)
15069	Cornish Game Hen, rstd	3 oz	85	221	19	0	0	15	4.3	6.8	3.1	111	27
16294	Duck, domesticated, whole, rstd, chpd	1 cup	140	472	27	0	0	40	13.5	18.1	5.1	118	88
16065	Goose, whole, w/o skin, raw	4 oz	113	183	26	0	0	8	3.2	2.1	1.0	95	14

PAGE KEY: 52 Granola Bars, Cereal Bars, Diet Bars, Scones, and Tarts 52 Meals and Dishes 56 Meats 62 Nuts, Seeds, and Products 64 Poultry
66 Salad Dressings, Dips, and Mayonnaise 66 Salads 68 Sandwiches 70 Sauces and Gravies 70 Snack Foods—Chips, Pretzels, Popcorn
72 Soups, Stews, and Chilis 74 Spices, Flavors, and Seasonings 76 Sports Bars and Drinks 76 Supplemental Foods and Formulas
78 Sweeteners and Sweet Substitutes 78 Vegetables and Legumes 92 Weight Loss Bars and Drinks 94 Miscellaneous

Thia (mg)	Ribo (mg)	Niac (mg NE)	Vit B6 (mg)	Vit B12 (μg)	Fol (μg)	Vit C (mg)	Vit D (IU)	Vit E (mg AT)	Cal (mg)	Iron (mg)	Magn (mg)	Phos (mg)	Pota (mg)	Sodi (mg)	Zinc (mg)	Wat (%)	Alco (g)	Caff (mg)
0.02	0.07	2.25	0.25	0.00	75.8	0.4	—	8.4	22	1.22	41.3	370	272	131	1.7	1	0.00	0.00
0.02	0.07	2.25	0.25	0.00	75.8	0.4	—	8.4	22	1.22	41.3	370	272	1	1.7	1	0.00	0.00
0.43	0.37	5.57	1.07	0.00	315.9	1.5	—	49.0	117	5.78	171.4	1538	652	4	7.0	2	0.00	0.00
0.10	0.09	1.38	0.27	0.00	79.0	0.4	—	12.3	29	1.44	42.9	384	163	138	1.8	2	0.00	0.00
—	—	—	—	0.00	—	0.0	—	—	105	3.20	—	—	—	—	—	2	0.00	0.00
0.07	0.15	6.25	0.30	0.34	15.3	0.0	—	0.8	31	0.76	19.6	160	295	509	0.8	46	0.00	0.00
—	—	—	—	—	—	0.0	—	—	0	1.08	—	—	—	410	—	—	0.00	0.00
0.00	0.00	1.44	0.05	0.03	0.4	0.0	—	0.0	3	0.12	3.8	25	28	457	0.1	77	0.00	0.00
0.05	0.07	3.08	0.18	0.07	5.8	12.1	—	0.7	15	0.83	20.8	75	185	506	0.7	79	0.00	0.00
0.05	0.12	5.82	0.31	0.18	8.1	2.1	—	0.2	18	1.13	23.4	132	205	1118	1.3	67	0.56	0.00
0.07	0.10	12.56	0.54	0.31	3.4	0.0	—	0.4	14	0.97	26.4	209	235	67	0.9	60	0.00	0.00
0.05	0.10	11.65	0.50	0.28	3.4	0.0	—	0.2	13	0.87	24.7	194	218	63	0.9	65	0.00	0.00
0.03	0.10	7.19	0.28	0.20	2.6	0.0	—	0.2	11	0.75	20.4	140	159	54	0.8	68	0.00	0.00
0.10	0.11	8.94	0.37	0.25	12.8	0.0	—	0.9	17	1.05	20.4	157	171	234	0.8	52	0.00	0.00
0.07	0.10	11.68	0.49	0.28	5.1	0.0	—	0.5	14	1.00	25.5	198	220	65	0.9	57	0.00	0.00
0.05	0.10	10.81	0.47	0.27	3.4	0.0	—	0.2	12	0.91	23.0	182	208	60	0.9	62	0.00	0.00
0.10	0.18	4.76	0.20	0.23	15.3	0.0	—	1.0	18	1.22	17.0	123	157	251	1.8	49	0.00	0.00
0.07	0.20	5.82	0.27	0.25	9.4	0.0	—	0.7	14	1.27	20.4	150	196	76	2.2	51	0.00	0.00
0.05	0.18	5.40	0.25	0.25	6.0	0.0	—	0.5	13	1.15	18.7	143	187	74	2.1	59	0.00	0.00
0.00	0.01	1.02	0.07	0.03	0.5	0.0	1.9	0.1	2	0.20	3.0	24	29	13	0.3	53	0.00	0.00
0.07	0.25	4.13	0.18	0.47	14.5	0.0	—	0.8	20	0.92	21.3	138	256	434	1.9	49	0.00	0.00
—	—	—	—	—	—	0.0	—	—	0	0.00	—	—	—	65	—	—	0.00	0.00
0.07	0.10	4.90	0.23	0.21	8.0	0.3	8.8	1.4	12	0.91	14.6	146	180	388	0.8	49	0.00	0.00
0.07	0.10	5.03	0.23	0.23	8.2	0.3	9.0	1.5	12	0.93	15.0	150	184	399	0.8	49	0.00	0.00
0.07	0.20	6.67	0.36	0.38	10.2	0.0	—	0.2	10	1.29	23.8	202	257	108	1.9	75	0.00	0.00
0.07	0.10	11.59	0.62	0.43	4.5	0.0	—	0.2	12	1.00	28.4	253	286	58	0.7	74	0.00	0.00
—	—	—	—	—	—	0.0	—	—	0	0.72	—	—	—	480	—	—	0.00	0.00
—	—	—	—	—	—	0.0	—	—	20	0.72	—	—	—	450	—	—	0.00	0.00
0.05	0.10	5.40	0.40	0.31	5.1	0.0	—	0.2	18	1.19	23.0	179	245	54	1.7	63	0.00	0.00
0.05	0.20	3.09	0.31	0.31	7.7	0.0	—	0.5	27	1.98	20.4	174	247	67	3.8	63	0.00	0.00
0.05	0.20	3.00	0.27	0.31	7.7	0.0	—	0.5	28	1.92	19.6	167	233	65	3.5	60	0.00	0.00
0.05	0.10	5.82	0.46	0.31	5.1	0.0	—	0.1	16	1.14	23.8	186	259	54	1.7	66	0.00	0.00
0.05	0.10	5.34	0.40	0.30	5.1	0.0	—	0.1	18	1.20	22.1	177	242	54	1.7	63	0.00	0.00
0.10	0.72	13.17	0.40	1.19	19.8	0.0	—	2.6	174	8.88	79.4	680	794	263	10.3	40	0.00	0.00
0.05	0.15	4.63	0.38	0.31	6.0	0.0	—	0.3	21	1.50	22.1	181	253	60	2.6	65	0.00	0.00
—	—	—	—	—	—	0.0	—	—	22	1.28	22.9	140	207	109	2.5	71	0.00	0.00
—	—	—	—	—	—	0.0	—	—	0	1.44	—	—	—	65	—	—	0.00	0.00
—	—	—	—	—	—	0.0	—	—	20	1.08	—	—	—	550	—	31	0.00	0.00
0.05	0.17	5.01	0.25	0.23	1.7	0.4	10.2	0.2	11	0.76	15.3	124	208	54	1.3	59	0.00	0.00
0.23	0.37	6.75	0.25	0.41	8.4	0.0	—	1.0	15	3.77	22.4	218	286	83	2.6	52	0.00	0.00
0.15	0.43	4.84	0.73	0.56	35.2	8.2	—	1.3	15	2.91	27.2	354	476	99	2.7	68	0.00	0.00

Code	Food Name	Unit/ Amt	Wt (g)	Energy (kcal)	Prot (g)	Carb (g)	Fiber (g)	Fat (g)	Sat (g)	Mono (g)	Poly (g)	Chol (mg)	Vit A (RE)
16064	Goose, whole, w/skin, raw	4 oz	113	421	18	0	0	38	11.1	20.2	4.3	91	19
81168	Ostrich, ground, brld	3 oz	85	149	22	0	0	6	1.5	1.8	0.6	71	0
51148	Pheasant, whole, ckd	3 oz	85	210	28	0	0	10	3.0	4.8	1.3	76	48

SALAD DRESSINGS, DIPS, MAYONNAISE, OR SPREADS

Dips

Code	Food Name	Unit/ Amt	Wt (g)	Energy (kcal)	Prot (g)	Carb (g)	Fiber (g)	Fat (g)	Sat (g)	Mono (g)	Poly (g)	Chol (mg)	Vit A (RE)
53685	Dip, bean	2 Tbs	35	40	2	6	0	1	0.5	—	—	5	0
27138	Dip, creamy ranch	2 Tbs	31	60	1	3	0	4	3.0	—	—	0	0
53554	Dip, French onion	2 Tbs	33	60	1	4	0	5	3.0	—	—	15	20
27136	Dip, green onion	2 Tbs	31	60	1	4	0	4	3.0	—	—	0	0
27132	Dip, guacamole	2 Tbs	32	60	1	4	0	4	3.0	—	—	0	0
90861	Dip, salsa con queso, medium	2 Tbs	32	42	1	5	1	2	0.5	—	—	5	19
44415	Dip, salsa, grande	2 Tbs	28	50	1	1	0	5	3.0	—	—	15	40
27143	Dip, spinach	2 Tbs	28	140	0	3	0	14	2.0	—	—	10	80
44414	Dip, Veggie	2 Tbs	28	50	1	2	0	5	3.0	—	—	15	60
44425	Guacamole, med	2 Tbs	28	57	1	3	2	5	1.0	—	—	0	10

Mayonnaise

Code	Food Name	Unit/ Amt	Wt (g)	Energy (kcal)	Prot (g)	Carb (g)	Fiber (g)	Fat (g)	Sat (g)	Mono (g)	Poly (g)	Chol (mg)	Vit A (RE)
8069	Mayonnaise, fat free	1 Tbs	16	11	0	2	0	0	0.1	—	—	2	3
4070	Mayonnaise, light	1 Tbs	15	50	0	2		5	0.0	2.5	1.5	5	0
44719	Mayonnaise, rducd cal, cholest free	1 Tbs	15	49	0	1	0	5	0.7	1.1	2.8	0	0
8503	Mayonnaise, real	1 Tbs	14	100	0	0	0	11	1.5	—	—	5	0

Salad Dressings—Lower Calorie/Fat/Sodium/Cholest

Code	Food Name	Unit/ Amt	Wt (g)	Energy (kcal)	Prot (g)	Carb (g)	Fiber (g)	Fat (g)	Sat (g)	Mono (g)	Poly (g)	Chol (mg)	Vit A (RE)
44731	Dip, hummus, low fat, dry mix	2 Tbs	15	75	3	8	2	3	0.0	—	—	0	0
44727	Salad Dressing, blue cheese, fat free	1 Tbs	17	20	0	4	1	0	0.0	0.0	0.1	1	1
44722	Salad Dressing, blue cheese, rducd cal	1 Tbs	16	14	0	2	0	0	0.1	0.2	0.1	2	11
44465	Salad Dressing, buttermilk, light	3.6 oz	100	225	1	16	1	17	1.3	5.4	4.3	21	19
8138	Salad Dressing, caesar, low cal	1 Tbs	15	16	0	3	0	1	0.1	0.2	0.4	0	0
44729	Salad Dressing, French, rducd cal	1 Tbs	16	32	0	4	0	2	0.3	0.5	1.2	0	3
44699	Salad Dressing, Italian	2 Tbs	31	70	0	0	0	8	1.0	—	—	0	0
44498	Salad Dressing, Italian, fat free	1 Tbs	14	7	0	1	0	0	0.0	0.0	0.0	0	1
44720	Salad Dressing, Italian, rducd cal	1 Tbs	14	28	0	1	0	3	0.4	0.7	1.6	0	0
44497	Salad Dressing, thousand island, fat free	1 Tbs	16	21	0	5	1	0	0.0	0.1	0.1	1	0
8545	Salad Dressing, vinaigrette, Italian, fat free	2 Tbs	35	35	0	8	0	0	0.0	0.0	0.0	0	0
8546	Salad Dressing, vinaigrette, raspberry, fat free	2 Tbs	35	35	0	8	0	0	0.0	0.0	0.0	0	0

Salad Dressings—Regular

Code	Food Name	Unit/ Amt	Wt (g)	Energy (kcal)	Prot (g)	Carb (g)	Fiber (g)	Fat (g)	Sat (g)	Mono (g)	Poly (g)	Chol (mg)	Vit A (RE)
44705	Salad Dressing, caesar	2 Tbs	29	155	0	1	0	17	2.6	4.0	9.7	1	1
8015	Salad Dressing, French, cmrcl	2 Tbs	31	143	0	5	0	14	1.8	2.6	6.6	0	14
8569	Salad Dressing, French, creamy	2 Tbs	32	160	0	5	0	15	2.5	—	—	0	250
8579	Salad Dressing, honey dijon	2 Tbs	31	110	0	6	0	10	1.5	—	—	0	0
8612	Salad Dressing, Italian, zesty	2 Tbs	31	109	0	2	0	11	1.2	—	—	0	2
8479	Salad Dressing, Miracle Whip	1 Tbs	15	70	0	2	0	7	1.0	—	—	5	0
44590	Salad Dressing, ranch, cmrcl	1 oz	28	137	0	2	0	15	2.3	3.2	8.0	9	3
8024	Salad Dressing, thousand island, cmrcl	1 Tbs	16	58	0	2	0	5	0.8	1.2	2.8	4	4

SPREADS—CRACKER OR SANDWICH

Salads

Code	Food Name	Unit/ Amt	Wt (g)	Energy (kcal)	Prot (g)	Carb (g)	Fiber (g)	Fat (g)	Sat (g)	Mono (g)	Poly (g)	Chol (mg)	Vit A (RE)
57482	Cole Slaw, prep f/recipe	0.5 cup	60	41	1	7	1	2	0.2	0.4	0.8	5	39
56118	Salad, bean, three	0.5 cup	75	70	2	7	3	4	0.6	0.9	2.2	0	10

Thia (mg)	Ribo (mg)	Niac (mg NE)	Vit B6 (mg)	Vit B12 (μg)	Fol (μg)	Vit C (mg)	Vit D (IU)	Vit E (mg AT)	Cal (mg)	Iron (mg)	Magn (mg)	Phos (mg)	Pota (mg)	Sodi (mg)	Zinc (mg)	Wat (%)	Alco (g)	Caff (mg)
0.10	0.28	4.09	0.43	0.38	4.5	4.8	—	2.0	14	2.83	20.4	265	349	83	2.0	50	0.00	0.00
0.18	0.23	5.57	0.43	4.88	11.9	0.0	—	0.2	7	2.92	19.6	191	275	68	3.7	67	0.00	0.00
0.05	0.15	6.40	0.63	0.61	4.3	2.0	—	0.2	14	1.22	18.7	206	230	37	1.2	54	0.00	0.00
—	—	—	—	—	—	0.0	—	—	0	0.36	—	—	—	140	—	70	0.00	0.00
—	—	—	—	—	—	0.0	—	—	0	0.00	—	—	20	210	—	—	0.00	0.00
—	—	—	—	—	—	0.0	—	—	0	0.00	—	—	—	230	—	—	0.00	0.00
—	—	—	—	—	—	0.0	—	—	0	0.00	—	0	20	190	—	—	0.00	0.00
—	—	—	—	—	—	0.0	—	—	0	0.00	—	0	25	240	—	—	0.00	0.00
—	—	—	—	—	—	0.0	—	—	19	0.00	—	—	—	254	—	—	0.00	0.00
—	—	—	—	—	—	1.2	—	—	20	0.00	—	—	—	130	—	—	0.00	0.00
—	—	—	—	—	—	0.0	—	—	0	0.36	—	—	—	200	—	—	0.00	0.00
—	—	—	—	—	—	0.0	—	—	20	0.00	—	—	—	125	—	—	0.00	0.00
—	—	—	—	—	—	1.8	—	—	10	0.18	—	—	—	147	—	66	0.00	0.00
—	—	—	—	—	—	0.0	—	0.5	1	0.01	—	4	8	120	—	82	0.00	0.00
—	—	—	—	—	—	—	—	0.6	—	—	—	—	—	125	—	51	0.00	0.00
0.00	0.00	0.00	0.00	0.00	0.0	0.0	—	0.9	0	0.00	0.0	0	10	107	0.0	56	0.00	0.00
—	—	—	—	—	—	0.0	—	0.4	0	0.00	—	0	0	75	—	20	0.00	0.00
—	—	—	—	—	—	0.0	—	—	0	0.54	—	—	—	240	—	—	0.00	0.00
0.00	0.01	0.00	0.00	0.03	1.0	0.0	—	0.0	12	0.00	1.5	18	33	136	0.0	68	0.00	0.00
0.00	0.00	0.00	0.00	0.01	4.5	0.0	—	0.1	11	0.01	0.6	8	8	258	0.0	78	0.00	0.00
0.01	0.02	0.00	0.02	0.00	4.0	0.7	4.9	1.6	125	0.87	6.0	193	132	932	0.6	62	0.00	0.00
0.00	0.00	0.00	0.00	0.00	0.3	0.0	—	0.1	4	0.02	0.3	3	4	162	0.0	73	0.00	0.00
0.00	0.00	0.00	0.00	0.00	0.3	0.0	—	0.5	2	0.05	0.0	2	13	160	0.0	59	0.00	0.00
—	—	—	—	—	—	0.0	—	—	0	0.00	—	—	—	350	—	71	0.00	0.00
0.00	0.00	0.01	0.00	0.03	1.7	0.1	—	0.1	4	0.05	0.7	15	14	158	0.1	86	0.00	0.00
0.00	0.00	0.00	0.00	0.00	0.4	0.1	—	0.1	1	0.01	0.3	1	5	199	0.0	70	0.00	0.00
0.03	0.00	0.03	0.00	0.00	1.9	0.0	—	0.1	2	0.03	0.6	0	20	117	0.0	66	0.00	0.00
—	—	—	—	—	—	0.0	—	—	0	0.00	—	—	—	280	—	—	0.00	0.00
—	—	—	—	—	—	0.0	—	—	0	0.00	—	—	—	35	—	—	0.00	0.00
0.00	0.00	0.00	0.00	0.00	0.9	0.0	—	1.5	7	0.05	0.6	6	9	317	0.0	34	0.00	0.00
0.00	0.01	0.05	0.00	0.03	0.0	0.0	—	1.6	7	0.25	1.6	6	21	261	0.1	37	0.00	0.00
—	—	—	—	—	—	0.0	—	—	0	0.00	—	0	20	270	—	35	0.00	0.00
—	—	—	—	—	—	0.0	—	—	0	0.00	—	0	35	210	—	—	0.00	0.00
—	—	—	—	—	—	0.2	—	—	1	0.05	—	4	9	505	—	53	0.00	0.00
—	—	—	—	—	—	0.0	—	0.0	0	0.00	—	0	0	95	—	—	0.00	0.00
0.02	0.01	0.00	0.00	0.09	1.1	1.0	0.8	1.3	9	0.18	1.4	46	18	231	0.1	38	0.00	0.00
0.23	0.00	0.07	0.00	0.00	0.0	0.0	—	0.6	3	0.18	1.2	4	17	135	0.0	47	0.00	0.00
0.03	0.03	0.15	0.07	0.00	16.2	19.6	—	0.1	27	0.34	6.0	19	109	14	0.1	82	0.00	0.00
0.03	0.05	0.21	0.01	0.00	28.0	2.0	—	0.9	18	0.74	13.7	38	123	260	0.3	81	0.00	0.00

Code	Food Name	Unit/ Amt	Wt (g)	Energy (kcal)	Prot (g)	Carb (g)	Fiber (g)	Fat (g)	Sat (g)	Mono (g)	Poly (g)	Chol (mg)	Vit A (RE)
52061	Salad, chicken	0.5 cup	100	250	10	9	2	20	4.0	—	—	55	20
56253	Salad, crab	1 cup	208	282	27	11	1	14	2.0	3.5	7.1	142	37
56003	Salad, egg	1 cup	183	584	17	3	0	56	10.5	17.4	23.9	581	263
3312	Salad, fruit, w/citrus, fresh	1 cup	175	99	1	25	3	1	0.1	0.0	0.1	0	14
3311	Salad, fruit, w/o citrus, fresh	1 cup	175	101	1	26	4	1	0.1	0.1	0.2	0	34
69160	Salad, gelatin, fruity, prep f/recipe	1 ea	192	376	5	41	2	22	9.5	—	—	35	94
52029	Salad, macaroni, elbow, classic	0.5 cup	106	197	3	25	2	9	1.5	—	—	8	—
69196	Salad, Mediterranean Blend	2 cup	100	90	1	5	1	8	1.0	—	—	0	225
5637	Salad, mixed greens, raw	1 cup	55	9	1	2	1	0	0.0	0.0	0.1	0	150
4839	Salad, pasta, Greek, w/feta cheese	0.66 cup	140	200	6	27	3	8	2.0	—	—	5	—
56005	Salad, potato, prep f/recipe	0.5 cup	125	179	3	14	2	10	1.8	3.1	4.7	85	44
56257	Salad, seafood	0.5 cup	104	164	13	2	0	11	1.6	8.0	1.2	66	25
56256	Salad, shrimp	1 cup	182	282	27	6	1	17	2.6	4.5	8.4	206	42
5537	Salad, spinach, w/o dressing	1 cup	74	108	5	11	2	5	1.4	2.2	0.7	77	176
56643	Salad, taco	1.5 cup	198	279	13	24	—	15	6.8	5.2	1.7	44	93
52060	Salad, tuna	0.5 cup	100	260	12	9	2	19	3.0	—	—	30	20

SANDWICHES

Code	Food Name	Unit/ Amt	Wt (g)	Energy (kcal)	Prot (g)	Carb (g)	Fiber (g)	Fat (g)	Sat (g)	Mono (g)	Poly (g)	Chol (mg)	Vit A (RE)
56647	Cheeseburger, reg, w/condiments	1 ea	113	295	16	27	—	14	6.3	5.3	1.1	37	97
66004	Hot Dog, plain, w/bun	1 ea	98	242	10	18	—	15	5.1	6.9	1.7	44	0
56667	Hot Dog, w/chili & bun	1 ea	114	296	14	31	—	13	4.9	6.6	1.2	51	7
56009	Sandwich, BLT, w/white	1 ea	124	318	10	29	2	18	4.1	—	—	20	49
56010	Sandwich, BLT, w/whole wheat	1 ea	137	339	12	29	5	20	4.9	—	—	23	56
56281	Sandwich, bologna	1 ea	83	256	7	26	1	13	4.1	6.3	2.1	16	37
56000	Sandwich, chicken, fillet, plain	1 ea	182	515	24	39	—	29	8.5	10.4	8.4	60	31
70755	Sandwich, egg cheese, medium	1 ea	119	350	12	30	1	20	8.0	—	—	110	0
56657	Sandwich, egg cheese, large	1 ea	146	340	16	26	—	19	6.6	8.3	2.6	291	201
66010	Sandwich, fish, w/tartar sauce	1 ea	158	431	17	41	0	23	5.2	7.7	8.2	55	33
56013	Sandwich, grilled cheese, w/white	1 ea	119	399	17	30	1	23	11.9	—	—	53	167
56014	Sandwich, grilled cheese, w/whole wheat	1 ea	132	431	20	30	4	27	13.8	—	—	60	192
56272	Sandwich, gyro	1 ea	105	170	12	21	1	4	1.5	1.4	0.4	34	11
56664	Sandwich, ham cheese	1 ea	146	352	21	33	—	15	6.4	6.7	1.4	58	96
56274	Sandwich, ham cheese, grilled	1 ea	141	381	21	30	1	20	7.9	7.9	2.4	54	106
56029	Sandwich, ham, w/white	1 ea	157	365	24	30	2	16	3.3	—	—	54	6
56030	Sandwich, ham, w/whole wheat	1 ea	169	379	27	29	4	18	3.9	—	—	59	7
56267	Sandwich, pastrami	1 ea	134	331	14	27	2	18	6.2	8.7	1.0	51	3
56040	Sandwich, peanut butter & jam, w/white	1 ea	101	348	11	47	3	14	2.7	—	—	1	0
56041	Sandwich, peanut butter & jam, w/whole wheat	1 ea	114	398	13	51	5	17	3.6	—	—	0	1
56277	Sandwich, pork	1 ea	136	324	26	32	1	9	2.9	4.1	1.0	62	1
56266	Sandwich, reuben	1 ea	181	464	21	30	3	29	9.9	9.7	6.7	82	94
66003	Sandwich, roast beef, plain	1 ea	139	346	22	33	—	14	3.6	6.8	1.7	51	22
56669	Sandwich, roast beef, w/cheese	1 ea	176	473	32	45	—	18	9.0	3.7	3.5	77	58
56286	Sandwich, salami	1 ea	82	234	8	25	1	11	3.4	5.2	1.9	19	35
56261	Sandwich, sloppy joe, w/bun	1 ea	186	358	18	36	2	15	5.0	6.6	1.4	46	73
56670	Sandwich, steak	1 ea	204	459	30	52	—	14	3.8	5.3	3.3	73	39
56048	Sandwich, tuna salad, w/white	1 ea	122	326	13	35	1	14	1.9	—	—	13	15
56052	Sandwich, turkey, w/white	1 ea	156	346	24	29	1	14	1.9	—	—	43	8
56053	Sandwich, turkey, w/whole wheat	1 ea	169	360	27	29	4	16	2.3	—	—	47	8

Thia (mg)	Ribo (mg)	Niac (mg NE)	Vit B6 (mg)	Vit B12 (µg)	Fol (µg)	Vit C (mg)	Vit D (IU)	Vit E (mg AT)	Cal (mg)	Iron (mg)	Magn (mg)	Phos (mg)	Pota (mg)	Sodi (mg)	Zinc (mg)	Wat (%)	Alco (g)	Caff (mg)
—	—	—	—	—	1.2	—	—	—	40	0.36	—	—	—	600	—	—	0.00	0.00
0.15	0.09	4.50	0.28	9.76	79.4	6.9	—	2.8	157	1.45	48.6	292	536	700	5.7	74	0.00	0.00
0.09	0.66	0.09	0.46	1.57	61.1	0.0	—	7.7	74	1.80	13.5	238	181	464	1.4	57	0.00	0.00
0.07	0.05	0.41	0.23	0.00	14.1	29.2	0.0	0.6	16	0.31	17.4	18	309	1	0.1	84	0.00	0.00
0.07	0.07	0.88	0.20	0.00	13.7	14.5	0.0	0.7	13	0.41	19.7	21	328	1	0.2	84	0.00	0.00
0.09	0.07	0.18	0.03	0.14	7.1	8.0	2.3	0.8	36	0.99	17.8	70	91	149	0.8	64	0.00	0.00
—	—	—	—	—	—	—	—	—	—	—	—	—	—	560	—	—	0.00	0.00
—	—	—	—	—	—	18.0	—	—	40	0.72	—	—	—	180	—	—	0.00	0.00
0.03	0.05	0.23	0.03	0.00	63.6	8.9	0.0	0.4	30	0.72	13.2	18	174	14	0.2	94	0.00	0.00
—	—	—	—	—	—	—	—	—	—	—	—	—	—	780	—	—	0.00	0.00
0.10	0.07	1.11	0.18	0.00	8.8	12.5	—	2.3	24	0.81	18.8	65	318	661	0.4	76	0.00	0.00
0.03	0.05	1.17	0.09	0.92	15.7	6.2	—	2.0	46	0.99	27.1	141	251	176	1.7	73	0.00	0.00
0.05	0.05	3.25	0.27	1.30	15.5	5.7	—	3.4	87	3.39	51.6	280	367	392	1.5	72	0.00	0.00
0.12	0.28	1.66	0.10	0.20	59.9	6.7	0.0	0.9	46	1.46	27.1	83	242	227	0.6	70	0.00	0.00
0.10	0.36	2.46	0.21	0.62	83.2	3.6	—	—	192	2.27	51.5	143	416	762	2.7	72	0.00	0.00
—	—	—	—	—	—	0.0	—	—	20	0.36	—	—	—	580	—	—	0.00	0.00
0.25	0.23	3.72	0.10	0.93	54.2	1.9	—	0.5	111	2.43	20.3	176	223	616	2.1	48	0.00	0.00
0.23	0.27	3.65	0.05	0.50	48.0	0.1	—	0.3	24	2.30	12.7	97	143	670	2.0	54	0.00	0.00
0.21	0.40	3.74	0.05	0.30	73.0	2.7	—	—	19	3.27	10.3	192	166	480	0.8	48	0.00	0.00
0.40	0.25	3.69	0.15	0.34	66.3	6.0	6.8	2.3	68	2.20	22.0	123	239	631	1.0	52	0.00	0.00
0.37	0.20	3.97	0.25	0.37	45.0	6.8	7.5	2.9	51	2.53	60.7	216	346	690	1.9	52	0.00	0.00
0.28	0.20	2.73	0.07	0.37	18.7	0.0	—	0.8	60	1.96	15.4	74	112	598	0.9	41	0.00	0.00
0.33	0.23	6.80	0.20	0.37	100.1	8.9	—	—	60	4.67	34.6	233	353	957	1.9	47	0.00	0.00
—	—	—	—	—	—	1.2	—	—	150	1.79	—	—	—	890	—	45	0.00	0.00
0.25	0.56	2.06	0.12	1.13	97.8	1.5	—	—	225	2.98	21.9	302	188	804	1.6	56	0.00	0.00
0.33	0.21	3.40	0.10	1.07	85.3	2.8	—	0.9	84	2.60	33.2	212	340	615	1.0	47	0.00	0.00
0.28	0.40	2.36	0.07	0.40	60.4	0.0	9.7	1.0	407	2.00	26.5	470	162	1155	2.0	37	0.00	0.00
0.23	0.36	2.46	0.15	0.46	36.6	0.0	10.8	1.4	439	2.31	68.2	619	264	1291	3.1	38	0.00	0.00
0.23	0.20	3.14	0.12	0.89	17.8	3.8	—	0.3	46	1.85	20.9	116	209	272	2.3	64	0.00	0.00
0.31	0.47	2.69	0.20	0.54	75.9	2.8	—	0.3	130	3.24	16.1	152	291	771	1.4	51	0.00	0.00
0.70	0.43	5.01	0.27	0.81	16.4	0.0	—	1.1	233	2.41	32.4	343	337	1465	2.5	47	0.00	0.00
0.89	0.43	6.82	0.38	0.61	59.8	0.1	25.1	2.5	76	3.09	32.1	270	384	1237	2.6	52	0.00	0.00
0.89	0.38	7.30	0.50	0.66	34.6	0.2	27.5	3.1	58	3.47	72.4	378	502	1339	3.7	53	0.00	0.00
0.28	0.27	4.76	0.12	0.97	21.2	2.0	—	0.3	68	2.64	23.1	135	243	1335	2.7	53	0.00	0.00
0.28	0.23	5.44	0.15	0.01	79.0	1.7	4.9	2.6	76	2.28	51.8	143	240	429	1.1	27	0.00	0.00
0.28	0.20	6.42	0.20	0.00	76.3	2.1	0.0	3.2	80	2.66	75.2	201	336	465	1.5	27	0.00	0.00
0.91	0.46	6.25	0.34	0.55	26.4	0.2	—	0.4	85	2.75	34.1	229	343	392	2.5	49	0.00	0.00
0.23	0.34	3.45	0.21	1.34	37.2	4.1	—	0.8	299	2.92	38.7	291	261	1348	4.0	53	0.00	0.00
0.37	0.31	5.86	0.25	1.22	57.0	2.1	—	0.2	54	4.23	30.6	239	316	792	3.4	49	0.00	0.00
0.38	0.46	5.90	0.33	2.05	63.4	0.0	—	—	183	5.05	40.5	401	345	1633	5.4	44	0.00	0.00
0.30	0.28	2.96	0.09	1.07	17.2	0.0	—	0.7	58	2.25	16.1	80	117	612	0.9	44	0.00	0.00
0.28	0.27	5.73	0.23	1.51	21.8	5.8	—	1.3	92	3.63	35.5	149	368	1008	3.2	61	0.00	0.00
0.40	0.37	7.30	0.37	1.57	89.8	5.5	—	—	92	5.15	49.0	298	524	798	4.5	51	0.00	0.00
0.30	0.23	5.88	0.12	0.66	62.5	1.1	72.0	2.8	76	2.40	24.5	152	168	588	0.7	46	0.00	0.00
0.31	0.28	9.27	0.41	1.74	60.3	0.0	15.0	3.3	72	2.18	30.9	250	306	1586	1.3	54	0.00	0.00
0.25	0.21	10.06	0.52	1.91	35.4	0.0	16.4	3.9	53	2.46	71.2	356	417	1734	2.2	54	0.00	0.00

Code	Food Name	Unit/ Amt	Wt (g)	Energy (kcal)	Prot (g)	Carb (g)	Fiber (g)	Fat (g)	Sat (g)	Mono (g)	Poly (g)	Chol (mg)	Vit A (RE)
SAUCES AND GRAVIES													
Gravies													
53564	Gravy, beef, fat free	0.25 cup	60	20	0	5	0	0	0.0	0.0	0.0	5	0
53006	Gravy, beef, prep f/recipe	0.5 cup	135	107	3	7	1	8	1.9	3.4	2.0	3	150
53022	Gravy, chicken, can	0.25 cup	60	47	1	3	0	3	0.8	1.5	0.9	1	1
53565	Gravy, chicken, fat free	0.25 cup	60	15	1	3	0	0	0.0	0.0	0.0	5	20
53401	Gravy, country, dry mix	1 Tbs	6	22	1	4	0	1	0.1	0.4	0.0	0	0
53038	Gravy, mushroom, dry mix, svg	1 ea	21	70	2	14	1	1	0.5	0.3	0.0	1	0
53403	Gravy, onion, dry mix	1 Tbs	5	18	1	3	1	0	0.1	0.2	0.0	0	0
53044	Gravy, turkey, dry mix, svg	1 ea	7	26	1	5	—	1	0.1	0.2	0.2	1	1
Sauces													
53591	Marinade, cooking sauce, mesquite	1 Tbs	17	10	0	3	0	0	0.0	0.0	0.0	0	0
53587	Marinade, cooking sauce, teriyaki	1 Tbs	18	25	1	5	0	0	0.0	0.0	0.0	0	0
9559	Sauce, alfredo	0.25 cup	61	110	1	2	0	10	3.5	—	—	30	40
53000	Sauce, barbecue	1 cup	250	188	4	32	3	4	0.7	1.9	1.7	0	5
53320	Sauce, barbecue, sweet & sour	2 Tbs	34	45	0	10	0	0	0.0	0.0	0.0	0	0
53420	Sauce, barbecue, teriyaki	2 Tbs	36	60	0	12	0	0	0.0	0.0	0.0	0	0
9558	Sauce, cheese, cheddar, rts	0.25 cup	61	90	2	2	0	8	2.5	—	—	25	20
53523	Sauce, cheese, rts	0.25 cup	63	110	4	4	0	8	3.8	2.4	1.6	18	52
53474	Sauce, fish, rts	2 Tbs	36	13	2	1	0	0	0.0	0.0	0.0	0	1
53356	Sauce, Italian, rts	1 ea	1956	1917	33	362	27	37	5.1	23.3	5.3	0	1545
9425	Sauce, pasta, alfredo, classic	0.25 cup	61	110	1	3	0	10	3.5	—	—	25	100
53627	Sauce, pasta, garlic & herb, cnd	0.5 cup	126	50	2	10	2	0	0.0	0.0	0.0	0	40
53623	Sauce, pasta, garlic & onion, cnd	0.5 cup	125	40	2	9	2	0	0.0	0.0	0.0	0	30
53629	Sauce, pasta, traditional, cnd	0.5 cup	126	50	2	11	2	0	0.0	0.0	0.0	0	30
53540	Sauce, peanut	1 cup	240	749	31	29	8	63	12.8	30.0	17.1	0	1
7479	Sauce, picante, mild	2 Tbs	32	10	0	2	1	0	0.0	0.0	0.0	0	20
53284	Sauce, picante, med	2 Tbs	30	10	0	2	0	0	0.0	0.0	0.0	0	20
53221	Sauce, picante, hot	2 Tbs	30	10	0	2	0	0	0.0	0.0	0.0	0	0
53363	Sauce, pizza, deluxe, rts	0.25 cup	63	34	1	5	1	1	0.3	0.3	0.1	2	42
53425	Sauce, sloppy joe, cnd	0.25 cup	73	50	2	11	2	0	0.0	0.0	0.0	0	150
1709	Sauce, spaghetti, meatless, USDA, cnd	3.6 oz	100	48	1	9	—	1	0.2	0.2	0.5	0	34
51016	Sauce, spaghetti, traditional, cnd	0.5 cup	125	60	2	15	3	1	0.0	—	—	0	75
53011	Sauce, spaghetti, w/meat, cnd	1 cup	250	178	7	19	4	8	1.8	3.3	1.8	15	176
53524	Sauce, spaghetti/marinara, rts	0.5 cup	125	92	2	14	0	3	0.4	1.0	1.2	0	68
92310	Sauce, steak	1 Tbs	16	5	0	1	0	0	0.0	0.0	0.0	0	0
53352	Sauce, stir fry, all purpose, rts	1 Tbs	15	16	0	2	0	1	0.1	0.2	0.3	0	1
8983	Sauce, tartar	2 Tbs	28	139	0	1	0	15	2.7	0.7	2.3	11	6
90268	Sauce, white, dehyd, svg	1 ea	20	92	2	10	1	5	1.3	2.4	1.4	0	0
5181	Tomato Paste, unsalted, 6 oz can	1 ea	170	139	7	32	8	1	0.2	0.1	0.3	0	259
5180	Tomato Sauce, cnd	0.5 cup	122	39	2	9	2	0	0.0	0.0	0.1	0	42
SNACK FOODS—CHIPS, PRETZELS, POPCORN													
44061	Chips, bagel	5 pce	70	298	6	52	4	7	1.3	2.1	3.4	0	0
44256	Chips, corn, original	11 pce	28	140	2	19	2	6	0.5	—	—	0	0
44278	Chips, corn, original	32 pce	28	158	2	15	1	10	1.0	2.5	6.4	0	0
61236	Chips, potato, bkd	1 oz	28	133	1	20	1	5	0.7	2.8	1.2	0	0
43703	Chips, potato, classic	20 pce	28	150	2	15	1	10	3.0	—	—	0	0

Thia (mg)	Ribo (mg)	Niac (mg NE)	Vit B6 (mg)	Vit B12 (µg)	Fol (µg)	Vit C (mg)	Vit D (IU)	Vit E (mg AT)	Cal (mg)	Iron (mg)	Magn (mg)	Phos (mg)	Pota (mg)	Sodi (mg)	Zinc (mg)	Wat (%)	Alco (g)	Caff (mg)
—	—	—	—	—	—	0.0	—	—	0	0.00	—	—	—	308	—	90	0.00	0.00
0.01	0.05	0.60	0.00	0.14	2.7	0.0	1.0	0.2	27	0.62	2.7	39	147	779	1.1	85	0.00	0.00
0.00	0.02	0.25	0.00	0.05	1.2	0.0	—	0.1	12	0.28	1.2	17	65	343	0.5	85	0.00	0.00
—	—	—	—	—	—	0.0	—	—	0	0.00	—	—	—	318	—	92	0.00	0.00
0.00	0.00	0.00	0.00	0.00	—	0.0	—	—	1	0.02	—	7	7	249	0.0	7	0.00	0.00
0.03	0.09	0.79	0.01	0.15	6.6	1.5	—	0.0	49	0.20	7.2	43	56	1402	0.3	3	0.00	0.00
0.02	0.01	0.00	0.01	0.00	—	0.0	—	—	1	0.10	—	10	25	229	0.0	8	0.00	0.00
0.00	0.02	0.18	0.00	0.03	5.7	0.0	—	0.0	10	0.23	3.1	18	30	307	0.1	5	0.00	0.00
—	—	—	—	—	—	1.8	—	—	0	0.00	—	—	25	400	—	—	0.00	0.00
—	—	—	—	—	—	3.0	—	—	0	0.00	—	—	40	480	—	64	0.00	0.00
—	—	—	—	—	—	0.0	—	—	40	0.00	—	—	—	390	—	76	0.00	0.00
0.07	0.05	2.25	0.18	0.00	10.0	17.5	—	0.0	48	2.25	45.0	50	435	2038	0.5	81	0.00	0.00
—	—	—	—	—	—	0.0	—	—	0	0.00	—	—	—	420	—	—	0.00	0.00
—	—	—	—	—	—	0.0	—	—	0	0.36	—	—	—	440	—	63	0.00	0.00
—	—	—	—	—	—	0.0	—	—	60	0.00	—	—	—	480	—	78	0.00	0.00
0.00	0.07	0.01	0.00	0.09	2.5	0.3	—	0.2	116	0.12	5.7	99	19	522	0.6	70	0.00	0.00
0.00	0.01	0.82	0.14	0.17	18.4	0.2	—	0.0	15	0.28	63.0	3	104	2779	0.1	71	0.00	0.00
2.41	1.42	35.63	5.40	0.00	508.6	131.1	—	37.8	1076	12.13	625.9	1350	11892	9584	8.2	76	0.00	0.00
—	—	—	—	—	—	0.0	—	—	40	—	—	—	—	340	—	75	0.00	0.00
—	—	—	—	—	—	6.0	—	—	40	1.08	—	—	—	390	—	88	0.00	0.00
—	—	—	—	—	—	6.0	—	—	40	1.08	—	—	—	390	—	89	0.00	0.00
—	—	—	—	—	—	6.0	—	—	40	1.08	—	—	—	390	—	87	0.00	0.00
0.11	0.14	16.63	0.58	0.00	99.2	27.1	—	12.4	52	2.29	200.9	460	901	580	3.7	47	0.00	0.00
—	—	—	—	—	—	0.0	—	—	0	0.00	—	—	—	230	—	92	0.00	0.00
—	—	—	—	—	—	0.0	—	—	0	0.00	—	—	—	230	—	91	0.00	0.00
—	—	—	—	—	—	19.8	—	—	0	0.00	—	—	—	260	—	91	0.00	0.00
0.03	0.02	0.89	0.09	0.00	6.3	7.1	—	1.6	34	0.56	13.2	32	223	117	0.2	87	0.00	0.00
—	—	—	—	—	—	0.0	—	—	0	0.72	—	—	—	420	—	—	0.00	0.00
0.02	0.11	0.73	0.05	0.00	—	3.9	—	—	20	0.89	13.0	25	292	590	0.2	87	0.00	0.00
—	—	—	—	—	—	9.0	—	—	40	1.44	—	—	—	590	—	84	0.00	0.00
0.12	0.11	3.47	0.31	0.49	25.0	18.8	1.2	3.0	54	2.09	43.2	104	742	982	1.3	85	0.00	0.00
0.02	0.07	4.90	0.21	0.00	13.8	3.9	—	2.5	34	1.05	26.2	45	470	601	0.7	82	0.00	0.00
—	—	—	—	—	—	0.0	—	—	0	0.00	—	—	—	200	—	90	0.00	0.00
0.00	0.00	0.14	0.00	0.00	0.6	0.7	—	0.0	2	0.10	1.5	4	8	233	0.0	74	0.00	0.00
—	—	—	—	—	—	0.7	—	—	6	0.14	—	—	38	153	—	39	0.00	0.00
0.03	0.07	0.14	0.01	0.15	6.7	0.6	—	0.1	133	0.10	7.7	49	73	675	0.2	2	0.00	0.00
0.10	0.25	5.23	0.37	0.00	20.4	37.3	—	7.3	61	5.07	71.4	141	1725	167	1.1	74	0.00	0.00
0.02	0.07	1.19	0.11	0.00	11.0	8.6	—	2.5	16	1.25	19.6	32	405	642	0.2	89	0.00	0.00
0.12	0.11	1.62	0.15	0.00	46.0	0.0	—	1.7	9	1.38	39.2	145	167	419	0.9	3	0.00	0.00
0.05	0.15	0.50	—	—	—	0.0	—	—	0	0.36	—	70	75	115	0.0	2	0.00	0.00
0.00	0.03	0.33	—	—	—	0.0	—	—	44	0.37	—	54	54	104	0.0	3	0.00	0.00
0.10	0.01	1.15	0.14	0.00	0.0	0.0	—	0.6	35	0.23	12.2	78	204	260	0.1	1	0.00	0.00
—	—	—	—	—	—	6.0	—	—	0	0.00	—	—	—	180	—	1	0.00	0.00

Code	Food Name	Unit/Amt	Wt (g)	Energy (kcal)	Prot (g)	Carb (g)	Fiber (g)	Fat (g)	Sat (g)	Mono (g)	Poly (g)	Chol (mg)	Vit A (RE)
61253	Chips, potato, fat free	100 g	100	379	10	84	8	1	0.2	0.0	0.3	0	2
44230	Chips, potato, original	18 pce	28	148	2	15	1	10	3.0	1.9	5.0	0	0
44241	Chips, potato, rducd fat	16 pce	28	128	2	18	1	7	1.0	1.6	4.1	0	0
44238	Chips, potato, unsalted	19 pce	28	158	2	16	1	10	3.0	—	—	0	0
44301	Chips, tortilla, blue corn	18 pce	28	110	3	22	2	2	0.0	—	—	0	0
44224	Chips, tortilla, cooler ranch	15 pce	28	138	2	18	1	7	1.5	1.9	2.2	0	0
61156	Chips, tortilla, light, bkd	10 ea	16	74	1	12	1	2	0.5	1.0	0.8	0	1
44225	Chips, tortilla, nacho cheesier	15 pce	28	138	2	17	1	7	1.5	1.9	2.2	0	0
4039	Chips, tortilla, salsa verde	12 pce	28	150	2	19	1	7	1.5	3.0	2.5	0	0
44223	Chips, tortilla, tstd corn	13 pce	28	138	2	18	1	7	1.5	—	—	0	0
44298	Chips, tortilla, yellow corn	18 pce	28	110	3	22	2	2	0.0	—	—	0	0
44087	Corn Cake, butter flvr	1 ea	9	34	1	7	0	0	0.1	0.1	0.1	0	4
44308	Corn Cake, caramel flvrd	1 ea	13	50	1	12	0	0	0.0	0.1	0.1	0	4
44031	Corn Nuts, plain	1 oz	28	126	2	20	2	4	0.7	2.7	0.9	0	0
44212	Fruit Leather, bar	1 ea	23	81	0	18	1	1	0.9	0.1	0.0	0	3
23404	Fruit Leather, roll, lrg	1 ea	21	78	0	18	1	1	0.1	0.3	0.1	0	3
44022	Popcorn Cake	1 ea	10	38	1	8	0	0	0.0	0.1	0.1	0	1
44014	Popcorn, caramel coated, w/o peanuts	1 oz	28	122	1	22	1	4	1.0	0.8	1.3	1	1
44038	Popcorn, cheese flvrd	1 cup	11	58	1	6	1	4	0.7	1.1	1.7	1	5
43701	Popcorn, Cracker Jacks, original	0.5 cup	28	120	2	23	1	2	0.0	—	—	0	0
44065	Popcorn, microw	1 ea	87	435	8	50	9	24	4.3	7.1	11.7	0	13
44013	Popcorn, oil popped	1 cup	11	55	1	6	1	3	0.5	0.9	1.5	0	2
44072	Popcorn, white, air popped	1 cup	8	31	1	6	1	0	0.0	0.1	0.2	0	0
44015	Pretzels, hard	5 pce	30	114	3	24	1	1	0.2	0.4	0.4	0	0
44215	Pretzels, hard, chocolate coated	1 ea	11	50	1	8	0	2	0.8	0.6	0.2	0	0
61182	Pretzels, soft, med	1 ea	115	389	9	80	2	4	0.8	1.2	1.1	3	0
60899	Rice Cake, brown	1 ea	20	74	1	16	0	0	0.1	0.2	0.2	—	0
44017	Rice Cake, caramel corn, mini	1 ea	3	13	0	3	0	0	0.1	0.0	0.0	0	1
44016	Rice Cake, plain	1 ea	9	35	1	7	0	0	0.1	0.1	0.1	0	0
44032	Snack Mix, Chex	1 cup	42	181	5	28	2	7	2.4	3.9	1.1	0	6
57096	Snack, cheese n' crackers, pkg	1 ea	27	100	2	10	0	6	2.0	—	—	10	20
44248	Snack, cheese puffs, Cheetos	29 pce	28	158	2	15	1	10	2.5	2.7	3.1	0	0
44058	Trail Mix, regular	0.25 cup	38	173	5	17	2	11	2.1	4.7	3.6	0	1
44060	Trail Mix, tropical	1 cup	140	570	9	92	9	24	11.9	3.5	7.2	0	6
44059	Trail Mix, w/chocolate chips, salted nuts & seeds	0.25 cup	36	175	5	16	2	12	2.2	4.9	4.1	1	1

SOUPS, STEWS AND CHILIS

Canned/Frozen/Prepared Soups, Stews and Chilis

Code	Food Name	Unit/Amt	Wt (g)	Energy (kcal)	Prot (g)	Carb (g)	Fiber (g)	Fat (g)	Sat (g)	Mono (g)	Poly (g)	Chol (mg)	Vit A (RE)
50595	Bouillon/Broth, beef, clear, cnd	1 cup	198	15	2	0	0	0	0.0	—	—	0	0
50596	Broth, chicken, clear, rts, cnd	1 cup	198	15	1	1	0	0	0.0	—	—	5	0
50312	Chili, con carne	1 cup	253	256	25	22	—	8	3.4	3.4	0.5	134	167
7760	Chili, vegetarian, cnd	1 cup	230	176	16	26	13	1	0.2	0.2	0.5	1	47
56001	Chili, w/beans, cnd	1 cup	256	287	15	30	11	14	6.0	6.0	0.9	44	87
50901	Chili, w/beef, rts, cnd	1 cup	245	190	16	34	8	2	0.5	—	—	5	100
28167	Chili, w/o beans, cnd	100 g	100	118	8	6	—	7	2.3	2.5	0.5	21	—
50406	Chowder, clam, New England, rts, cnd	1 cup	244	117	5	20	1	2	0.5	0.7	0.4	5	49

Thia (mg)	Ribo (mg)	Niac (mg NE)	Vit B6 (mg)	Vit B12 (μg)	Fol (μg)	Vit C (mg)	Vit D (IU)	Vit E (mg AT)	Cal (mg)	Iron (mg)	Magn (mg)	Phos (mg)	Pota (mg)	Sodi (mg)	Zinc (mg)	Wat (%)	Alco (g)	Caff (mg)
1.08	0.11	6.44	0.80	0.00	45.0	9.3	—	0.0	35	3.56	70.0	167	1628	643	0.7	2	0.00	0.00
0.05	0.03	1.09	—	0.00	—	5.9	—	—	6	0.44	—	44	489	178	0.4	2	0.00	0.00
0.03	0.05	1.09	—	0.00	—	5.9	—	—	0	0.36	—	45	356	158	0.3	2	0.00	0.00
—	—	—	—	0.00	—	5.9	—	—	0	0.00	—	—	—	15	—	—	0.00	0.00
—	—	—	—	—	—	0.0	—	—	60	0.36	—	—	—	140	—	4	0.00	—
0.02	0.02	0.49	—	—	—	0.0	—	—	40	0.41	—	64	69	168	0.0	2	0.00	0.00
0.03	0.03	0.07	0.02	0.00	2.6	0.0	—	0.6	25	0.25	15.5	51	44	160	0.2	1	0.00	0.00
0.02	0.02	0.40	—	—	—	0.0	—	—	43	0.41	—	59	64	188	0.0	6	0.00	0.00
0.02	0.00	0.43	—	—	—	0.0	—	—	20	0.00	—	18	38	210	0.2	—	0.00	0.00
—	—	—	—	—	—	0.0	—	—	40	0.00	—	—	—	119	—	2	0.00	0.00
—	—	—	—	—	—	0.0	—	—	60	0.36	—	—	—	160	—	3	0.00	—
0.01	0.00	0.34	0.02	0.00	3.0	0.0	0.0	0.0	1	0.07	8.9	20	17	45	0.1	6	0.00	0.00
0.02	0.00	0.31	0.03	0.00	3.0	0.0	—	0.0	1	0.07	8.9	20	15	28	0.1	3	0.00	0.00
0.00	0.03	0.47	0.05	0.00	0.0	0.0	—	0.6	3	0.46	32.0	78	79	156	0.5	1	0.00	0.00
0.00	0.00	0.01	0.07	0.00	0.9	16.1	—	0.1	7	0.18	5.1	13	32	18	0.0	14	0.00	0.00
0.01	0.00	0.01	0.05	0.00	0.8	25.2	—	0.1	7	0.20	4.2	7	62	67	0.0	10	0.00	0.00
0.00	0.01	0.60	0.01	0.00	1.8	0.0	—	0.0	1	0.18	15.9	28	33	29	0.4	5	0.00	0.00
0.01	0.01	0.62	0.00	0.00	1.4	0.0	—	0.3	12	0.49	9.9	24	31	58	0.2	3	0.00	0.00
0.00	0.02	0.15	0.02	0.05	1.2	0.1	—	0.0	12	0.25	10.0	40	29	98	0.2	2	0.00	0.00
—	—	—	—	—	—	0.0	—	—	0	0.00	—	—	—	70	—	—	0.00	0.00
0.11	0.11	1.35	0.18	0.00	14.8	0.3	—	0.1	9	2.42	94.0	218	196	769	2.3	3	0.00	0.00
0.00	0.00	0.17	0.01	0.00	1.9	0.0	—	0.6	1	0.31	11.9	28	25	97	0.3	3	0.00	0.00
0.01	0.01	0.15	0.01	0.00	1.8	0.0	—	0.0	1	0.20	10.5	24	24	0	0.3	4	0.00	0.00
0.14	0.18	1.58	0.02	0.00	51.3	0.0	—	0.1	11	1.29	10.5	34	44	514	0.3	3	0.00	0.00
0.00	0.01	0.09	0.01	0.00	1.0	0.1	—	0.0	8	0.21	4.5	16	25	63	0.1	2	0.00	—
0.46	0.33	4.90	0.01	0.00	27.6	0.0	—	0.6	26	4.51	24.1	91	101	1615	1.1	15	0.00	0.00
—	—	—	—	—	—	0.0	—	—	5	0.15	—	—	67	57	—	5	0.00	0.00
0.00	0.00	0.10	0.00	0.00	0.6	0.0	0.0	0.0	1	0.02	2.6	6	6	14	0.0	2	0.00	0.00
0.03	0.00	0.58	0.05	0.00	1.8	0.0	0.0	0.0	1	0.12	14.2	33	25	14	2.0	3	0.00	0.00
0.66	0.20	7.15	0.66	5.26	21.2	20.2	—	0.1	15	10.50	26.8	79	114	432	0.9	4	0.00	0.00
—	—	—	—	—	—	0.0	—	—	60	0.36	—	—	—	331	—	—	0.00	0.00
0.10	0.05	0.72	—	—	—	0.0	—	—	22	0.58	—	15	20	365	0.0	2	0.00	0.00
0.17	0.07	1.76	0.10	0.00	26.6	0.5	—	1.3	29	1.13	59.2	129	257	86	1.2	9	0.00	0.00
0.62	0.15	2.06	0.46	0.00	58.8	10.6	—	3.1	80	3.70	134.4	260	993	14	1.6	9	0.00	0.00
0.15	0.07	1.60	0.09	0.00	23.6	0.5	—	3.9	40	1.23	58.4	140	235	44	1.1	7	0.00	2.18
—	—	—	—	—	—	0.0	—	—	0	0.00	—	—	—	890	—	98	0.00	0.00
—	—	—	—	—	—	0.0	—	—	0	0.00	—	—	—	960	—	—	0.00	0.00
0.12	1.13	2.48	0.33	1.13	45.5	1.5	—	1.6	68	5.19	45.5	197	691	1007	3.6	77	0.00	0.00
0.00	0.15	0.00	—	0.00	—	0.0	—	—	40	3.68	—	237	645	1144	0.6	79	0.00	0.00
0.11	0.27	0.92	0.34	0.00	58.9	4.4	—	1.5	120	8.77	115.2	394	934	1336	5.1	76	0.00	0.00
—	—	—	—	—	—	2.4	—	—	100	4.50	—	—	—	480	—	—	0.00	0.00
0.02	0.10	1.25	0.12	1.01	—	1.8	—	—	30	2.00	20.0	77	185	389	1.1	78	0.00	0.00
0.05	0.09	0.86	0.09	6.17	29.3	5.1	—	0.6	17	0.89	12.2	59	283	529	0.4	89	0.00	0.00

PAGE KEY: 2 Beverage and Beverage Mixes   4 Other Beverages   4 Beverages, Alcoholic   6 Candies and Confections, Gum   10 Cereals, Breakfast Type
14 Cheese and Cheese Substitutes   16 Dairy Products and Substitutes   18 Desserts   24 Dessert Toppings   24 Eggs, Substitutes, and Egg Dishes   26 Ethnic Foods
30 Fast Foods/Restaurants   44 Fats, Oils, Margarines, Shortenings, and Substitutes   44 Fish, Seafood, and Shellfish   46 Food Additives
46 Fruit, Vegetable, or Blended Juices   48 Grains, Flours, and Fractions   48 Grain Products, Prepared and Baked Goods

Code	Food Name	Unit/ Amt	Wt (g)	Energy (kcal)	Prot (g)	Carb (g)	Fiber (g)	Fat (g)	Sat (g)	Mono (g)	Poly (g)	Chol (mg)	Vit A (RE)
50907	Chowder, clam, New England, rts, cnd	1 cup	251	120	5	24	4	2	1.0	—	—	10	0
50647	Soup, bean & pork, cond, cnd, cmrcl	1 cup	269	347	16	46	16	12	3.1	4.4	3.7	5	180
50003	Soup, beef noodle, prep f/cnd w/water, cmrcl	1 cup	244	83	5	9	1	3	1.1	1.2	0.5	5	12
50399	Soup, beef vegetable, rts, cnd	1 cup	241	154	10	25	6	2	0.6	0.6	0.2	14	415
50686	Soup, chicken mushroom, cond, cnd, cmrcl	1 cup	251	274	9	19	1	18	4.8	8.1	4.6	20	25
50080	Soup, chicken mushroom, prep f/cnd w/water, cmrcl	1 cup	244	132	4	9	0	9	2.4	4.0	2.3	10	112
50982	Soup, chicken noodle, chunky, rts, cnd, svg	1 ea	243	114	8	14	—	3	0.8	1.2	0.6	24	262
50400	Soup, chicken noodle, rts, cnd	1 cup	237	76	6	9	1	2	0.4	0.6	0.4	19	182
50020	Soup, chicken rice, prep f/cnd w/water, cmrcl	1 cup	241	60	4	7	1	2	0.5	0.9	0.4	7	43
50091	Soup, chicken vegetable, prep f/cnd w/water, cmrcl	1 cup	241	75	4	9	1	3	0.8	1.3	0.6	10	193
50402	Soup, cream of broccoli, rts, cnd	1 cup	244	88	2	13	2	3	0.7	0.9	0.6	5	59
50654	Soup, cream of chicken, cond, cnd, cmrcl	1 cup	251	223	6	18	0	14	4.0	5.1	2.6	20	113
50666	Soup, cream of mushroom, cond, cnd, cmrcl	1 cup	251	213	4	17	0	15	3.4	2.8	3.6	0	20
50049	Soup, cream of mushroom, prep f/cnd w/water, cmrcl	1 cup	244	129	2	9	0	9	2.4	1.7	4.2	2	17
50197	Soup, cream of potato, prep f/cnd w/water, cmrcl	1 cup	244	73	2	11	0	2	1.2	0.6	0.4	5	76
50999	Soup, gumbo, zesty, rts, cnd	1 cup	244	100	6	15	3	2	1.0	—	—	10	40
50404	Soup, lentil, rts, cnd	1 cup	242	126	8	20	6	2	0.3	0.8	0.2	0	191
50405	Soup, minestrone, rts, cnd	1 cup	241	123	5	20	1	3	0.4	0.9	1.0	0	272
50486	Soup, onion, French, cond, cnd	0.5 cup	119	45	2	6	1	2	0.5	—	—	5	0
50403	Soup, pasta & garlic, rts, cnd	1 cup	243	100	4	20	3	1	0.3	0.4	0.5	5	311
50050	Soup, pea, green, prep f/cnd w/water, cmrcl	1 cup	250	165	9	26	3	3	1.4	1.0	0.4	0	20
50407	Soup, split pea, rts, cnd	1 cup	253	180	10	30	5	2	0.8	0.9	0.4	5	142
50504	Soup, tomato, cond, cnd	0.5 cup	122	90	2	20	1	0	0.0	0.0	0.0	0	100
50409	Soup, vegetable, rts, cnd	1 cup	238	81	4	13	1	1	0.3	0.4	0.3	5	640
57659	Stew, beef, cnd, svg	1 ea	232	218	11	16	3	12	5.2	5.5	0.5	37	385
7559	Stew, vegetarian	1 cup	247	304	42	17	3	7	1.2	1.8	3.8	0	232
Dry and Prepared Soups and Chilis													
90243	Broth, beef, dry cube, svg	1.33 ea	5	8	1	1	0	0	0.1	0.1	0.0	0	0
90247	Broth, chicken, cube, dry svg	1 ea	6	13	1	2	0	0	0.1	0.1	0.1	1	0
50037	Soup, chicken noodle, prep f/dehyd w/water	1 cup	252	58	2	9	0	1	0.3	0.5	0.4	10	5
50036	Soup, cream of chicken, prep f/dehyd w/water	1 cup	261	107	2	13	0	5	3.4	1.2	0.4	3	42
90346	Soup, minestrone, prep f/pkt w/water	1 ea	1142	354	20	54	—	8	3.7	3.3	0.5	11	137
50039	Soup, mushroom, prep f/dehyd w/water, pkt	1 ea	194	74	2	9	1	4	0.6	1.7	1.2	0	14
50040	Soup, onion, prep f/dehyd w/water, pkt	1 ea	184	20	1	4	1	0	0.1	0.2	0.1	0	0
92163	Soup, ramen noodle, any flvr, dry	3.6 oz	100	453	9	66	2	17	7.6	6.4	2.6	0	2
50042	Soup, tomato, prep f/dry w/water, pkt	1 ea	199	78	2	15	0	2	0.8	0.7	0.2	0	66
50044	Soup, vegetable beef, prep f/dry w/water	1 cup	253	53	3	8	1	1	0.6	0.5	0.1	0	25
Homemade/Generic Soups and Chilis													
50709	Broth, vegetable	1 cup	235	16	2	2	0	0	—	—	—	0	1
92757	Chili, con carne, w/beans & chicken	1 cup	254	217	17	27	7	5	1.2	1.9	1.5	33	124
50211	Chowder, fish	1 cup	244	194	24	12	1	5	2.4	1.9	0.6	56	63
50077	Soup, chicken gumbo, prep f/cnd w/water, cmrcl	1 cup	244	56	3	8	2	1	0.3	0.7	0.3	5	15
SPICES, FLAVORS, AND SEASONINGS													
90622	Salt Substitute, Mrs. Dash, original blend	0.25 tsp	1	0	0	0	0	0	0.0	0.0	0.0	0	0
26632	Salt Substitute, Nu-Salt, no sod, pkt	1 g	1	0	0	0	0	0	0.0	0.0	0.0	0	0
26014	Salt, table	0.25 tsp	2	0	0	0	0	0	0.0	0.0	0.0	0	0

Thia (mg)	Ribo (mg)	Niac (mg NE)	Vit B6 (mg)	Vit B12 (µg)	Fol (µg)	Vit C (mg)	Vit D (IU)	Vit E (mg AT)	Cal (mg)	Iron (mg)	Magn (mg)	Phos (mg)	Pota (mg)	Sodi (mg)	Zinc (mg)	Wat (%)	Alco (g)	Caff (mg)
—	—	—	—	—	4.8	—	—	—	20	0.72	—	—	—	480	—	86	0.00	0.00
0.17	0.07	1.12	0.07	0.07	64.6	3.2	—	2.3	161	4.11	88.8	264	807	1907	2.1	70	0.00	0.00
0.07	0.05	1.07	0.03	0.20	19.5	0.2	—	0.7	15	1.10	4.9	46	100	952	1.5	92	0.00	0.00
0.10	0.11	2.80	0.25	0.31	24.1	4.6	—	0.5	14	1.77	31.3	99	605	405	1.3	85	0.00	0.00
0.05	0.23	3.25	0.10	0.12	5.0	0.0	—	1.6	58	1.75	17.6	55	316	1940	2.0	80	0.00	0.00
0.01	0.10	1.62	0.05	0.05	0.0	0.0	—	1.2	29	0.87	9.8	27	154	942	1.0	90	0.00	0.00
—	—	—	—	—	—	—	—	—	—	1.19	—	—	—	875	—	89	0.00	0.00
0.10	0.10	3.44	0.05	0.20	33.2	0.7	—	0.1	19	1.11	9.5	85	209	460	0.4	92	0.00	0.00
0.01	0.01	1.12	0.01	0.14	0.0	0.2	—	0.1	17	0.75	0.0	22	101	815	0.3	94	0.00	0.00
0.03	0.05	1.23	0.05	0.11	4.8	1.0	—	0.4	17	0.87	7.2	41	154	945	0.4	93	0.00	0.00
0.02	0.05	0.31	0.07	0.00	29.3	5.9	—	0.4	41	1.22	14.6	39	161	578	0.3	92	0.00	0.00
0.02	0.11	0.98	0.00	0.00	5.0	0.3	—	1.4	35	2.66	10.0	78	123	1644	0.7	83	0.00	0.00
0.10	0.10	1.05	0.00	0.00	5.0	0.0	—	2.0	30	2.78	10.0	65	156	1619	0.5	84	0.00	0.00
0.05	0.09	0.72	0.00	0.05	4.9	1.0	—	1.0	46	0.50	4.9	49	100	881	0.6	90	0.00	0.00
0.02	0.03	0.54	0.03	0.05	2.4	0.0	—	0.0	20	0.49	2.4	46	137	1000	0.6	92	0.00	0.00
—	—	—	—	—	—	3.6	—	—	40	0.72	—	—	—	480	—	88	0.00	0.00
0.10	0.09	0.69	0.15	0.00	101.6	1.0	—	0.6	41	2.66	41.1	128	336	443	1.0	88	0.00	0.00
0.15	0.07	1.02	0.14	0.00	60.3	0.7	—	0.7	39	1.69	31.3	87	306	470	0.7	87	0.00	0.00
—	—	—	—	—	—	0.0	—	—	20	0.00	—	—	—	900	—	90	0.00	0.00
0.23	0.12	2.03	0.10	0.00	63.2	0.0	—	0.5	51	0.87	34.0	87	299	450	0.6	88	0.00	0.00
0.10	0.07	1.24	0.05	0.00	2.5	1.8	—	0.4	28	1.95	40.0	125	190	918	1.7	83	0.00	0.00
0.18	0.07	1.15	0.18	0.02	50.6	0.0	—	0.5	43	1.95	35.4	137	463	420	1.0	82	0.00	0.00
—	—	—	—	—	—	6.0	—	—	0	0.72	—	—	—	710	—	80	0.00	0.00
0.07	0.07	1.83	0.07	0.07	28.6	1.4	—	0.1	31	1.51	21.4	74	290	466	0.4	91	0.00	0.00
0.17	0.14	2.85	0.30	0.86	25.5	10.2	—	0.2	28	1.64	32.5	128	404	947	1.9	82	0.00	0.00
1.73	1.48	29.63	2.72	5.42	254.4	0.0	—	1.2	77	3.21	313.7	543	296	988	2.7	70	0.00	0.00
0.00	0.00	0.15	0.00	0.05	1.5	0.0	—	0.0	3	0.10	2.4	11	19	1152	0.0	3	0.00	0.00
0.00	0.01	0.25	0.00	0.01	2.0	0.1	0.0	0.0	12	0.11	3.6	12	24	1536	0.0	2	0.00	0.00
0.20	0.07	1.09	0.02	0.05	17.7	0.0	—	0.1	5	0.50	7.6	30	33	578	0.2	94	0.00	0.00
0.10	0.20	2.60	0.05	0.25	5.2	0.5	—	0.6	76	0.25	5.2	97	214	1185	1.6	91	0.00	0.00
0.34	0.23	4.57	0.46	0.00	159.9	4.6	—	0.2	171	4.57	34.3	274	1531	4616	3.4	92	0.00	0.00
0.21	0.09	0.37	0.01	0.18	3.9	0.8	—	0.4	50	0.38	3.9	58	153	782	0.1	92	0.00	0.00
0.01	0.03	0.36	0.00	0.00	1.8	0.2	—	0.0	9	0.10	3.7	22	48	635	0.0	96	0.00	0.00
0.66	0.43	5.40	0.05	0.00	147.0	0.0	—	2.0	16	4.26	24.0	108	120	1160	0.6	5	0.00	0.00
0.05	0.03	0.58	0.07	0.05	6.0	3.4	—	0.4	40	0.31	9.9	50	221	708	0.2	90	0.00	0.00
0.02	0.03	0.46	0.05	0.25	7.6	1.3	—	0.2	13	0.86	22.8	35	76	1002	0.3	94	0.00	0.00
0.00	0.01	0.54	0.01	0.11	3.8	0.0	—	0.0	7	0.11	7.0	38	54	3114	0.0	95	0.00	0.00
0.21	0.23	5.17	0.36	0.11	58.0	21.4	—	1.7	58	2.68	53.1	195	682	874	1.5	79	0.00	0.00
0.17	0.25	2.88	0.36	1.25	16.3	7.3	—	0.4	148	0.70	49.1	298	711	180	1.1	83	0.00	0.00
0.01	0.05	0.66	0.05	0.01	4.9	4.9	—	0.4	24	0.89	4.9	24	76	954	0.4	94	0.00	0.00
—	—	—	—	0.00	—	0.0	—	—	0	0.00	—	—	—	0	—	—	0.00	0.00
—	—	—	—	—	—	0.0	—	0.0	0	—	0.0	—	530	0	—	—	0.00	0.00
0.00	0.00	0.00	0.00	0.00	0.0	0.0	—	0.0	0	0.00	0.0	0	0	581	0.0	0	0.00	0.00

PAGE KEY: 2 Beverage and Beverage Mixes 4 Other Beverages 4 Beverages, Alcoholic 6 Candies and Confections, Gum 10 Cereals, Breakfast Type
14 Cheese and Cheese Substitutes 16 Dairy Products and Substitutes 18 Desserts 24 Dessert Toppings 24 Eggs, Substitutes, and Egg Dishes 26 Ethnic Foods
30 Fast Foods/Restaurants 44 Fats, Oils, Margarines, Shortenings, and Substitutes 44 Fish, Seafood, and Shellfish 46 Food Additives
46 Fruit, Vegetable, or Blended Juices 48 Grains, Flours, and Fractions 48 Grain Products, Prepared and Baked Goods

Code	Food Name	Unit/ Amt	Wt (g)	Energy (kcal)	Prot (g)	Carb (g)	Fiber (g)	Fat (g)	Sat (g)	Mono (g)	Poly (g)	Chol (mg)	Vit A (RE)
53439	Sea Salt	100 g	100	0	0	0	0	0	0.0	0.0	0.0	0	0
669	Seasoning, garlic salt	0.25 tsp	1	0	0	0	0	0	0.0	0.0	0.0	—	—
26604	Seasoning, lemon pepper	1 tsp	2	2	0	0	0	0	0.0	0.0	0.0	0	0
26028	Seasoning, poultry	1 tsp	2	5	0	1	0	0	0.0	0.0	0.0	0	4
26004	Spice Blend, curry, pwd	1 tsp	2	6	0	1	1	0	0.0	0.1	0.1	0	2
26001	Spice, basil, ground	1 tsp	1	4	0	1	1	0	0.0	0.0	0.0	0	13
26524	Spice, chili pepper, ground, domestic	1 tsp	2	6	0	1	1	0	—	—	—	—	42
26002	Spice, chili pepper, pwd	1 tsp	3	8	0	1	1	0	0.1	0.1	0.2	0	77
7395	Spice, cilantro, dehyd	100 g	100	265	31	34	11	8	0.2	3.7	0.5	0	3670
26003	Spice, cinnamon, ground	1 tsp	2	6	0	2	1	0	0.0	0.0	0.0	0	1
26019	Spice, clove, ground	1 tsp	2	7	0	1	1	0	0.1	0.0	0.1	0	1
26109	Spice, dill seed	1 tsp	2	6	0	1	0	0	0.0	0.2	0.0	0	0
26065	Spice, garlic powder	1 tsp	3	8	0	2	1	0	—	—	—	0	0
26008	Spice, onion, powder	1 tsp	2	7	0	2	0	0	0.0	0.0	0.0	0	0
26009	Spice, oregano, ground	1 tsp	2	5	0	1	1	0	0.0	0.0	0.1	0	10
26010	Spice, paprika	1 tsp	2	6	0	1	1	0	0.0	0.0	0.2	0	111
26522	Spice, pepper, black, ground	1 tsp	2	7	0	1	1	0	—	—	—	—	2
26628	Spice, peppermint, fresh	2 Tbs	3	2	0	0	0	0	0.0	0.0	0.0	0	14
26015	Spice, poppy seed	1 tsp	3	15	1	1	0	1	0.1	0.2	0.9	0	0
26631	Spice, spearmint, dried	1 Tbs	2	5	0	1	0	0	0.0	0.0	0.1	0	17
26033	Spice, thyme, ground	1 tsp	1	4	0	1	1	0	0.0	0.0	0.0	0	5
SPORTS BARS AND DRINKS													
62275	Bar, energy, apple cinnamon	1 ea	65	230	10	45	3	2	0.5	1.5	0.5	0	0
62714	Bar, energy, carrot cake	1 ea	68	234	10	41	5	4	1.8	—	—	0	884
62278	Bar, energy, chocolate	1 ea	65	230	10	45	3	2	0.5	0.5	1.0	0	0
62715	Bar, energy, chocolate almond fudge	1 ea	68	231	10	38	5	5	0.9	—	—	0	276
62709	Bar, energy, chocolate chip	1 ea	68	238	10	42	5	4	0.9	—	—	0	278
62831	Bar, energy, chocolate fudge brownie	1 ea	78	290	24	38	4	5	4.0	—	—	5	0
62561	Bar, energy, chocolate peanut butter	1 ea	65	230	10	45	3	3	0.5	1.5	1.0	0	0
62716	Bar, energy, cookies & cream	1 ea	68	225	10	39	5	4	1.5	—	—	0	277
62725	Bar, energy, honey peanut	1 ea	50	200	14	22	1	6	3.5	—	—	3	500
62710	Bar, energy, peanut butter	1 ea	68	240	12	38	5	5	0.8	—	—	0	277
62205	Bar, energy, peanut butter, Tiger's Milk	1 ea	35	140	6	18	1	5	1.0	—	—	0	150
62821	Bar, energy, vanilla crisp	1 ea	65	230	9	45	3	2	0.5	1.5	0.5	0	0
62833	Carbohydrate Gel, chocolate, pkt	1 ea	41	120	0	28	0	2	1.0	—	—	0	0
63031	Drink, protein, Max Whey, all flvrs, pwd, scoop	1 ea	27	88	20	3	0	1	—	—	—	25	0
62995	Formula, Myoplex Pro, vanilla, rtd	0.33 ea	250	110	15	8	2	2	0.5	—	—	13	168
20142	Sports Drink, btld	1 cup	241	60	0	15	0	0	0.0	0.0	0.0	0	0
20558	Sports Drink, grape, can/btl	1 cup	247	73	0	19	0	0	0.0	0.0	0.0	0	0
20559	Sports Drink, lemon lime, can/btl	1 cup	247	72	0	19	0	0	0.0	0.0	0.0	0	0
SUPPLEMENTAL FOODS AND FORMULAS—CHILD/ADULT													
Medical Nutritionals													
63162	Instant Breakfast, supplement, chocolate, rtu	1 ea	260	390	12	44	0	12	2.0	—	—	5	250
62761	Instant Breakfast, supplement, straw, liquid, rts	8 fl-oz	250	250	12	33	0	8	—	—	—	18	250
62760	Instant Breakfast, supplement, van, liquid, rts	8 fl-oz	250	250	12	33	0	8	—	—	—	18	250

PAGE KEY: 52 Granola Bars, Cereal Bars, Diet Bars, Scones, and Tarts   52 Meals and Dishes   56 Meats   62 Nuts, Seeds, and Products   64 Poultry
66 Salad Dressings, Dips, and Mayonnaise   66 Salads   68 Sandwiches   70 Sauces and Gravies   70 Snack Foods—Chips, Pretzels, Popcorn
72 Soups, Stews, and Chilis   74 Spices, Flavors, and Seasonings   76 Sports Bars and Drinks   76 Supplemental Foods and Formulas
78 Sweeteners and Sweet Substitutes   78 Vegetables and Legumes   92 Weight Loss Bars and Drinks   94 Miscellaneous

Thia (mg)	Ribo (mg)	Niac (mg NE)	Vit B6 (mg)	Vit B12 (µg)	Fol (µg)	Vit C (mg)	Vit D (IU)	Vit E (mg AT)	Cal (mg)	Iron (mg)	Magn (mg)	Phos (mg)	Pota (mg)	Sodi (mg)	Zinc (mg)	Wat (%)	Alco (g)	Caff (mg)
0.00	0.00	0.00	0.00	0.00	0.0	0.0	0.0	0.0	12	380.00	500.0	0	260	32000	870.0	7	0.00	0.00
—	—	—	—	0.00	—	—	—	—	—	—	—	—	—	240	—	11	0.00	0.00
0.00	0.00	0.00	0.00	0.00	0.0	0.0	0.0	0.0	3	0.10	0.8	1	6	461	0.0	2	0.00	0.00
0.00	0.00	0.03	0.01	0.00	2.1	0.2	0.0	0.0	15	0.52	3.4	3	10	0	0.0	9	0.00	0.00
0.00	0.00	0.07	0.01	0.00	3.1	0.2	0.0	0.4	10	0.58	5.1	7	31	1	0.1	10	0.00	0.00
0.00	0.00	0.10	0.02	0.00	3.8	0.9	0.0	0.1	30	0.58	5.9	7	48	0	0.1	6	0.00	0.00
—	—	—	—	0.00	—	0.7	—	—	4	0.23	—	—	—	3	—	14	0.00	0.00
0.00	0.01	0.20	0.10	0.00	2.6	1.7	0.0	0.8	7	0.37	4.4	8	50	26	0.1	8	0.00	0.00
0.93	1.59	9.68	1.46	0.00	137.0	139.0	—	—	1300	25.89	345.0	478	7189	371	6.0	4	0.00	0.00
0.00	0.00	0.02	0.00	0.00	0.7	0.7	0.0	0.0	28	0.87	1.3	1	12	1	0.0	10	0.00	0.00
0.00	0.00	0.02	0.00	0.00	2.0	1.7	0.0	0.2	14	0.18	5.5	2	23	5	0.0	7	0.00	0.00
0.00	0.00	0.05	0.00	0.00	0.2	0.4	0.0	0.0	32	0.34	5.4	6	25	0	0.1	8	0.00	0.00
0.00	0.00	0.01	—	0.00	—	0.1	—	—	3	0.01	—	—	38	1	—	6	0.00	0.00
0.00	0.00	0.00	0.02	0.00	3.5	0.3	0.0	0.0	8	0.05	2.6	7	20	1	0.0	5	0.00	0.00
0.00	0.00	0.09	0.01	0.00	4.1	0.8	0.0	0.3	24	0.66	4.0	3	25	0	0.1	7	0.00	0.00
0.00	0.03	0.31	0.07	0.00	2.2	1.5	0.0	0.6	4	0.50	3.9	7	49	1	0.1	10	0.00	0.00
—	—	—	—	0.00	—	0.0	—	—	8	0.15	—	—	—	0	—	12	0.00	0.00
0.00	0.00	0.05	0.00	0.00	3.6	1.0	—	0.0	8	0.15	2.6	2	18	1	0.0	79	0.00	0.00
0.01	0.00	0.02	0.00	0.00	1.6	0.1	0.0	0.0	41	0.25	9.3	24	20	1	0.3	7	0.00	0.00
0.00	0.01	0.10	0.03	0.00	8.5	0.0	—	0.0	24	1.39	9.6	4	31	6	0.0	11	0.00	0.00
0.00	0.00	0.07	0.00	0.00	3.8	0.7	0.0	0.1	26	1.73	3.1	3	11	1	0.1	8	0.00	0.00
1.50	1.70	20.00	2.00	6.00	400.0	60.0	—	18.4	300	6.30	140.0	350	110	90	5.2	—	0.00	0.00
0.37	0.28	3.54	0.41	0.98	87.0	67.1	—	20.2	275	5.32	103.2	298	246	170	3.2	17	0.00	0.00
1.50	1.70	20.00	2.00	6.00	400.0	60.0	—	18.4	300	6.30	140.0	350	145	90	5.2	—	0.00	15.00
0.38	0.31	3.63	0.43	0.98	84.6	65.7	—	20.8	278	5.73	128.3	304	232	139	3.7	19	0.00	0.00
0.34	0.28	3.49	0.38	0.98	85.6	66.1	—	20.3	265	5.21	95.5	286	206	76	3.5	15	0.00	—
1.50	1.70	20.00	2.00	6.00	400.0	60.0	—	18.3	300	6.30	140.0	350	—	150	5.2	—	0.00	—
1.50	1.70	20.00	2.00	6.00	400.0	60.0	—	18.3	300	6.30	140.0	350	140	95	5.2	—	0.00	—
0.34	0.27	3.45	0.43	0.98	85.1	66.2	—	20.3	279	5.23	102.6	266	212	179	3.2	20	0.00	0.00
0.60	0.50	9.00	0.60	1.20	80.0	60.0	80.0	13.6	100	3.59	40.0	100	115	220	3.0	—	0.00	—
0.40	0.30	6.25	0.41	0.98	96.2	65.8	—	20.4	268	5.30	113.7	305	301	289	3.6	15	0.00	0.00
1.26	0.60	3.00	0.60	1.50	—	6.0	60.0	—	300	2.70	100.0	100	—	75	—	—	0.00	0.00
1.50	1.70	20.00	2.00	6.00	400.0	60.0	—	18.3	300	6.30	140.0	350	110	90	5.2	—	0.00	0.00
—	—	—	—	—	—	9.0	—	2.8	0	0.00	—	—	40	50	—	—	0.00	25.00
—	—	—	—	—	—	0.0	—	—	0	0.00	—	—	—	35	—	10	0.00	—
0.25	0.33	3.32	0.33	1.33	120.0	15.0	66.7	4.5	116	—	59.3	141	167	177	2.5	—	0.00	0.00
0.00	0.00	0.00	0.00	0.00	0.0	0.0	0.0	0.0	0	0.11	2.4	22	26	96	0.0	94	0.00	0.00
—	—	—	—	—	—	0.0	—	—	0	0.00	—	—	32	28	—	—	0.00	0.00
—	—	—	—	—	—	0.0	—	—	0	0.00	—	—	32	28	—	—	0.00	0.00
0.37	0.43	5.00	0.50	1.50	100.0	15.0	—	—	250	4.50	100.0	250	430	120	3.8	—	0.00	—
0.37	0.43	5.00	0.50	1.50	1000.0	15.0	100.0	3.4	300	4.50	60.0	300	480	190	3.8	—	0.00	0.00
0.37	0.43	5.00	0.50	1.50	1000.0	15.0	100.0	3.4	300	4.50	60.0	300	480	190	3.8	—	0.00	0.00

PAGE KEY: 2 Beverage and Beverage Mixes 4 Other Beverages 4 Beverages, Alcoholic 6 Candies and Confections, Gum 10 Cereals, Breakfast Type
14 Cheese and Cheese Substitutes 16 Dairy Products and Substitutes 18 Desserts 24 Dessert Toppings 24 Eggs, Substitutes, and Egg Dishes 26 Ethnic Foods
30 Fast Foods/Restaurants 44 Fats, Oils, Margarines, Shortenings, and Substitutes 44 Fish, Seafood, and Shellfish 46 Food Additives
46 Fruit, Vegetable, or Blended Juices 48 Grains, Flours, and Fractions 48 Grain Products, Prepared and Baked Goods

Code	Food Name	Unit/ Amt	Wt (g)	Energy (kcal)	Prot (g)	Carb (g)	Fiber (g)	Fat (g)	Sat (g)	Mono (g)	Poly (g)	Chol (mg)	Vit A (RE)
62136	Pudding, supplement, rtu, 5 oz can	1 ea	142	240	7	32	0	9	1.5	—	—	5	150
62795	Supplement Drink, Hi Protein, vanilla, rtu	1 cup	256	240	15	33	0	6	0.5	—	—	10	250
62796	Supplement Drink, Plus, vanilla, rtu	8 fl-oz	260	360	14	45	1	14	1.5	—	—	10	250
62162	Supplement Drink, vanilla, rtu	1 cup	256	240	10	41	0	4	0.5	—	—	5	250

Soy Nutritionals

SWEETENERS AND SWEET SUBSTITUTES

Jams and Jellies

Code	Food Name	Unit/ Amt	Wt (g)	Energy (kcal)	Prot (g)	Carb (g)	Fiber (g)	Fat (g)	Sat (g)	Mono (g)	Poly (g)	Chol (mg)	Vit A (RE)
90974	Fruit Spread, apricot, 100% fruit	1 Tbs	19	40	0	10	0	0	0.0	0.0	0.0	0	0
90976	Fruit Spread, blueberry, 100% fruit	1 Tbs	19	40	0	10	0	0	0.0	0.0	0.0	0	0
90984	Fruit Spread, concord grape, 100% fruit	1 Tbs	19	40	0	10	0	0	0.0	0.0	0.0	0	0
90978	Fruit Spread, red raspberry, 100% fruit	1 Tbs	19	40	0	10	0	0	0.0	0.0	0.0	0	0
90979	Fruit Spread, strawberry, 100% fruit	1 Tbs	19	40	0	10	0	0	0.0	0.0	0.0	0	0
23054	Jam	1 Tbs	20	56	0	14	0	0	0.0	0.0	0.0	0	0
23205	Jam, apricot	1 Tbs	20	48	0	13	0	0	0.0	0.0	0.0	0	6
23288	Jam, concord grape	1 Tbs	20	50	0	13	0	0	0.0	0.0	0.0	0	0
92262	Jam, red raspberry	1 Tbs	20	50	0	13	0	0	0.0	0.0	0.0	0	0
23286	Jam, strawberry	1 Tbs	20	50	0	13	0	0	0.0	0.0	0.0	0	0
23003	Jelly	1 Tbs	19	51	0	13	0	0	0.0	0.0	0.0	0	0
23285	Jelly, apple	1 Tbs	20	50	0	13	0	0	0.0	0.0	0.0	0	0
23293	Jelly, concord grape	1 Tbs	20	50	0	13	0	0	0.0	0.0	0.0	0	0
90881	Jelly, mixed fruit	1 Tbs	20	50	0	13	0	0	0.0	0.0	0.0	0	0
23294	Jelly, strawberry	1 Tbs	20	50	0	13	0	0	0.0	0.0	0.0	0	0
23005	Marmalade, orange	1 Tbs	20	49	0	13	0	0	0.0	0.0	0.0	0	1
92229	Preserves	1 Tbs	20	56	0	14	0	0	0.0	0.0	0.0	0	0
92232	Preserves, apricot	1 Tbs	20	48	0	13	0	0	0.0	0.0	0.0	0	6
90891	Preserves, blueberry	1 Tbs	20	50	0	13	0	0	0.0	0.0	0.0	0	0
23297	Preserves, red raspberry	1 Tbs	20	50	0	13	0	0	0.0	0.0	0.0	0	0
23301	Preserves, strawberry	1 Tbs	20	50	0	13	0	0	0.0	0.0	0.0	0	0

Sugars, Sugar Substitutes, and Syrups

Code	Food Name	Unit/ Amt	Wt (g)	Energy (kcal)	Prot (g)	Carb (g)	Fiber (g)	Fat (g)	Sat (g)	Mono (g)	Poly (g)	Chol (mg)	Vit A (RE)
25309	Honey, light	1 Tbs	21	64	0	17	0	0	0.0	0.0	0.0	0	0
25003	Molasses	1 Tbs	20	59	0	15	0	0	0.0	0.0	0.0	0	0
25201	Sugar, brown, unpacked	1 cup	145	547	0	141	0	0	0.0	0.0	0.0	0	0
63415	Sugar, powdered	0.25 cup	37	140	0	37	0	0	0.0	0.0	0.0	0	0
25006	Sugar, white, granulated	1 tsp	4	16	0	4	0	0	0.0	0.0	0.0	0	0
25007	Sugar, white, granulated, pkt	1 ea	6	23	0	6	0	0	0.0	0.0	0.0	0	0
25010	Syrup, corn, dark	2 Tbs	41	117	0	32	0	0	0.0	0.0	0.0	0	0
25000	Syrup, corn, light	1 cup	328	961	0	261	0	0	0.0	0.0	0.0	0	0
63334	Syrup, dietetic	1 Tbs	15	6	0	7	0	0	0.0	0.0	0.0	0	0
23042	Syrup, pancake	1 Tbs	20	47	0	12	0	0	0.0	0.0	0.0	0	0
23090	Syrup, pancake, w/butter	1 cup	315	932	0	233	0	5	3.2	1.5	0.2	13	47

VEGETABLES AND LEGUMES

VEGETABLES

Fresh Vegetables

Code	Food Name	Unit/ Amt	Wt (g)	Energy (kcal)	Prot (g)	Carb (g)	Fiber (g)	Fat (g)	Sat (g)	Mono (g)	Poly (g)	Chol (mg)	Vit A (RE)
5010	Alfalfa Sprouts, fresh	0.5 cup	16	5	1	1	0	0	0.0	0.0	0.1	0	3
7440	Artichokes, Calif, fresh	1 ea	340	85	7	20	10	0	0.0	0.0	0.0	0	0
5001	Asparagus, fresh	0.5 cup	67	13	1	3	1	0	0.0	0.0	0.1	0	51

Thia (mg)	Ribo (mg)	Niac (mg NE)	Vit B6 (mg)	Vit B12 (μg)	Fol (μg)	Vit C (mg)	Vit D (IU)	Vit E (mg AT)	Cal (mg)	Iron (mg)	Magn (mg)	Phos (mg)	Pota (mg)	Sodi (mg)	Zinc (mg)	Wat (%)	Alco (g)	Caff (mg)
0.23	0.25	3.00	0.30	0.89	60.0	9.0	60.0	2.0	230	2.70	60.0	230	320	120	2.3	65	0.00	0.00
0.37	0.43	5.00	0.69	2.09	140.0	60.0	150.0	13.6	330	4.50	105.0	310	380	170	4.5	78	0.00	0.00
0.37	0.43	5.00	0.69	2.09	140.0	60.0	150.0	13.6	330	4.50	105.0	310	380	170	4.5	72	0.00	0.00
0.37	0.43	5.00	0.69	2.09	140.0	60.0	100.0	13.6	300	3.59	100.0	250	400	130	4.5	78	0.00	0.00
—	—	—	—	—	—	0.0	—	—	0	0.00	—	—	—	0	—	47	0.00	0.00
—	—	—	—	—	—	0.0	—	—	0	0.00	—	—	—	0	—	47	0.00	0.00
—	—	—	—	—	—	0.0	—	—	0	0.00	—	—	—	0	—	47	0.00	0.00
—	—	—	—	—	—	0.0	—	—	0	0.00	—	—	—	0	—	47	0.00	0.00
—	—	—	—	—	—	0.0	—	—	0	0.00	—	—	—	0	—	47	0.00	0.00
0.00	0.01	0.00	0.00	0.00	2.2	1.8	—	0.0	4	0.10	0.8	4	15	6	0.0	30	0.00	0.00
0.00	0.00	0.00	0.00	0.00	6.6	1.8	—	0.0	4	0.10	0.8	2	15	8	0.0	34	0.00	0.00
—	—	—	—	—	—	0.0	—	—	0	0.00	—	—	—	0	—	35	0.00	0.00
—	—	—	—	—	—	0.0	—	—	0	0.00	—	—	—	0	—	35	0.00	0.00
—	—	—	—	—	—	0.0	—	—	0	0.00	—	—	—	0	—	35	0.00	0.00
0.00	0.00	0.00	0.00	0.00	0.4	0.2	—	0.0	1	0.03	1.1	1	10	6	0.0	30	0.00	0.00
—	—	—	—	—	—	0.0	—	—	0	0.00	—	—	—	0	—	35	0.00	0.00
—	—	—	—	—	—	0.0	—	—	0	0.00	—	—	—	0	—	35	0.00	0.00
—	—	—	—	—	—	0.0	—	—	0	0.00	—	—	—	0	—	35	0.00	0.00
—	—	—	—	—	—	0.0	—	—	0	0.00	—	—	—	0	—	35	0.00	0.00
0.00	0.00	0.00	0.00	0.00	1.8	1.0	—	0.0	8	0.02	0.4	1	7	11	0.0	33	0.00	0.00
0.00	0.01	0.00	0.00	0.00	2.2	1.8	—	0.0	4	0.10	0.8	4	15	6	0.0	30	0.00	0.00
0.00	0.00	0.00	0.00	0.00	6.6	1.8	—	0.0	4	0.10	0.8	2	15	8	0.0	34	0.00	0.00
—	—	—	—	—	—	0.0	—	—	0	0.00	—	—	—	0	—	35	0.00	0.00
—	—	—	—	—	—	0.0	—	—	0	0.00	—	—	—	0	—	35	0.00	0.00
—	—	—	—	—	—	0.0	—	—	0	0.00	—	—	—	0	—	35	0.00	0.00
0.00	0.05	0.05	0.00	0.00	2.1	0.1	0.0	0.0	1	0.05	0.4	1	10	1	0.0	17	0.00	0.00
0.00	0.00	0.18	0.14	0.00	0.0	0.0	—	0.0	42	0.97	49.6	6	300	8	0.1	22	0.00	0.00
0.00	0.00	0.11	0.03	0.00	1.5	0.0	—	0.0	123	2.76	42.1	32	502	57	0.3	2	0.00	0.00
—	—	—	—	—	—	—	—	—	—	—	—	—	—	0	—	0	0.00	0.00
0.00	0.00	0.00	0.00	0.00	0.0	0.0	—	0.0	0	0.00	0.0	0	0	0	0.0	0	0.00	0.00
0.00	0.00	0.00	0.00	0.00	0.0	0.0	—	0.0	0	0.00	0.0	0	0	0	0.0	0	0.00	0.00
0.00	0.00	0.00	0.00	0.00	0.0	0.0	0.0	0.0	7	0.15	3.3	5	18	64	0.0	22	0.00	0.00
0.03	0.02	0.07	0.02	0.00	0.0	0.0	0.0	0.0	10	0.15	6.6	7	13	397	0.1	20	0.00	0.00
0.00	0.00	0.00	0.00	0.00	0.0	0.0	—	0.0	0	0.00	0.0	0	0	3	0.0	50	0.00	0.00
0.00	0.00	0.00	0.00	0.00	0.0	0.0	—	0.0	1	0.00	0.4	2	3	16	0.0	38	0.00	0.00
0.02	0.02	0.05	0.00	0.00	0.0	0.0	—	0.1	6	0.28	6.3	32	9	309	0.1	24	0.00	0.00
0.00	0.01	0.07	0.00	0.00	5.9	1.4	—	0.0	5	0.15	4.5	12	13	1	0.2	91	0.00	0.00
0.10	0.11	2.72	0.14	—	136.0	20.4	—	1.4	68	2.45	136.0	204	578	255	—	91	0.00	0.00
0.10	0.09	0.66	0.05	0.00	34.8	3.8	—	0.8	16	1.42	9.4	35	135	1	0.4	93	0.00	0.00

Code	Food Name	Unit/ Amt	Wt (g)	Energy (kcal)	Prot (g)	Carb (g)	Fiber (g)	Fat (g)	Sat (g)	Mono (g)	Poly (g)	Chol (mg)	Vit A (RE)
5572	Beets, fresh, whole, 2"	1 ea	82	35	1	8	2	0	0.0	0.0	0.1	0	3
5678	Broccoflower, fresh	1 cup	100	32	3	6	3	0	0.0	0.0	0.1	0	7
6757	Broccoli, fresh	1 cup	71	24	2	5	2	0	0.0	0.0	0.0	0	47
5036	Cabbage, fresh, shredded	1 cup	70	17	1	4	2	0	0.0	0.0	0.0	0	13
5042	Cabbage, red, fresh, shredded	0.5 cup	35	11	1	3	1	0	0.0	0.0	0.0	0	39
9329	Carrots, baby, fresh	0.75 cup	85	40	1	9	2	0	0.0	0.0	0.0	0	1250
90429	Carrots, fresh, slices	1 pce	3	1	0	0	0	0	0.0	0.0	0.0	0	36
5049	Cauliflower, fresh	0.5 cup	50	12	1	3	1	0	0.0	0.0	0.0	0	1
90436	Celery, stalk, sml, 5" long, fresh	1 ea	17	2	0	1	0	0	0.0	0.0	0.0	0	7
7927	Chili Peppers, banana, fresh	1 cup	124	33	2	7	4	1	0.1	0.0	0.3	0	42
5359	Chives, fresh	1 Tbs	3	1	0	0	0	0	0.0	0.0	0.0	0	13
5560	Corn, white, sweet, kernels f/one ear, ckd, drained	1 ea	77	83	3	19	2	1	0.2	0.3	0.5	0	0
6015	Corn, white, sweet, kernels, fresh	1 cup	154	132	5	29	4	2	0.3	0.5	0.9	0	0
5379	Corn, yellow, sweet, kernels, ckd, drained	0.5 cup	82	89	3	21	2	1	0.2	0.3	0.5	0	21
5378	Corn, yellow, sweet, kernels, fresh	0.5 cup	77	66	2	15	2	1	0.1	0.3	0.4	0	15
7921	Cucumber, w/o skin, fresh, sliced	1 pce	7	1	0	0	0	0	0.0	0.0	0.0	0	1
5071	Cucumber, w/skin, fresh, slices	0.5 cup	52	8	0	2	0	0	0.0	0.0	0.0	0	5
5371	Eggplant, fresh, cubes	1 cup	82	20	1	5	3	0	0.0	0.0	0.1	0	2
26005	Garlic, cloves, fresh	4 ea	12	18	1	4	0	0	0.0	0.0	0.0	0	0
7081	Hummus, prep f/recipe	1 cup	246	435	12	49	10	21	2.8	12.1	5.1	0	1
5208	Kale, fresh, chpd	1 cup	67	34	2	7	1	0	0.1	0.0	0.2	0	1030
4851	Lettuce, crisphead, fresh, chpd	1 cup	55	8	0	2	1	0	0.0	0.0	0.0	0	28
5083	Lettuce, iceberg, fresh, chpd	1 cup	55	8	0	2	1	0	0.0	0.0	0.0	0	28
9316	Lettuce, iceberg, shredded	1.5 cup	100	15	1	3	1	0	0.0	0.0	0.0	0	20
5088	Lettuce, romaine, fresh, chpd	1 cup	56	10	1	2	1	0	0.0	0.0	0.1	0	325
5090	Mushrooms, fresh, pces/slices	0.5 cup	35	8	1	1	0	0	0.0	0.0	0.0	0	0
6494	Mushrooms, fresh, whole	1 cup	96	21	3	3	1	0	0.0	0.0	0.1	0	0
5099	Okra, ckd, drained, slices	0.5 cup	80	18	1	4	2	0	0.0	0.0	0.0	0	22
5775	Okra, fresh	0.5 cup	50	16	1	4	2	0	0.0	0.0	0.0	0	19
7498	Onion, red, fresh, chpd	1 cup	160	67	1	16	2	0	0.0	0.0	0.1	0	0
9548	Onion, sweet, fresh	100 g	100	32	1	8	1	0	—	—	—	0	0
5101	Onion, white, fresh, chpd	0.5 cup	80	34	1	8	1	0	0.0	0.0	0.0	0	0
7499	Onion, yellow, fresh, chpd	0.5 cup	80	34	1	8	1	0	0.0	0.0	0.0	0	0
26012	Parsley, fresh, chpd	0.5 cup	30	11	1	2	1	0	0.0	0.1	0.0	0	253
5124	Peppers, bell, green, sweet, fresh, chpd	0.5 cup	74	15	1	3	1	0	0.0	0.0	0.0	0	27
5128	Peppers, bell, red, sweet, fresh, chpd	0.5 cup	74	19	1	4	1	0	0.0	0.0	0.1	0	234
9242	Peppers, bell, yellow, sweet, fresh, chpd	0.5 cup	74	20	1	5	1	0	0.0	0.0	0.1	0	15
5143	Radishes, fresh, med, 3/4" to 1"	10 ea	45	7	0	2	1	0	0.0	0.0	0.0	0	0
7214	Rutabaga, fresh, cubes	0.5 cup	70	25	1	6	2	0	0.0	0.0	0.1	0	0
6861	Soybean Sprouts, mature, fresh	10 ea	10	12	1	1	0	1	0.1	0.2	0.4	0	0
5146	Spinach, fresh, chpd	1 cup	30	7	1	1	1	0	0.0	0.0	0.0	0	281
6863	Spinach, fresh, leaf	1 ea	10	2	0	0	0	0	0.0	0.0	0.0	0	94
7369	Squash, banana, fresh	0.75 cup	85	30	1	7	1	0	0.0	0.0	0.0	0	350
5801	Squash, butternut, fresh, cubes	0.5 cup	120	54	1	14	2	0	0.0	0.0	0.1	0	1277
90537	Squash, summer, all types, fresh, med	1 ea	196	31	2	7	2	0	0.1	0.0	0.2	0	39

Thia (mg)	Ribo (mg)	Niac (mg NE)	Vit B6 (mg)	Vit B12 (µg)	Fol (µg)	Vit C (mg)	Vit D (IU)	Vit E (mg AT)	Cal (mg)	Iron (mg)	Magn (mg)	Phos (mg)	Pota (mg)	Sodi (mg)	Zinc (mg)	Wat (%)	Alco (g)	Caff (mg)
0.02	0.02	0.27	0.05	0.00	89.4	4.0	—	0.0	13	0.66	18.9	33	266	64	0.3	88	0.00	0.00
0.07	0.10	0.80	0.20	0.00	57.0	74.0	0.0	0.3	32	0.07	20.0	64	322	23	0.5	90	0.00	0.00
0.05	0.07	0.44	0.11	0.00	44.7	63.3	—	0.6	33	0.51	14.9	47	224	23	0.3	89	0.00	0.00
0.03	0.02	0.20	0.07	0.00	30.1	22.5	—	0.1	33	0.40	10.5	16	172	13	0.1	92	0.00	0.00
0.01	0.01	0.15	0.07	0.00	6.3	19.9	—	0.0	16	0.28	5.6	10	85	9	0.1	90	0.00	0.00
—	—	—	—	—	—	6.0	—	—	20	0.00	—	—	—	45	—	88	0.00	0.00
0.00	0.00	0.02	0.00	0.00	0.6	0.2	—	0.0	1	0.00	0.4	1	10	2	0.0	88	0.00	0.00
0.02	0.02	0.25	0.10	0.00	28.5	23.2	—	0.0	11	0.21	7.5	22	152	15	0.1	92	0.00	0.00
0.00	0.00	0.05	0.00	0.00	6.1	0.5	—	0.0	7	0.02	1.9	4	44	14	0.0	95	0.00	0.00
0.10	0.07	1.53	0.43	0.00	36.0	102.5	—	0.9	17	0.56	21.1	40	317	16	0.3	92	0.00	0.00
0.00	0.00	0.01	0.00	0.00	3.1	1.7	—	0.0	3	0.05	1.3	2	9	0	0.0	91	0.00	0.00
0.17	0.05	1.24	0.05	0.00	35.4	4.8	0.0	0.1	2	0.46	24.6	79	192	13	0.4	70	0.00	0.00
0.31	0.09	2.61	0.07	0.00	70.8	10.5	—	0.1	3	0.80	57.0	137	416	23	0.7	76	0.00	0.00
0.18	0.05	1.32	0.05	0.00	37.7	5.1	—	0.1	2	0.50	26.2	84	204	14	0.4	70	0.00	0.00
0.15	0.05	1.30	0.03	0.00	35.4	5.2	—	0.1	2	0.40	28.5	69	208	12	0.3	76	0.00	0.00
0.00	0.00	0.00	0.00	0.00	1.0	0.2	—	0.0	1	0.01	0.8	1	10	0	0.0	97	0.00	0.00
0.00	0.01	0.05	0.01	0.00	3.6	1.5	—	0.0	8	0.15	6.8	12	76	1	0.1	95	0.00	0.00
0.02	0.02	0.52	0.07	0.00	18.0	1.8	—	0.2	7	0.20	11.5	20	189	2	0.1	92	0.00	0.00
0.01	0.00	0.07	0.15	0.00	0.4	3.7	—	0.0	22	0.20	3.0	18	48	2	0.1	59	0.00	0.00
0.21	0.12	0.98	0.98	0.00	145.1	19.4	—	1.8	121	3.85	71.3	271	426	595	2.7	65	0.00	0.00
0.07	0.09	0.67	0.18	0.00	19.4	80.4	—	0.5	90	1.13	22.8	38	299	29	0.3	84	0.00	0.00
0.01	0.00	0.07	0.01	0.00	16.0	1.5	—	0.1	10	0.23	3.9	11	78	6	0.1	96	0.00	0.00
0.01	0.00	0.07	0.01	0.00	16.0	1.5	—	0.1	10	0.23	3.9	11	78	6	0.1	96	0.00	0.00
—	—	—	—	—	—	3.6	—	—	0	0.00	—	—	—	10	—	96	0.00	0.00
0.03	0.03	0.18	0.03	0.00	76.2	13.4	—	0.1	18	0.54	7.8	17	138	4	0.1	95	0.00	0.00
0.02	0.15	1.35	0.03	0.00	5.6	0.8	26.6	0.0	1	0.18	3.1	30	110	1	0.2	92	0.00	0.00
0.09	0.40	3.70	0.10	0.03	15.4	2.3	73.0	0.0	3	0.50	8.6	82	301	4	0.5	92	0.00	0.00
0.10	0.03	0.69	0.15	0.00	36.8	13.0	—	0.2	62	0.21	28.8	26	108	5	0.3	93	0.00	0.00
0.10	0.02	0.50	0.10	0.00	44.0	10.6	—	0.2	40	0.40	28.5	32	152	4	0.3	90	0.00	0.00
0.07	0.03	0.12	0.23	0.00	30.4	10.2	—	0.0	35	0.30	16.0	43	230	5	0.3	89	0.00	0.00
0.03	0.01	0.12	0.12	—	23.0	4.8	—	0.0	20	0.25	9.0	27	119	8	0.1	91	0.00	0.00
0.03	0.01	0.07	0.11	0.00	15.2	5.1	—	0.0	18	0.15	8.0	22	115	2	0.1	89	0.00	0.00
0.03	0.01	0.07	0.11	0.00	15.2	5.1	—	0.0	18	0.15	8.0	22	115	2	0.1	89	0.00	0.00
0.02	0.02	0.38	0.02	0.00	45.6	39.9	—	0.2	41	1.86	15.0	17	166	17	0.3	88	0.00	0.00
0.03	0.01	0.36	0.17	0.00	8.2	59.9	—	0.3	7	0.25	7.4	15	130	2	0.1	94	0.00	0.00
0.03	0.05	0.73	0.21	0.00	13.4	141.6	—	1.2	5	0.31	8.9	19	157	1	0.2	92	0.00	0.00
0.01	0.01	0.66	0.12	0.00	19.4	136.7	0.0	0.5	8	0.34	8.9	18	158	1	0.1	92	0.00	0.00
0.00	0.01	0.10	0.02	0.00	11.2	6.7	—	0.0	11	0.15	4.5	9	105	18	0.1	95	0.00	0.00
0.05	0.02	0.49	0.07	0.00	14.7	17.5	—	0.2	33	0.36	16.1	41	236	14	0.2	90	0.00	0.00
0.02	0.00	0.10	0.01	0.00	17.2	1.5	—	0.0	7	0.20	7.2	16	48	1	0.1	69	0.00	0.00
0.01	0.05	0.21	0.05	0.00	58.2	8.4	—	0.6	30	0.81	23.7	15	167	24	0.2	91	0.00	0.00
0.00	0.01	0.07	0.01	0.00	19.4	2.8	—	0.2	10	0.27	7.9	5	56	8	0.1	91	0.00	0.00
—	—	—	—	0.00	—	9.0	—	—	20	0.36	—	—	—	0	—	90	0.00	0.00
0.11	0.01	1.44	0.18	0.00	32.4	25.2	—	1.7	58	0.83	40.8	40	422	5	0.2	86	0.00	0.00
0.09	0.28	0.94	0.43	0.00	56.8	33.3	—	0.2	29	0.68	33.3	74	514	4	0.6	95	0.00	0.00

Code	Food Name	Unit/ Amt	Wt (g)	Energy (kcal)	Prot (g)	Carb (g)	Fiber (g)	Fat (g)	Sat (g)	Mono (g)	Poly (g)	Chol (mg)	Vit A (RE)
90538	Squash, summer, all types, fresh, sml	1 ea	118	19	1	4	1	0	0.1	0.0	0.1	0	24
5833	Squash, winter, all types, fresh, cubes	0.5 cup	58	20	1	5	1	0	0.0	0.0	0.0	0	79
90604	Squash, zucchini, baby, med, fresh	1 ea	11	2	0	0	0	0	0.0	0.0	0.0	0	0
5519	Tomatoes, green, fresh, chpd	0.5 cup	90	21	1	5	1	0	0.0	0.0	0.1	0	58
3973	Tomatoes, orange, fresh	1 ea	111	18	1	4	1	0	0.0	0.0	0.1	0	166
90530	Tomatoes, red, cherry, fresh, year round avg	1 ea	17	3	0	1	0	0	0.0	0.0	0.0	0	14
5178	Tomatoes, red, ckd f/fresh w/o salt	0.5 cup	120	22	1	5	1	0	0.0	0.0	0.1	0	58
5177	Tomatoes, red, ckd f/fresh w/o salt, med	1 ea	123	22	1	5	1	0	0.0	0.0	0.1	0	59
5170	Tomatoes, red, fresh, year round avg, chpd/sliced	0.5 cup	90	16	1	4	1	0	0.0	0.0	0.1	0	76
6492	Tomatoes, roma, fresh, year round avg, fresh	1 ea	62	11	1	2	1	0	0.0	0.0	0.1	0	52
5547	Turnip Greens, chpd, fresh	1 cup	55	18	1	4	2	0	0.0	0.0	0.1	0	0
5183	Turnips, ckd, drained, cubes	0.5 cup	78	17	1	4	2	0	0.0	0.0	0.0	0	0
5306	Yams, fresh, cubes	0.5 cup	75	88	1	21	3	0	0.0	0.0	0.1	0	10
Cooked Vegetables													
4437	Artichokes, French, hearts, ckd, drained	0.5 cup	84	42	3	9	5	0	0.0	0.0	0.1	0	15
5000	Artichokes, globe, ckd, drained, med	1 ea	120	60	4	13	6	0	0.0	0.0	0.1	0	22
5003	Asparagus, ckd, drained	0.5 cup	90	20	2	4	2	0	0.1	0.0	0.1	0	90
5249	Bamboo Shoots, slices, ckd, drained	1 cup	120	14	2	2	1	0	0.1	0.0	0.1	0	0
5025	Beet Greens, ckd, drained	1 cup	144	39	4	8	4	0	0.0	0.1	0.1	0	1103
5022	Beets, ckd, drained, sliced	0.5 cup	85	37	1	8	2	0	0.0	0.0	0.1	0	3
5407	Borage, ckd, drained	100 g	100	25	2	4	1	1	0.2	0.2	0.1	0	438
5028	Broccoli, chpd, ckd, drained	0.5 cup	78	27	2	6	3	0	0.1	0.0	0.1	0	153
6092	Broccoli, spears, ckd f/fzn w/salt, drained	0.5 cup	92	26	3	5	3	0	0.0	0.0	0.1	0	103
5234	Broccoli, spears, ckd f/fzn, drained	0.5 cup	92	26	3	5	3	0	0.0	0.0	0.1	0	103
5653	Broccoli, stmd	1 cup	156	44	5	8	5	1	0.1	0.0	0.3	0	228
5033	Brussels Sprouts, ckd, drained, cup	0.5 cup	78	28	2	6	2	0	0.1	0.0	0.2	0	61
5038	Cabbage, ckd, drained, shredded	1 cup	150	33	2	7	3	1	0.1	0.0	0.3	0	21
5238	Cabbage, red, ckd, drained, shredded	0.5 cup	75	22	1	5	2	0	0.0	0.0	0.0	0	3
5358	Carrots, ckd f/fzn w/o salt, drained, slices	0.5 cup	73	27	0	6	2	0	0.1	0.0	0.2	0	1213
5889	Carrots, ckd f/fzn w/salt, drained, slices	0.5 cup	73	27	0	6	2	0	0.1	0.0	0.2	0	1213
5656	Carrots, stir fried	1 cup	156	67	2	16	5	0	0.0	0.0	0.1	0	3955
5655	Carrots, stmd	1 cup	156	67	2	16	5	0	0.0	0.0	0.1	0	3955
5052	Cauliflower, florets, ckd, drained	3 ea	54	12	1	2	1	0	0.0	0.0	0.1	0	1
7266	Cauliflower, green, ckd, head	0.2 ea	90	29	3	6	3	0	0.0	0.0	0.1	0	13
5894	Celery, ckd w/salt, drained, diced	0.5 cup	75	14	1	3	1	0	0.0	0.0	0.1	0	44
5056	Celery, ckd, drained, diced	1 cup	150	27	1	6	2	0	0.1	0.0	0.1	0	87
6093	Collards, chpd, ckd w/salt, drained	1 cup	190	49	4	9	5	1	0.1	0.0	0.3	0	1543
5061	Collards, chpd, ckd, drained	0.5 cup	80	21	2	4	2	0	0.0	0.0	0.1	0	650
6917	Corn, white, sweet, cob, ckd f/fzn w/salt, drained	1 ea	63	59	2	14	1	0	0.1	0.1	0.2	0	0
5567	Corn, white, sweet, cob, ckd f/fzn, drained	1 ea	63	59	2	14	1	0	0.1	0.1	0.2	0	0
6019	Corn, white, sweet, kernels, ckd f/fzn w/salt, drained	0.5 cup	82	66	2	16	2	0	0.1	0.1	0.2	0	0
5393	Corn, white, sweet, kernels, ckd f/fzn, drained	0.5 cup	82	66	2	16	2	0	0.1	0.1	0.2	0	0
6964	Corn, yellow, sweet, kernels, ckd f/fzn cob w/salt, drnd	0.5 cup	82	76	3	18	2	1	0.1	0.2	0.3	0	20
5365	Corn, yellow, sweet, kernels, ckd f/fzn cob, drained	0.5 cup	82	76	3	18	2	1	0.1	0.2	0.3	0	20
5639	Cucumber, ckd	1 cup	180	29	2	6	2	0	0.1	0.0	0.1	0	42
5456	Dish, broccoli, w/cheese sauce, ckd	0.5 cup	114	115	7	6	2	8	3.6	2.5	1.1	16	152

Thia (mg)	Ribo (mg)	Niac (mg NE)	Vit B6 (mg)	Vit B12 (µg)	Fol (µg)	Vit C (mg)	Vit D (IU)	Vit E (mg AT)	Cal (mg)	Iron (mg)	Magn (mg)	Phos (mg)	Pota (mg)	Sodi (mg)	Zinc (mg)	Wat (%)	Alco (g)	Caff (mg)
0.05	0.17	0.56	0.25	0.00	34.2	20.1	—	0.1	18	0.40	20.1	45	309	2	0.3	95	0.00	0.00
0.01	0.03	0.28	0.09	0.00	13.9	7.1	—	0.1	16	0.34	8.1	13	203	2	0.1	90	0.00	0.00
0.00	0.00	0.07	0.01	0.00	2.2	3.8	0.0	0.0	2	0.09	3.6	10	50	0	0.1	93	0.00	0.00
0.05	0.03	0.44	0.07	0.00	8.1	21.1	—	0.3	12	0.46	9.0	25	184	12	0.1	93	0.00	0.00
0.05	0.03	0.66	0.07	0.00	32.2	17.8	—	—	6	0.51	8.9	32	235	47	0.2	95	0.00	0.00
0.00	0.00	0.10	0.00	0.00	2.5	2.2	—	0.1	2	0.05	1.9	4	40	1	0.0	94	0.00	0.00
0.03	0.02	0.63	0.09	0.00	15.6	27.4	—	0.7	13	0.81	10.8	34	262	13	0.2	94	0.00	0.00
0.03	0.02	0.64	0.10	0.00	16.0	28.0	—	0.7	14	0.83	11.1	34	268	14	0.2	94	0.00	0.00
0.02	0.01	0.52	0.07	0.00	13.5	11.4	—	0.5	9	0.23	9.9	22	213	4	0.2	94	0.00	0.00
0.01	0.00	0.37	0.05	0.00	9.3	7.9	—	0.3	6	0.17	6.8	15	147	3	0.1	94	0.00	0.00
0.03	0.05	0.33	0.14	0.00	106.7	33.0	—	1.6	104	0.61	17.1	23	163	22	0.1	90	0.00	0.00
0.01	0.01	0.23	0.05	0.00	7.0	9.0	—	0.0	26	0.14	7.0	20	138	12	0.1	94	0.00	0.00
0.07	0.01	0.40	0.21	0.00	17.2	12.8	—	0.3	13	0.40	15.8	41	612	7	0.2	70	0.00	0.00
0.05	0.05	0.83	0.09	0.00	42.8	8.4	—	0.2	38	1.08	50.4	72	297	80	0.4	84	0.00	0.00
0.07	0.07	1.20	0.12	0.00	61.2	12.0	—	0.2	54	1.54	72.0	103	425	114	0.6	84	0.00	0.00
0.15	0.12	0.98	0.07	0.00	134.1	6.9	—	1.3	21	0.81	12.6	49	202	13	0.5	93	0.00	0.00
0.01	0.05	0.36	0.11	0.00	2.4	0.0	—	0.8	14	0.28	3.6	24	640	5	0.6	96	0.00	0.00
0.17	0.41	0.72	0.18	0.00	20.2	35.9	—	2.6	164	2.74	97.9	59	1309	347	0.7	89	0.00	0.00
0.01	0.02	0.28	0.05	0.00	68.0	3.1	—	0.0	14	0.67	19.6	32	259	65	0.3	87	0.00	0.00
0.05	0.17	0.93	0.09	0.00	10.0	32.5	—	—	102	3.64	57.0	55	491	88	0.2	92	0.00	0.00
0.05	0.10	0.43	0.15	0.00	84.2	50.6	—	1.1	31	0.51	16.4	52	229	32	0.4	89	0.00	0.00
0.05	0.07	0.41	0.11	0.00	27.6	36.9	—	1.2	47	0.56	18.4	51	166	239	0.3	91	0.00	0.00
0.05	0.07	0.41	0.11	0.00	27.6	36.9	—	1.2	47	0.56	18.4	51	166	22	0.3	91	0.00	0.00
0.09	0.18	0.93	0.21	0.00	93.9	123.4	0.0	0.7	75	1.37	39.0	103	505	42	0.6	91	0.00	0.00
0.07	0.05	0.46	0.14	0.00	46.8	48.4	—	0.3	28	0.93	15.6	44	247	16	0.3	89	0.00	0.00
0.09	0.07	0.41	0.17	0.00	30.0	30.2	—	0.2	46	0.25	12.0	22	146	12	0.1	94	0.00	0.00
0.05	0.03	0.28	0.17	0.00	18.0	8.1	—	0.1	32	0.50	12.8	25	196	6	0.2	91	0.00	0.00
0.01	0.02	0.30	0.05	0.00	8.0	1.7	—	0.7	26	0.38	8.0	23	140	43	0.3	90	0.00	0.00
0.01	0.02	0.30	0.05	0.00	8.0	1.7	0.0	0.3	26	0.38	8.0	23	140	215	0.3	90	0.00	0.00
0.14	0.09	1.37	0.21	0.00	20.7	11.6	0.0	0.7	42	0.77	23.4	69	504	55	0.3	88	0.00	0.00
0.14	0.09	1.37	0.21	0.00	20.7	10.9	0.0	0.7	42	0.77	23.4	69	504	55	0.3	88	0.00	0.00
0.01	0.02	0.21	0.09	0.00	23.8	23.9	—	0.0	9	0.18	4.9	17	77	8	0.1	93	0.00	0.00
0.05	0.09	0.61	0.18	0.00	36.9	65.3	—	0.0	29	0.64	17.1	51	250	21	0.6	89	0.00	0.00
0.02	0.03	0.23	0.05	0.00	16.5	4.6	0.0	0.3	32	0.31	9.0	19	213	245	0.1	94	0.00	0.00
0.05	0.07	0.47	0.12	0.00	33.0	9.1	—	0.5	63	0.62	18.0	38	426	136	0.2	94	0.00	0.00
0.07	0.20	1.09	0.23	0.00	176.7	34.6	0.0	1.7	266	2.20	38.0	57	220	479	0.4	92	0.00	0.00
0.02	0.07	0.46	0.10	0.00	74.4	14.6	—	0.7	112	0.93	16.0	24	93	13	0.2	92	0.00	0.00
0.10	0.03	0.95	0.14	0.00	19.5	3.0	—	0.0	2	0.37	18.3	47	158	151	0.4	73	0.00	0.00
0.10	0.03	0.95	0.14	0.00	19.5	3.0	—	0.0	2	0.37	18.3	47	158	3	0.4	73	0.00	0.00
0.07	0.05	1.07	0.10	0.00	25.4	2.5	—	0.1	3	0.28	15.6	47	121	201	0.3	77	0.00	0.00
0.07	0.05	1.07	0.10	0.00	25.4	2.5	—	0.1	3	0.28	15.6	47	121	4	0.3	77	0.00	0.00
0.14	0.05	1.24	0.18	0.00	25.4	3.9	—	0.1	2	0.50	23.8	62	206	197	0.5	73	0.00	0.00
0.14	0.05	1.24	0.18	0.00	25.4	3.9	—	0.1	2	0.50	23.8	62	206	3	0.5	73	0.00	0.00
0.03	0.05	0.43	0.07	0.00	20.2	9.4	0.0	0.2	30	0.55	23.2	40	288	4	0.4	95	0.00	0.00
0.05	0.18	0.54	0.11	0.14	39.4	54.0	—	1.7	161	0.79	25.0	138	268	202	0.8	81	0.00	0.00

Code	Food Name	Unit/ Amt	Wt (g)	Energy (kcal)	Prot (g)	Carb (g)	Fiber (g)	Fat (g)	Sat (g)	Mono (g)	Poly (g)	Chol (mg)	Vit A (RE)
5457	Dish, broccoli, w/cream sauce, ckd	0.5 cup	114	87	4	8	2	5	1.3	2.0	1.4	3	154
5989	Dish, succotash, ckd w/salt, drained	0.5 cup	96	110	5	23	5	1	0.1	0.1	0.4	0	29
5642	Eggplant, batter dipped, fried	1 pce	50	75	1	6	1	5	1.1	2.3	1.7	8	4
5072	Eggplant, ckd, drained, 1" cubes	0.5 cup	50	17	0	4	1	0	0.0	0.0	0.0	0	2
5673	Eggplant, stmd	1 cup	96	25	1	6	2	0	0.0	0.0	0.1	0	8
5640	Hominy, ckd	1 cup	165	119	2	24	4	1	0.2	0.4	0.7	0	0
7957	Hummus, cmrcl	1 cup	250	415	20	36	15	24	3.6	10.1	9.0	0	10
5075	Kale, ckd, drained	0.5 cup	65	18	1	4	1	0	0.0	0.0	0.1	0	885
5514	Mushrooms, batter dipped, fried	5 ea	70	156	2	11	1	12	1.5	3.6	6.0	2	6
5924	Mushrooms, ckd w/salt, drained, pieces	0.5 cup	78	22	2	4	2	0	0.0	0.0	0.1	0	0
5092	Mushrooms, ckd, drained	0.5 cup	78	22	2	4	2	0	0.0	0.0	0.1	0	0
5384	Mushrooms, shiitake, ckd, whole	4 ea	72	40	1	10	2	0	0.0	0.0	0.0	0	0
5657	Mushrooms, stmd	1 cup	156	39	3	7	2	1	0.1	0.0	0.3	0	0
5643	Mushrooms, stuffed	2 ea	48	138	5	13	1	7	2.2	3.1	1.6	6	50
5096	Mustard Greens, ckd, drained	1 cup	140	21	3	3	3	0	0.0	0.2	0.1	0	885
5644	Okra, batter dipped, fried	1 cup	92	175	2	14	2	13	1.7	3.1	7.1	2	39
5932	Okra, ckd f/fzn w/salt, drained, slices	0.5 cup	92	26	2	5	3	0	0.1	0.0	0.1	0	31
70623	Onion Rings	6 ea	88	222	3	27	—	12	1.9	4.1	5.1	0	9
6074	Onion, ckd w/salt, drained	0.5 cup	105	46	1	11	1	0	0.0	0.0	0.1	0	0
5529	Onion, pearl, ckd, whole	3 ea	45	20	1	5	1	0	0.0	0.0	0.0	0	0
7811	Onion, red, ckd, drained, chpd	0.5 cup	105	46	1	11	1	0	0.0	0.0	0.1	0	0
5650	Onion, stir fried	1 cup	210	80	2	18	4	0	0.1	0.0	0.1	0	0
5649	Onion, stmd	1 cup	210	80	2	18	4	0	0.1	0.0	0.1	0	0
5108	Onion, white, ckd, drained, chpd	0.5 cup	105	46	1	11	1	0	0.0	0.0	0.1	0	0
7812	Onion, yellow, ckd, drained, chpd	0.5 cup	105	46	1	11	1	0	0.0	0.0	0.1	0	0
5212	Parsnips, ckd, drained	1 cup	156	111	2	27	6	0	0.1	0.2	0.1	0	0
5662	Peppers, bell, green, sweet, chpd, stir fried	0.5 cup	68	18	1	4	1	0	0.0	0.0	0.1	0	39
5661	Peppers, bell, green, sweet, chpd, stmd	0.5 cup	68	18	1	4	1	0	0.0	0.0	0.1	0	41
9549	Peppers, bell, green, sweet, sauteed	100 g	100	127	1	4	2	12	1.6	2.3	5.9	0	28
5663	Peppers, bell, red, sweet, chpd, stmd	0.5 cup	68	18	1	4	1	0	0.0	0.0	0.1	0	368
5229	Poi	0.5 cup	120	134	0	33	0	0	0.0	0.0	0.1	0	7
9366	Potatoes, white, baby, ckd	0.5 cup	85	70	2	15	1	0	0.0	0.0	0.0	0	0
9368	Potatoes, yukon gold, ckd	0.5 cup	85	70	2	15	1	0	0.0	0.0	0.0	0	0
5426	Purslane, ckd, drained	0.5 cup	58	10	1	2	—	0	0.0	0.0	0.0	0	107
7226	Rutabaga, ckd, drained, mashed	0.5 cup	120	47	2	10	2	0	0.0	0.0	0.1	0	0
5459	Soybean Sprouts, mature, stmd	0.5 cup	47	38	4	3	0	2	0.3	0.5	1.2	0	2
6227	Spinach, chpd, fzn	0.33 cup	85	20	3	3	2	0	0.1	—	—	0	681
5972	Spinach, ckd w/salt, drained	0.5 cup	90	21	3	3	2	0	0.0	0.0	0.1	0	943
5147	Spinach, ckd, drained	0.5 cup	90	21	3	3	2	0	0.0	0.0	0.1	0	943
5670	Spinach, stmd	0.5 cup	95	21	3	3	3	0	0.1	0.0	0.1	0	607
5316	Squash, acorn, ckd, mashed	0.5 cup	122	42	1	11	3	0	0.0	0.0	0.0	0	100
5317	Squash, butternut, bkd, cubes	0.5 cup	102	41	1	11	3	0	0.0	0.0	0.0	0	1144
5455	Squash, spaghetti, bkd/ckd, drained	0.5 cup	78	21	1	5	1	0	0.0	0.0	0.1	0	9
6922	Squash, spaghetti, ckd w/salt, drained	0.5 cup	78	21	1	5	1	0	0.0	0.0	0.1	0	9
5975	Squash, summer, all types, ckd w/salt, drained	0.5 cup	90	18	1	4	1	0	0.1	0.0	0.1	0	20

PAGE KEY: 52 Granola Bars, Cereal Bars, Diet Bars, Scones, and Tarts   52 Meals and Dishes   56 Meats   62 Nuts, Seeds, and Products   64 Poultry   66 Salad Dressings, Dips, and Mayonnaise   66 Salads   68 Sandwiches   70 Sauces and Gravies   70 Snack Foods—Chips, Pretzels, Popcorn   72 Soups, Stews, and Chilis   74 Spices, Flavors, and Seasonings   76 Sports Bars and Drinks   76 Supplemental Foods and Formulas   78 Sweeteners and Sweet Substitutes   78 Vegetables and Legumes   92 Weight Loss Bars and Drinks   94 Miscellaneous

Thia (mg)	Ribo (mg)	Niac (mg NE)	Vit B6 (mg)	Vit B12 (µg)	Fol (µg)	Vit C (mg)	Vit D (IU)	Vit E (mg AT)	Cal (mg)	Iron (mg)	Magn (mg)	Phos (mg)	Pota (mg)	Sodi (mg)	Zinc (mg)	Wat (%)	Alco (g)	Caff (mg)
0.07	0.14	0.50	0.10	0.12	22.7	27.6	—	1.3	89	0.56	20.0	83	194	180	0.4	84	0.00	0.00
0.15	0.09	1.26	0.10	0.00	31.7	7.9	—	0.3	16	1.46	50.9	112	394	243	0.6	68	0.00	0.00
0.05	0.03	0.46	0.03	0.02	7.4	0.6	—	0.8	14	0.34	7.6	23	106	15	0.1	74	0.00	0.00
0.03	0.00	0.30	0.03	0.00	6.9	0.6	—	0.2	3	0.11	5.4	7	61	0	0.1	90	0.00	0.00
0.05	0.02	0.55	0.07	0.00	15.5	1.4	0.0	0.0	7	0.25	13.4	21	208	3	0.1	92	0.00	0.00
0.00	0.00	0.05	0.00	0.00	1.6	0.0	0.0	0.1	16	1.01	26.4	58	15	346	1.7	83	0.00	0.00
0.44	0.15	1.46	0.50	0.00	207.5	0.0	—	—	95	6.09	177.5	440	570	948	4.6	67	0.00	0.00
0.02	0.05	0.31	0.09	0.00	8.4	26.6	0.0	0.6	47	0.57	11.7	18	148	15	0.2	91	0.00	0.00
0.10	0.25	2.25	0.03	0.02	8.3	1.2	—	2.3	15	1.22	6.8	119	154	112	0.4	63	0.00	0.00
0.05	0.23	3.48	0.07	0.00	14.0	3.1	59.3	0.0	5	1.36	9.4	68	278	186	0.7	91	0.00	0.00
0.05	0.23	3.48	0.07	0.00	14.0	3.1	—	0.0	5	1.36	9.4	68	278	2	0.7	91	0.00	0.00
0.02	0.11	1.08	0.10	0.00	15.1	0.2	—	0.0	2	0.31	10.1	21	84	3	1.0	83	0.00	0.00
0.14	0.67	6.13	0.14	0.00	28.1	4.7	0.0	0.2	8	1.92	15.6	162	577	6	1.1	92	0.00	0.00
0.15	0.25	2.64	0.07	0.10	11.0	2.8	25.0	0.8	100	1.49	14.3	107	209	298	0.7	43	0.07	0.00
0.05	0.09	0.61	0.14	0.00	102.2	35.4	—	1.7	104	0.98	21.0	57	283	22	0.2	94	0.00	0.00
0.18	0.14	1.44	0.11	0.03	38.1	10.3	11.0	3.0	61	1.25	35.8	122	190	122	0.5	67	0.00	0.00
0.09	0.10	0.72	0.03	0.00	134.3	11.2	—	0.3	88	0.62	46.9	42	215	220	0.6	91	0.00	0.00
0.07	0.03	1.05	—	0.00	—	4.2	—	—	18	0.82	—	—	161	200	—	52	0.00	0.00
0.03	0.01	0.17	0.14	0.00	15.7	5.5	—	0.0	23	0.25	11.5	37	174	251	0.2	88	0.00	0.00
0.01	0.00	0.07	0.05	0.00	6.8	2.3	0.0	0.1	10	0.10	4.9	16	75	1	0.1	88	0.00	0.00
0.03	0.01	0.17	0.14	0.00	15.7	5.5	—	0.0	23	0.25	11.5	37	174	3	0.2	88	0.00	0.00
0.07	0.03	0.30	0.23	0.00	32.3	10.9	0.0	0.7	42	0.46	21.0	69	330	6	0.4	90	0.00	0.00
0.07	0.03	0.30	0.23	0.00	32.3	10.2	0.0	0.7	42	0.46	21.0	69	330	6	0.4	90	0.00	0.00
0.03	0.01	0.17	0.14	0.00	15.7	5.5	—	0.0	23	0.25	11.5	37	174	3	0.2	88	0.00	0.00
0.03	0.01	0.17	0.14	0.00	15.7	5.5	—	0.0	23	0.25	11.5	37	174	3	0.2	88	0.00	0.00
0.12	0.07	1.12	0.15	0.00	90.5	20.3	—	1.6	58	0.89	45.2	108	573	16	0.4	80	0.00	0.00
0.03	0.01	0.33	0.15	0.00	12.0	51.7	0.0	0.5	6	0.31	6.8	13	120	1	0.1	92	0.00	0.00
0.03	0.01	0.33	0.15	0.00	12.7	51.7	0.0	0.5	6	0.31	6.8	13	120	1	0.1	92	0.00	0.00
0.03	0.05	0.57	0.20	0.00	2.0	177.0	—	1.4	8	0.30	8.0	15	134	17	0.1	83	0.00	0.00
0.03	0.01	0.33	0.15	0.00	12.7	110.2	0.0	0.5	6	0.31	6.8	13	120	1	0.1	92	0.00	0.00
0.15	0.05	1.32	0.33	0.00	25.2	4.8	—	2.8	19	1.05	28.8	47	220	14	0.3	72	0.00	0.00
—	—	—	—	—	—	18.0	—	—	0	0.72	—	—	—	5	—	79	0.00	0.00
—	—	—	—	—	—	18.0	—	—	0	0.72	—	—	—	5	—	79	0.00	0.00
0.01	0.05	0.25	0.03	0.00	5.2	6.0	—	—	45	0.43	38.5	21	281	25	0.1	94	0.00	0.00
0.10	0.05	0.86	0.11	0.00	18.0	22.6	—	0.4	58	0.63	27.6	67	391	24	0.4	89	0.00	0.00
0.10	0.01	0.50	0.05	0.00	37.6	3.9	—	0.1	28	0.62	28.2	63	167	5	0.5	79	0.00	0.00
0.07	0.12	0.34	0.09	0.00	26.1	18.5	—	—	90	1.75	40.0	33	260	79	—	91	0.00	0.00
0.09	0.20	0.43	0.21	0.00	131.4	8.8	0.0	1.9	122	3.21	78.3	50	419	275	0.7	91	0.00	0.00
0.09	0.20	0.43	0.21	0.00	131.4	8.8	—	1.9	122	3.21	78.3	50	419	63	0.7	91	0.00	0.00
0.05	0.17	0.62	0.17	0.00	120.7	16.1	0.0	1.8	89	2.44	75.0	40	494	75	0.5	92	0.00	0.00
0.11	0.00	0.64	0.14	0.00	13.5	8.0	—	0.1	32	0.68	31.9	33	322	4	0.1	90	0.00	0.00
0.07	0.01	0.99	0.12	0.00	19.5	15.5	—	1.3	42	0.62	29.7	28	291	4	0.1	88	0.00	0.00
0.02	0.01	0.62	0.07	0.00	6.2	2.7	—	0.1	16	0.25	8.5	11	91	14	0.2	92	0.00	0.00
0.02	0.01	0.62	0.07	0.00	6.2	2.7	—	0.1	16	0.25	8.5	11	91	197	0.2	92	0.00	0.00
0.03	0.03	0.46	0.05	0.00	18.0	4.9	—	0.1	24	0.31	21.6	35	173	213	0.4	94	0.00	0.00

PAGE KEY: 2 Beverage and Beverage Mixes   4 Other Beverages   4 Beverages, Alcoholic   6 Candies and Confections, Gum   10 Cereals, Breakfast Type   14 Cheese and Cheese Substitutes   16 Dairy Products and Substitutes   18 Desserts   24 Dessert Toppings   24 Eggs, Substitutes, and Egg Dishes   26 Ethnic Foods   30 Fast Foods/Restaurants   44 Fats, Oils, Margarines, Shortenings, and Substitutes   44 Fish, Seafood, and Shellfish   46 Food Additives   46 Fruit, Vegetable, or Blended Juices   48 Grains, Flours, and Fractions   48 Grain Products, Prepared and Baked Goods

Code	Food Name	Unit/ Amt	Wt (g)	Energy (kcal)	Prot (g)	Carb (g)	Fiber (g)	Fat (g)	Sat (g)	Mono (g)	Poly (g)	Chol (mg)	Vit A (RE)
5152	Squash, summer, all types, ckd, drained, slices	0.5 cup	90	18	1	4	1	0	0.1	0.0	0.1	0	20
5153	Squash, winter, ckd w/salt	1 cup	240	94	2	21	7	2	0.3	0.1	0.6	0	854
5667	Squash, zucchini, slices, stmd	0.5 cup	90	13	1	3	1	0	0.0	0.0	0.1	0	29
5327	Squash, zucchini, w/skin, ckd, drained, slices	0.5 cup	90	14	1	4	1	0	0.0	0.0	0.0	0	101
5059	Swiss Chard, ckd, drained, chpd	0.5 cup	88	18	2	4	2	0	0.0	0.0	0.0	0	536
5544	Taro, ckd, slices, Tahitian, Colocassia	0.5 cup	68	30	3	5	1	0	0.1	0.0	0.2	0	121
7277	Tempeh, ckd	3.6 oz	100	197	18	9	—	11	3.4	3.7	2.6	—	—
5536	Tomatoes, green, ckd/frd	1 ea	144	284	5	19	1	22	4.6	9.4	6.4	41	82
5628	Tomatoes, red, fried	1 ea	101	168	3	12	1	13	2.7	5.5	3.8	24	57
5185	Turnip Greens, chpd, ckd, drained	0.5 cup	72	14	1	3	3	0	0.0	0.0	0.1	0	549
6004	Turnip Greens, ckd w/salt, drained, chpd	0.5 cup	72	14	1	3	3	0	0.0	0.0	0.1	0	549
6233	Vegetables, mixed, broccoli cauliflower carrots, fzn	0.5 cup	92	25	2	5	2	0	0.0	—	—	0	500
6644	Vegetables, mixed, broccoli cauliflower, fzn	0.5 cup	91	22	2	4	—	0	0.1	—	—	0	41
5187	Vegetables, mixed, ckd f/fzn w/o salt, drnd, 10 oz pkg	1 cup	182	118	5	24	8	0	0.1	0.0	0.1	0	779
6007	Vegetables, mixed, ckd f/fzn w/salt, drained	0.5 cup	91	54	3	12	4	0	0.0	0.0	0.1	0	389
6224	Vegetables, mixed, fzn	0.33 cup	85	52	2	12	3	0	0.1	—	—	0	582
6010	Yams, ckd/bkd w/salt, cubes	0.5 cup	68	79	1	19	3	0	0.0	0.0	0.0	0	8
5168	Yams, ckd/bkd, cubes	0.5 cup	68	79	1	19	3	0	0.0	0.0	0.0	0	8

Frozen, Dehydrated, and Dried Vegetables

Code	Food Name	Unit/ Amt	Wt (g)	Energy (kcal)	Prot (g)	Carb (g)	Fiber (g)	Fat (g)	Sat (g)	Mono (g)	Poly (g)	Chol (mg)	Vit A (RE)
5361	Asparagus, spears, fzn	4 pce	58	14	2	2	1	0	0.0	0.0	0.1	0	55
6388	Broccoli, cuts, fzn	0.66 cup	90	25	2	4	2	0	0.0	0.0	0.0	0	40
6551	Broccoli, florets, select, fzn	1.33 cup	83	25	2	4	2	0	0.0	0.0	0.0	0	50
5740	Carrots, fzn, slices	0.5 cup	64	23	0	5	2	0	0.0	0.0	0.2	0	719
70617	Corn, cob, fzn	1 ea	174	212	6	45	—	6	1.1	0.2	0.3	0	59
6706	Corn, cob, Nibblers, fzn	1 ea	61	70	2	14	1	0	0.0	—	—	0	0
56958	Corn, cream style, fzn	0.5 cup	118	110	2	23	2	1	0.0	—	—	0	0
6392	Corn, niblets, fzn	0.66 cup	96	80	3	17	3	0	0.0	—	—	0	0
6018	Corn, white, sweet, kernels, fzn	0.5 cup	82	72	2	17	2	1	0.1	0.2	0.3	0	0
338	Dish, mixed vegetables, skillet, fzn	0.66 cup	82	25	2	4	2	0	0.0	0.0	0.0	0	200
6558	Mushrooms, dehyd	100 g	100	285	24	53	9	5	0.7	0.1	2.0	0	0
90491	Onion Rings, breaded, par fried, heated f/fzn	1 cup	48	195	3	18	1	13	4.1	5.2	2.5	0	11
5492	Onion, green, dehyd	100 g	100	295	20	66	10	2	0.3	0.3	0.6	0	5900
1830	Spinach, 80% ckd, fzn	3 oz	85	20	2	3	2	0	0.0	0.0	0.0	0	600
5446	Tomatoes, sun dried	0.5 cup	27	70	4	15	3	1	0.1	0.1	0.3	0	24
5821	Turnip Greens, fzn, chpd/dices, 10 oz pkg	0.5 cup	82	18	2	3	2	0	0.1	0.0	0.1	0	507
6395	Vegetables, stew style, fzn	0.5 cup	65	38	1	8	0	0	0.0	0.0	0.0	0	49

Canned Vegetables

Code	Food Name	Unit/ Amt	Wt (g)	Energy (kcal)	Prot (g)	Carb (g)	Fiber (g)	Fat (g)	Sat (g)	Mono (g)	Poly (g)	Chol (mg)	Vit A (RE)
7867	Artichokes, hearts, cnd, pieces	3 pce	80	30	2	5	0	0	0.0	0.0	0.0	0	10
6261	Asparagus, spears, cnd	128 g	128	20	2	3	1	0	0.0	0.0	0.0	0	40
6607	Beets, slices, cnd	0.5 cup	121	35	1	8	2	0	0.0	0.0	0.0	0	0
5199	Carrots, cnd, drained, slices	1 ea	3	1	0	0	0	0	0.0	0.0	0.0	0	31
7933	Chili Peppers, green, cnd	0.5 cup	70	15	1	3	1	0	0.0	0.0	0.1	0	8
6268	Corn, cnd	0.33 cup	77	70	2	15	2	0	0.0	0.0	0.0	0	0
6265	Corn, cream style, cnd	0.5 cup	127	100	2	22	1	0	0.0	—	—	0	20
51031	Corn, golden, cream style, cnd	0.5 cup	125	90	2	20	2	1	0.0	—	—	0	0

PAGE KEY: 52 Granola Bars, Cereal Bars, Diet Bars, Scones, and Tarts 52 Meals and Dishes 56 Meats 62 Nuts, Seeds, and Products 64 Poultry 66 Salad Dressings, Dips, and Mayonnaise 66 Salads 68 Sandwiches 70 Sauces and Gravies 70 Snack Foods—Chips, Pretzels, Popcorn 72 Soups, Stews, and Chilis 74 Spices, Flavors, and Seasonings 76 Sports Bars and Drinks 76 Supplemental Foods and Formulas 78 Sweeteners and Sweet Substitutes 78 Vegetables and Legumes 92 Weight Loss Bars and Drinks 94 Miscellaneous

Thia (mg)	Ribo (mg)	Niac (mg NE)	Vit B6 (mg)	Vit B12 (µg)	Fol (µg)	Vit C (mg)	Vit D (IU)	Vit E (mg AT)	Cal (mg)	Iron (mg)	Magn (mg)	Phos (mg)	Pota (mg)	Sodi (mg)	Zinc (mg)	Wat (%)	Alco (g)	Caff (mg)
0.03	0.03	0.46	0.05	0.00	18.0	4.9	—	0.1	24	0.31	21.6	35	173	1	0.4	94	0.00	0.00
0.20	0.05	1.67	0.17	0.00	67.2	23.0	—	0.3	34	0.79	19.2	48	1049	2	0.6	89	0.00	0.00
0.05	0.02	0.34	0.07	0.00	16.9	6.9	0.0	0.1	14	0.37	19.8	29	223	3	0.2	95	0.00	0.00
0.03	0.03	0.38	0.07	0.00	15.3	4.1	—	0.1	12	0.31	19.8	36	228	3	0.2	95	0.00	0.00
0.02	0.07	0.31	0.07	0.00	7.9	15.8	—	1.7	51	1.98	75.2	29	480	157	0.3	93	0.00	0.00
0.02	0.14	0.33	0.07	0.00	4.8	26.0	—	1.8	102	1.07	34.9	46	427	37	0.1	86	0.00	0.00
0.05	0.36	2.13	0.20	0.14	21.0	—	—	—	96	2.13	77.0	253	401	14	1.6	60	0.00	0.00
0.15	0.18	1.36	0.10	0.14	12.7	20.9	9.2	3.0	101	1.50	17.1	102	254	134	0.4	68	0.00	0.00
0.10	0.11	0.97	0.07	0.07	11.8	13.4	6.5	1.8	55	0.93	12.6	62	200	78	0.2	72	0.00	0.00
0.02	0.05	0.30	0.12	0.00	85.0	19.7	—	1.4	99	0.57	15.8	21	146	21	0.1	93	0.00	0.00
0.02	0.05	0.30	0.12	0.00	85.0	19.7	0.0	1.4	99	0.57	15.8	21	146	191	0.1	93	0.00	0.00
0.05	0.07	0.46	0.15	0.00	50.0	43.7	—	—	31	0.51	12.9	39	192	28	—	—	0.00	0.00
—	—	—	—	0.00	—	—	54.7	—	29	0.44	—	—	—	22	—	—	0.00	0.00
0.12	0.21	1.54	0.12	0.00	34.6	5.8	—	0.8	46	1.49	40.0	93	308	64	0.9	83	0.00	0.00
0.05	0.10	0.76	0.07	0.00	17.3	2.9	0.0	0.3	23	0.75	20.0	46	154	247	0.4	83	0.00	0.00
0.09	0.05	1.01	0.11	0.00	23.8	7.6	—	—	20	0.72	16.1	47	167	37	—	83	0.00	0.00
0.05	0.01	0.37	0.15	0.00	10.9	8.2	—	0.3	10	0.34	12.2	33	456	166	0.1	70	0.00	0.00
0.05	0.01	0.37	0.15	0.00	10.9	8.2	—	0.3	10	0.34	12.2	33	456	5	0.1	70	0.00	0.00
0.07	0.07	0.69	0.05	0.00	110.8	18.4	—	1.2	14	0.41	8.1	37	147	5	0.3	92	0.00	0.00
—	—	—	—	0.00	—	42.0	—	—	20	0.72	—	—	—	150	—	93	0.00	0.00
—	—	—	—	—	—	36.0	—	—	0	0.00	—	—	—	20	—	92	0.00	0.00
0.02	0.01	0.30	0.05	0.00	6.4	1.6	—	0.5	23	0.28	7.7	21	150	44	0.2	90	0.00	0.00
0.14	0.14	4.30	—	0.00	—	14.9	—	—	—	1.66	—	—	532	26	—	67	0.00	0.00
—	—	—	—	0.00	—	2.4	—	—	0	0.00	—	—	—	5	—	72	0.00	0.00
—	—	—	—	—	—	40.0	—	—	0	0.00	—	—	—	330	—	—	0.00	0.00
—	—	—	—	0.00	—	1.2	—	—	0	0.36	—	—	—	60	—	78	0.00	0.00
0.07	0.05	1.41	0.15	0.00	29.5	5.2	0.0	0.0	3	0.34	14.8	57	172	2	0.3	75	0.00	0.00
—	—	—	—	—	—	18.0	—	—	0	0.00	—	—	—	30	—	—	0.00	0.00
1.13	5.13	47.00	1.13	0.00	241.0	40.0	—	—	57	14.19	114.0	1187	4224	46	8.3	6	0.00	0.00
0.12	0.07	1.73	0.03	0.00	31.7	0.7	—	0.3	15	0.81	9.1	39	62	180	0.2	28	0.00	0.00
0.82	1.64	2.35	0.00	0.00	162.0	531.0	—	—	708	22.29	236.0	390	3034	47	5.2	4	0.00	0.00
—	—	—	—	—	—	6.0	—	—	60	0.36	—	—	—	115	—	93	0.00	0.00
0.14	0.12	2.44	0.09	0.00	18.4	10.6	—	0.0	30	2.45	52.4	96	925	566	0.5	15	0.00	0.00
0.03	0.07	0.31	0.07	0.00	60.7	22.0	—	1.9	97	1.24	22.1	22	151	10	0.1	93	0.00	0.00
0.05	0.01	1.05	—	0.00	—	2.3	—	—	0	0.00	—	—	152	38	—	85	0.00	0.00
—	—	—	—	0.00	—	3.6	—	—	0	1.08	—	—	0	200	—	91	0.00	0.00
—	—	—	—	—	—	12.0	—	—	0	0.36	—	—	—	450	—	95	0.00	0.00
—	—	—	—	—	—	0.0	—	—	0	1.08	—	—	—	260	—	92	0.00	0.00
0.00	0.00	0.01	0.00	0.00	0.3	0.1	—	0.0	1	0.01	0.2	1	5	7	0.0	93	0.00	0.00
0.00	0.01	0.43	0.07	0.00	37.5	23.8	—	—	25	0.92	2.8	8	79	276	0.1	93	0.00	0.00
—	—	—	—	—	—	2.4	—	—	0	0.00	—	—	—	230	—	77	0.00	0.00
—	—	—	—	—	—	2.4	—	—	0	0.00	—	—	—	430	—	80	0.00	0.00
—	—	—	—	—	—	2.4	—	—	0	0.36	—	—	—	360	—	81	0.00	0.00

PAGE KEY: 2 Beverage and Beverage Mixes 4 Other Beverages 4 Beverages, Alcoholic 6 Candies and Confections, Gum 10 Cereals, Breakfast Type
14 Cheese and Cheese Substitutes 16 Dairy Products and Substitutes 18 Desserts 24 Dessert Toppings 24 Eggs, Substitutes, and Egg Dishes 26 Ethnic Foods
30 Fast Foods/Restaurants 44 Fats, Oils, Margarines, Shortenings, and Substitutes 44 Fish, Seafood, and Shellfish 46 Food Additives
46 Fruit, Vegetable, or Blended Juices 48 Grains, Flours, and Fractions 48 Grain Products, Prepared and Baked Goods

Code	Food Name	Unit/ Amt	Wt (g)	Energy (kcal)	Prot (g)	Carb (g)	Fiber (g)	Fat (g)	Sat (g)	Mono (g)	Poly (g)	Chol (mg)	Vit A (RE)
51059	Corn, golden, whole kernel, cnd	0.5 cup	125	90	2	18	3	1	0.0	—	—	0	0
7855	Corn, whole kernel, cnd	0.5 cup	125	90	2	14	2	1	0.0	—	—	0	0
38077	Hominy, white, cnd	0.5 cup	82	59	1	12	2	1	0.1	0.2	0.3	0	0
5094	Mushrooms, cnd, drained, pces/slices	0.5 cup	78	20	1	4	2	0	0.0	0.0	0.1	0	0
5095	Mushrooms, cnd, drained, whole, med	1 ea	12	3	0	1	0	0	0.0	0.0	0.0	0	0
27169	Olives, black, jumbo, cnd	1 ea	8	7	0	0	0	1	0.1	0.4	0.0	0	3
9539	Olives, green, pickled, cnd	100 g	100	145	1	4	3	15	2.0	11.3	1.3	0	40
92209	Pickles, bread & butter	1 ea	8	6	0	1	0	0	0.0	0.0	0.0	0	1
90583	Pickles, dill, chpd/diced	1 cup	143	26	1	6	2	0	0.1	0.0	0.1	0	26
27028	Pickles, dill, low sod, med	1 ea	65	12	0	3	1	0	0.0	0.0	0.1	0	21
27039	Pickles, dill, rducd salt	1 ea	65	7	0	1	1	0	0.0	0.0	0.1	0	10
27013	Pickles, dill, slices	5 pce	35	6	0	1	0	0	0.0	0.0	0.0	0	6
27025	Pickles, sour	1 cup	155	17	1	4	2	0	0.1	0.0	0.1	0	22
90585	Pickles, sweet, slices	1 ea	7	8	0	2	0	0	0.0	0.0	0.0	0	1
5227	Pimentos, cnd	1 Tbs	12	3	0	1	0	0	0.0	0.0	0.0	0	32
5142	Pumpkin, cnd, unsalted	0.5 cup	122	42	1	10	4	0	0.2	0.0	0.0	0	1906
5964	Pumpkin, cnd, w/salt	0.5 cup	122	42	1	10	4	0	0.2	0.0	0.0	0	2702
27063	Relish, pickle, hotdog	1 Tbs	15	18	0	4	0	0	0.0	0.0	0.1	0	1
27052	Relish, pickle, sweet	1 cup	245	318	1	86	3	1	0.1	0.5	0.3	0	44
6393	Sauerkraut, crisp	30 g	30	5	0	1	1	0	0.0	0.0	0.0	0	0
5595	Spinach, cnd, not drained	0.5 cup	117	22	2	3	2	0	0.1	0.0	0.2	0	753
5599	Squash, zucchini, Italian style, cnd	0.5 cup	114	33	1	8	2	0	0.0	0.0	0.1	0	61
51000	Tomatoes, chunky, chili style, cnd	0.5 cup	128	30	1	8	2	0	0.0	0.0	0.0	0	50
51001	Tomatoes, chunky, pasta style, cnd	0.5 cup	128	45	1	11	2	0	0.0	0.0	0.0	0	50
6927	Tomatoes, crushed, cnd	0.5 cup	50	16	1	4	1	0	0.0	0.0	0.1	0	35
51005	Tomatoes, dices, cnd	0.5 cup	126	25	1	6	2	0	0.0	0.0	0.0	0	50
5630	Tomatoes, green, pickled	0.5 cup	71	26	1	6	1	0	0.0	0.1	0.1	0	59
6394	Tomatoes, pickled, halves	1 oz	28	5	0	1	1	0	0.0	0.0	0.0	0	0
6293	Tomatoes, puree, cnd	0.25 cup	63	20	1	4	0	0	0.0	0.0	0.0	0	50
9169	Tomatoes, stwd, cnd	0.5 cup	121	35	1	8	1	0	0.0	0.0	0.0	0	30
51020	Tomatoes, stwd, Italian recipe, cnd	0.5 cup	126	30	1	8	2	0	0.0	0.0	0.0	0	50
51022	Tomatoes, stwd, original recipe, cnd	0.5 cup	126	35	1	9	2	0	0.0	0.0	0.0	0	50
7885	Tomatoes, stwd, unsalted, cnd	0.5 cup	123	35	1	7	2	0	0.0	0.0	0.0	0	50
7896	Tomatoes, whole, peeled, cnd	0.5 cup	121	25	1	4	1	0	0.0	0.0	0.0	0	50
9520	Turnip Greens, cnd, unsalted	1 cup	144	27	2	4	2	0	0.1	0.0	0.2	0	858
51044	Vegetables, mixed, cnd	0.5 cup	124	40	2	8	2	0	0.0	0.0	0.0	0	225
5305	Vegetables, mixed, cnd, drained	0.5 cup	82	40	2	8	2	0	0.0	0.0	0.1	0	949
9522	Vegetables, mixed, cnd, unsalted	1 cup	182	67	3	13	6	0	0.1	0.0	0.2	0	2118
7873	Vegetables, peas & carrots, cnd	0.5 cup	123	50	4	10	3	0	0.0	0.0	0.0	0	500

Legumes

Code	Food Name	Unit/ Amt	Wt (g)	Energy (kcal)	Prot (g)	Carb (g)	Fiber (g)	Fat (g)	Sat (g)	Mono (g)	Poly (g)	Chol (mg)	Vit A (RE)
7165	Beans, bbq	0.5 cup	100	160	6	32	6	2	0.5	—	—	—	—
7042	Beans, black turtle soup, mature, cnd	0.5 cup	120	109	7	20	8	0	0.1	0.0	0.2	0	0
7012	Beans, black, mature, ckd	1 cup	172	227	15	41	15	1	0.2	0.1	0.4	0	1
5213	Beans, blackeyed, immature, ckd, drained	0.5 cup	82	80	3	17	4	0	0.1	0.0	0.1	0	66
4450	Beans, blackeyed, mature, ckd	1 cup	172	200	13	36	11	1	0.2	0.1	0.4	0	3

Thia (mg)	Ribo (mg)	Niac (mg NE)	Vit B6 (mg)	Vit B12 (µg)	Fol (µg)	Vit C (mg)	Vit D (IU)	Vit E (mg AT)	Cal (mg)	Iron (mg)	Magn (mg)	Phos (mg)	Pota (mg)	Sodi (mg)	Zinc (mg)	Wat (%)	Alco (g)	Caff (mg)
—	—	—	—	—	—	3.6	—	—	0	0.36	—	—	—	360	—	82	0.00	0.00
—	—	—	—	0.00	—	2.4	—	—	0	0.36	—	—	0	340	—	85	0.00	0.00
0.00	0.00	0.02	0.00	0.00	0.8	0.0	—	0.0	8	0.50	13.2	29	7	173	0.9	83	0.00	0.00
0.07	0.01	1.24	0.05	0.00	9.4	0.0	—	0.0	9	0.62	11.7	51	101	332	0.6	91	0.00	0.00
0.00	0.00	0.18	0.00	0.00	1.4	0.0	—	0.0	1	0.09	1.8	8	15	51	0.1	91	0.00	0.00
0.00	0.00	0.00	0.00	0.00	0.0	0.1	0.0	0.1	8	0.28	0.3	0	1	75	0.0	84	0.00	0.00
0.01	0.00	0.23	0.02	0.00	3.0	0.0	—	3.8	52	0.49	11.0	4	42	1556	0.0	75	0.00	0.00
0.00	0.00	0.00	0.00	0.00	0.3	0.7	—	0.0	3	0.02	0.2	2	16	54	0.0	79	0.00	0.00
0.01	0.03	0.09	0.01	0.00	1.4	2.7	—	0.1	13	0.75	15.7	30	166	1833	0.2	92	0.00	0.00
0.00	0.01	0.03	0.00	0.00	0.6	1.2	—	0.1	6	0.34	7.1	14	75	12	0.1	92	0.00	0.00
0.00	0.00	0.00	0.00	0.00	0.5	0.6	0.0	0.0	0	0.25	2.6	9	15	12	0.0	94	0.00	0.00
0.00	0.00	0.01	0.00	0.00	0.3	0.7	—	0.0	3	0.18	3.8	7	41	449	0.0	92	0.00	0.00
0.00	0.01	0.00	0.00	0.00	1.5	1.5	—	0.1	0	0.62	6.2	22	36	1872	0.0	94	0.00	0.00
0.00	0.00	0.00	0.00	0.00	0.1	0.1	—	0.0	0	0.03	0.3	1	2	66	0.0	65	0.00	0.00
0.00	0.00	0.07	0.02	0.00	0.7	10.2	—	0.1	1	0.20	0.7	2	19	2	0.0	93	0.00	0.00
0.02	0.07	0.44	0.07	0.00	14.7	5.1	—	1.3	32	1.70	28.2	43	252	6	0.2	90	0.00	0.00
0.02	0.07	0.44	0.07	0.00	14.7	5.1	—	1.2	32	1.70	28.2	43	252	295	0.2	90	0.00	0.00
0.00	0.00	0.00	0.00	0.00	0.8	0.9	0.0	0.0	4	0.20	3.2	3	31	81	0.0	69	0.00	0.00
0.00	0.07	0.56	0.03	0.00	2.5	2.5	—	0.2	7	2.13	12.2	34	61	1987	0.3	62	0.00	0.00
—	—	—	—	—	—	3.6	—	—	0	0.00	—	—	—	220	—	94	0.00	0.00
0.01	0.11	0.31	0.09	0.00	67.9	15.8	—	1.3	97	1.85	65.5	37	269	373	0.5	93	0.00	0.00
0.05	0.05	0.60	0.17	0.00	34.0	2.6	0.0	0.1	19	0.76	15.9	33	311	424	0.3	91	0.00	0.00
—	—	—	—	—	—	9.0	—	—	20	0.36	—	—	—	670	—	92	0.00	0.00
—	—	—	—	—	—	9.0	—	—	20	0.36	—	—	—	560	—	—	0.00	0.00
0.03	0.02	0.62	0.07	0.00	6.6	4.6	—	0.3	17	0.66	10.1	16	148	67	0.1	89	0.00	0.00
—	—	—	—	—	—	9.0	—	—	20	0.36	—	—	—	160	—	—	0.00	0.00
0.03	0.01	0.28	0.05	0.00	5.3	20.0	0.0	0.2	11	0.36	7.5	19	128	89	0.1	90	0.00	0.00
—	—	—	—	—	—	0.0	—	—	0	0.00	—	—	—	324	—	—	0.00	0.00
—	—	—	—	—	—	9.0	—	—	0	0.36	—	—	—	15	—	91	0.00	0.00
—	—	—	—	—	—	15.0	—	—	60	1.08	—	—	—	390	—	—	0.00	0.00
—	—	—	—	—	—	9.0	—	—	20	0.36	—	—	—	420	—	—	0.00	0.00
—	—	—	—	—	—	9.0	—	—	20	0.36	—	—	—	360	—	—	0.00	0.00
—	—	—	—	0.00	—	12.0	—	—	40	1.44	—	—	150	15	—	93	0.00	0.00
—	—	—	—	0.00	—	12.0	—	—	20	0.72	—	—	200	220	—	95	0.00	0.00
0.00	0.09	0.51	0.05	0.00	132.5	22.3	—	2.1	170	2.17	28.8	30	203	42	0.3	95	0.00	0.00
—	—	—	—	—	—	2.4	—	—	20	0.72	—	—	—	360	—	91	0.00	0.00
0.03	0.03	0.46	0.05	0.00	19.6	4.1	—	0.3	22	0.86	13.0	34	237	121	0.3	87	0.00	0.00
0.05	0.07	0.87	0.15	0.00	32.8	6.9	—	0.6	38	1.17	27.3	67	251	47	0.9	90	0.00	0.00
—	—	—	—	0.00	—	9.0	—	—	20	1.08	—	—	0	330	—	88	0.00	0.00
—	—	—	—	—	—	—	—	—	—	—	—	—	—	640	—	—	0.00	0.00
0.17	0.14	0.74	0.07	0.00	73.2	3.2	—	0.3	42	2.27	42.0	130	370	461	0.6	76	0.00	0.00
0.41	0.10	0.87	0.11	0.00	256.3	0.0	—	0.1	46	3.60	120.4	241	611	2	1.9	66	0.00	0.00
0.07	0.11	1.15	0.05	0.00	104.8	1.8	—	0.2	106	0.92	42.9	42	345	3	0.8	75	0.00	0.00
0.34	0.09	0.85	0.17	0.00	357.8	0.7	—	0.5	41	4.32	91.2	268	478	7	2.2	70	0.00	0.00

Code	Food Name	Unit/ Amt	Wt (g)	Energy (kcal)	Prot (g)	Carb (g)	Fiber (g)	Fat (g)	Sat (g)	Mono (g)	Poly (g)	Chol (mg)	Vit A (RE)
7027	Beans, broad, mature, ckd	1 cup	170	187	13	33	9	1	0.1	0.1	0.3	0	3
7056	Beans, catjang cowpeas, ckd	1 cup	171	200	14	35	6	1	0.3	0.1	0.5	0	3
4441	Beans, chickpea, mature, ckd	0.5 cup	82	134	7	22	6	2	0.2	0.5	0.9	0	2
4465	Beans, cowpeas, immature, ckd, drained	1 cup	165	160	5	34	8	1	0.2	0.1	0.3	0	132
7018	Beans, cowpeas, mature, ckd	0.5 cup	86	100	7	18	6	0	0.1	0.0	0.2	0	2
4444	Beans, fava, mature, ckd	1 cup	170	187	13	33	9	1	0.1	0.1	0.3	0	3
7045	Beans, French, mature, ckd	1 cup	177	228	12	43	17	1	0.1	0.1	0.8	0	1
7175	Beans, garbanzo, cnd	0.5 cup	130	100	6	16	4	2	0.0	—	—	0	0
7001	Beans, garbanzo, mature, ckd	1 cup	164	269	15	45	12	4	0.4	1.0	1.9	0	3
7031	Beans, goa, mature, ckd	1 cup	172	253	18	26	4	10	1.4	3.7	2.7	0	0
7219	Beans, golden gram, mature, ckd	0.5 cup	101	106	7	19	8	0	0.1	0.1	0.1	0	2
7021	Beans, great northern, mature, ckd	1 cup	177	209	15	37	12	1	0.2	0.0	0.3	0	0
6219	Beans, green, cut, fzn	0.5 cup	83	25	1	6	2	0	0.0	—	—	0	44
6220	Beans, green, French cut, fzn	0.5 cup	83	25	1	6	2	0	0.0	—	—	0	38
5013	Beans, green, snap, ckd f/fzn, drained	1 cup	135	38	2	9	4	0	0.1	0.0	0.1	0	76
5856	Beans, green, snap, ckd w/salt, drained	1 cup	125	44	2	10	4	0	0.1	0.0	0.2	0	88
5009	Beans, green, snap, fresh	0.5 cup	55	17	1	4	2	0	0.0	0.0	0.0	0	38
6198	Beans, green, whole, deluxe, fzn	10 ea	40	11	1	2	1	0	0.0	—	—	0	27
6241	Beans, green, whole, fzn	21 ea	84	22	1	5	2	0	0.0	—	—	0	58
7008	Beans, kidney, all types, mature, ckd	1 cup	177	225	15	40	11	1	0.1	0.1	0.5	0	0
7047	Beans, kidney, red, mature, ckd	1 cup	177	225	15	40	13	1	0.1	0.1	0.5	0	0
7006	Beans, lentils, ckd f/dry w/o salt	0.5 cup	99	115	9	20	8	0	0.1	0.1	0.2	0	1
90019	Beans, lentils, mature, ckd w/salt	1 cup	198	230	18	40	16	1	0.1	0.1	0.3	0	2
6222	Beans, lima, baby, fzn	0.5 cup	94	126	7	24	6	0	0.1	—	—	0	22
7058	Beans, lima, baby, mature, ckd	0.5 cup	91	115	7	21	7	0	0.1	0.0	0.2	0	0
7010	Beans, lima, lrg, mature, ckd	1 cup	188	216	15	39	13	1	0.2	0.1	0.3	0	0
7059	Beans, mung, mature, ckd	0.5 cup	101	106	7	19	8	0	0.1	0.1	0.1	0	2
7022	Beans, navy, mature, ckd	1 cup	182	255	15	47	19	1	0.1	0.2	0.6	0	0
7050	Beans, pink, mature, ckd	1 cup	169	252	15	47	9	1	0.2	0.1	0.4	0	0
7013	Beans, pinto, mature, ckd	1 cup	171	245	15	45	15	1	0.2	0.2	0.3	0	0
7053	Beans, white, mature, ckd	1 cup	179	249	17	45	11	1	0.2	0.1	0.3	0	0
57290	Dish, green beans, French cut, w/toasted almonds, fzn	0.66 cup	81	51	2	6	2	3	0.3	—	—	0	33
5939	Peas, green, ckd f/fzn w/salt, drained	0.5 cup	80	62	4	11	4	0	0.0	0.0	0.1	0	53
5938	Peas, green, ckd w/salt, drained	0.5 cup	80	67	4	13	4	0	0.0	0.0	0.1	0	64
5116	Peas, green, fresh	1 cup	145	117	8	21	7	1	0.1	0.1	0.3	0	110
6226	Peas, green, fzn	0.5 cup	89	71	5	13	5	0	0.1	—	—	0	62
7020	Peas, split, ckd	1 cup	196	231	16	41	16	1	0.1	0.2	0.3	0	1
6364	Peas, sweet, fzn	0.66 cup	94	60	4	12	4	0	0.0	0.0	0.0	0	30
5971	Soybeans, green, ckd w/salt, drained	0.5 cup	90	127	11	10	4	6	0.7	1.1	2.7	0	14
7015	Soybeans, mature, ckd	1.25 cup	215	372	36	21	13	19	2.8	4.3	10.9	0	2
90028	Soybeans, mature, ckd w/salt	1.25 cup	215	372	36	21	13	19	2.8	4.3	10.9	0	2
5123	Vegetables, peas & carrots, ckd f/fzn, drnd	0.5 cup	80	38	2	8	2	0	0.1	0.0	0.2	0	749
Potatoes													
6179	Dish, baked potato & broccoli, w/cheese sauce	1 ea	339	403	14	47	—	21	8.5	7.7	4.2	20	315
5464	Dish, mashed potatoes, flakes, prep f/dry w/milk & butter	0.5 cup	105	102	2	11	1	5	2.9	1.2	0.1	15	46
5138	Dish, mashed potatoes, flakes, prep f/dry w/milk & margarine	0.5 cup	105	119	2	16	2	6	1.5	2.4	1.6	4	52

Thia (mg)	Ribo (mg)	Niac (mg NE)	Vit B6 (mg)	Vit B12 (μg)	Fol (μg)	Vit C (mg)	Vit D (IU)	Vit E (mg AT)	Cal (mg)	Iron (mg)	Magn (mg)	Phos (mg)	Pota (mg)	Sodi (mg)	Zinc (mg)	Wat (%)	Alco (g)	Caff (mg)
0.15	0.15	1.21	0.11	0.00	176.8	0.5	—	0.0	61	2.54	73.1	212	456	8	1.7	72	0.00	0.00
0.28	0.07	1.22	0.15	0.00	242.8	0.7	—	0.6	44	5.21	164.2	243	641	32	3.2	70	0.00	0.00
0.10	0.05	0.43	0.10	0.00	141.0	1.1	—	0.3	40	2.36	39.4	138	239	6	1.3	60	0.00	0.00
0.17	0.23	2.30	0.10	0.00	209.6	3.6	—	0.4	211	1.85	85.8	84	690	7	1.7	75	0.00	0.00
0.17	0.05	0.43	0.09	0.00	178.9	0.3	—	0.2	21	2.16	45.6	134	239	3	1.1	70	0.00	0.00
0.15	0.15	1.21	0.11	0.00	176.8	0.5	—	0.0	61	2.54	73.1	212	456	8	1.7	72	0.00	0.00
0.23	0.10	0.97	0.18	0.00	132.8	2.1	—	0.2	112	1.90	99.1	181	655	11	1.1	67	0.00	0.00
—	—	—	—	—	—	0.0	—	—	40	1.44	—	—	—	340	—	—	0.00	0.00
0.18	0.10	0.86	0.23	0.00	282.1	2.1	—	0.6	80	4.73	78.7	276	477	11	2.5	60	0.00	0.00
0.50	0.21	1.42	0.07	0.00	17.2	0.0	—	0.2	244	7.44	92.9	263	482	22	2.5	67	0.00	0.00
0.17	0.05	0.57	0.07	0.00	160.6	1.0	—	0.2	27	1.40	48.5	100	269	2	0.8	73	0.00	0.00
0.28	0.10	1.21	0.20	0.00	180.5	2.3	—	0.5	120	3.76	88.5	292	692	4	1.6	69	0.00	0.00
0.03	0.07	0.02	0.03	0.00	10.8	8.9	—	—	35	0.70	16.6	22	128	3	—	—	0.00	0.00
0.05	0.07	0.25	0.03	0.00	11.1	7.6	—	—	38	0.79	18.3	21	141	3	—	—	0.00	0.00
0.05	0.11	0.51	0.07	0.00	31.1	5.5	—	0.5	66	1.19	32.4	42	170	12	0.6	91	0.00	0.00
0.09	0.11	0.76	0.07	0.00	41.2	12.1	—	0.6	58	1.60	31.2	49	374	299	0.5	89	0.00	0.00
0.05	0.05	0.40	0.03	0.00	20.4	9.0	—	0.2	20	0.56	13.8	21	115	3	0.1	90	0.00	0.00
0.01	0.03	0.11	0.01	0.00	4.7	4.3	—	—	15	0.31	8.0	10	71	1	—	—	0.00	0.00
0.05	0.07	0.25	0.03	0.00	9.8	9.1	—	—	32	0.64	16.8	21	149	2	—	—	0.00	0.00
0.28	0.10	1.01	0.20	0.00	230.1	2.1	—	0.1	62	3.93	74.3	244	717	2	1.8	67	0.00	0.00
0.28	0.10	1.01	0.20	0.00	230.1	2.1	—	1.5	50	5.19	79.7	251	713	4	1.9	67	0.00	0.00
0.17	0.07	1.04	0.18	0.00	179.2	1.5	—	0.1	19	3.29	35.6	178	365	2	1.3	70	0.00	0.00
0.33	0.14	2.09	0.34	0.00	358.4	3.0	—	0.2	38	6.59	71.3	356	731	471	2.5	70	0.00	0.00
0.09	0.07	1.12	0.15	0.00	83.2	18.0	—	—	32	1.85	45.1	96	471	114	0.9	65	0.00	0.00
0.15	0.05	0.60	0.07	0.00	136.5	0.0	—	0.2	26	2.18	48.2	116	365	3	0.9	67	0.00	0.00
0.30	0.10	0.79	0.30	0.00	156.0	0.0	—	0.3	32	4.48	80.8	209	955	4	1.8	70	0.00	0.00
0.17	0.05	0.57	0.07	0.00	160.6	1.0	—	0.2	27	1.40	48.5	100	269	2	0.8	73	0.00	0.00
0.43	0.11	1.17	0.25	0.00	254.8	1.6	—	0.0	126	4.30	96.5	262	708	0	1.9	64	0.00	0.00
0.43	0.10	0.95	0.30	0.00	283.9	0.0	—	1.7	88	3.89	109.9	279	859	3	1.6	61	0.00	0.00
0.33	0.10	0.54	0.38	0.00	294.1	1.4	—	1.6	79	3.56	85.5	251	746	2	1.7	63	0.00	0.00
0.20	0.07	0.25	0.17	0.00	145.0	0.0	—	1.7	161	6.61	112.8	202	1004	11	2.5	63	0.00	0.00
—	—	—	—	0.00	—	6.6	—	—	42	1.08	—	—	—	347	—	—	0.00	0.00
0.23	0.07	1.17	0.09	0.00	47.2	7.9	—	0.1	19	1.25	23.2	72	134	258	0.8	80	0.00	0.00
0.20	0.11	1.62	0.17	0.00	50.4	11.4	—	0.1	22	1.23	31.2	94	217	191	1.0	78	0.00	0.00
0.38	0.18	3.02	0.25	0.00	94.2	58.0	—	0.2	36	2.13	47.9	157	354	7	1.8	79	0.00	0.00
0.28	0.09	1.96	0.11	0.00	49.2	17.8	—	—	21	1.41	22.2	79	152	125	0.9	79	0.00	0.00
0.37	0.10	1.74	0.09	0.00	127.4	0.8	—	0.1	27	2.52	70.6	194	710	4	2.0	69	0.00	0.00
—	—	—	—	0.00	—	6.0	—	—	0	1.08	—	—	—	200	—	—	0.00	0.00
0.23	0.14	1.12	0.05	0.00	99.9	15.3	—	0.0	130	2.25	54.0	142	485	225	0.8	69	0.00	0.00
0.33	0.61	0.86	0.50	0.00	116.1	3.7	—	0.8	219	11.05	184.9	527	1107	2	2.5	63	0.00	0.00
0.33	0.61	0.86	0.50	0.00	116.1	3.7	—	0.8	219	11.05	184.9	527	1107	510	2.5	63	0.00	0.00
0.18	0.05	0.92	0.07	0.00	20.8	6.5	—	0.4	18	0.75	12.8	39	126	54	0.4	86	0.00	0.00
0.27	0.27	3.58	0.77	0.34	61.0	48.5	—	—	336	3.31	78.0	346	1441	485	2.0	70	0.00	0.00
0.14	0.05	0.80	0.10	0.11	6.3	10.6	12.9	0.1	30	0.17	11.5	41	170	172	0.2	81	0.00	0.00
0.11	0.05	0.69	0.00	0.00	7.3	10.2	—	0.7	51	0.23	18.9	59	245	349	0.2	76	0.00	0.00

PAGE KEY: 2 Beverage and Beverage Mixes   4 Other Beverages   4 Beverages, Alcoholic   6 Candies and Confections, Gum   10 Cereals, Breakfast Type
14 Cheese and Cheese Substitutes   16 Dairy Products and Substitutes   18 Desserts   24 Dessert Toppings   24 Eggs, Substitutes, and Egg Dishes   26 Ethnic Foods
30 Fast Foods/Restaurants   44 Fats, Oils, Margarines, Shortenings, and Substitutes   44 Fish, Seafood, and Shellfish   46 Food Additives
46 Fruit, Vegetable, or Blended Juices   48 Grains, Flours, and Fractions   48 Grain Products, Prepared and Baked Goods

Code	Food Name	Unit/ Amt	Wt (g)	Energy (kcal)	Prot (g)	Carb (g)	Fiber (g)	Fat (g)	Sat (g)	Mono (g)	Poly (g)	Chol (mg)	Vit A (RE)
66107	Dish, mashed potatoes, real, premium, prep	0.5 cup	108	63	2	13	1	1	0.1	0.4	0.1	0	0
5137	Dish, mashed potatoes, w/whole milk	0.5 cup	105	87	2	18	2	1	0.3	0.1	0.1	2	4
5569	Dish, mashed potatoes, w/whole milk & butter	0.5 cup	105	119	2	18	2	4	1.8	1.3	0.2	12	38
5272	Dish, mashed potatoes, w/whole milk & margarine	0.5 cup	105	119	2	18	2	4	1.0	1.8	1.3	1	45
5786	Dish, potatoes au gratin, prep f/recipe w/butter	1 cup	245	323	12	28	4	19	11.6	5.3	0.7	56	164
5275	Dish, potatoes au gratin, prep f/recipe w/margarine	1 cup	245	323	12	28	4	19	8.6	6.3	2.6	37	167
70605	Dish, potatoes o'brien	0.5 cup	78	56	1	12	2	0	0.0	0.0	0.0	0	0
5787	Dish, potatoes o'brien, fzn	0.5 cup	97	74	2	17	2	0	0.0	0.0	0.1	—	14
5268	Dish, potatoes o'brien, prep f/recipe	1 cup	97	79	2	15	1	1	0.8	0.3	0.1	4	93
57362	Dish, potatoes, au gratin, prep f/dry	3 oz	85	90	3	14	—	2	—	—	—	—	—
70612	Dish, twice baked potatoes, w/butter	1 ea	143	204	4	27	4	9	3.1	3.1	0.5	0	86
5948	Potatoes, baked, peeled, salted	0.5 cup	61	57	1	13	1	0	0.0	0.0	0.0	0	0
5130	Potatoes, baked, peeled, unsalted	0.5 cup	61	57	1	13	1	0	0.0	0.0	0.0	0	0
6996	Potatoes, baked, salted	0.5 cup	61	57	2	13	1	0	0.0	0.0	0.0	0	1
5334	Potatoes, baked, unsalted, med, 2 1/4" to 3 1/4"	1 ea	173	161	4	37	4	0	0.1	0.0	0.1	0	3
7259	Potatoes, dehyd	100 g	100	367	8	81	3	1	—	—	—	—	0
5691	Potatoes, french fries, battered, shoestring, 80% ckd, fzn	3 oz	85	170	4	17	1	10	2.5	—	—	0	0
8900	Potatoes, french fries, crinkle, 1/2" x 1/2", 80% ckd, fzn	3 oz	85	170	3	24	2	7	2.0	—	—	0	0
5790	Potatoes, french fries, fzn	10 ea	65	101	2	16	2	4	0.6	2.4	0.4	0	0
5592	Potatoes, french fries, heated f/fzn w/o salt	10 ea	50	100	2	16	2	4	0.6	2.4	0.4	0	0
6413	Potatoes, french fries, waffle style	15 pce	84	140	2	22	2	5	1.5	2.0	0.0	0	0
6851	Potatoes, fresh, w/skin, med, 2 1/4" to 3 1/4"	1 ea	213	164	4	37	5	0	0.1	0.0	0.1	0	0
70611	Potatoes, hash browns, box, microw	3.6 oz	100	193	2	23	1	10	2.6	3.5	0.0	0	0
70603	Potatoes, hash browns, shredded	0.5 cup	78	62	2	14	1	5	1.9	2.1	0.6	0	0
6402	Potatoes, patty, golden	1 ea	71	140	1	16	1	7	1.5	3.5	0.5	0	0
9250	Potatoes, red, w/skin, baked, med, 2 1/4" to 3 1/4"	1 ea	173	154	4	34	3	0	0.0	0.0	0.1	0	3
5512	Potatoes, rstd	1 ea	93	132	3	30	3	0	0.0	0.0	0.1	0	0
57368	Potatoes, scalloped, prep	3 oz	85	90	2	16	—	2	—	—	—	—	—
5339	Potatoes, skin, bkd	1 ea	58	115	2	27	5	0	0.0	0.0	0.0	0	1
70598	Potatoes, tater tots	0.5 cup	62	107	1	16	1	6	1.1	1.8	0.0	0	0
9247	Potatoes, w/skin, baked, med, 2 1/4"–3 1/4"	1 ea	173	163	4	36	4	0	0.0	0.0	0.1	0	3
7906	Potatoes, wedges, USDA, fzn	3 oz	85	105	2	22	2	2	0.5	1.2	0.1	0	0
5162	Sweetpotatoes, mashed f/cnd	1 cup	256	259	5	59	4	1	0.1	0.0	0.2	0	0

WEIGHT LOSS BARS & DRINKS

Weight Loss Bars

Code	Food Name	Unit/ Amt	Wt (g)	Energy (kcal)	Prot (g)	Carb (g)	Fiber (g)	Fat (g)	Sat (g)	Mono (g)	Poly (g)	Chol (mg)	Vit A (RE)
63408	Bar, diet, chocolate chip	1 ea	50	200	16	17	0	8	4.0	—	—	3	350
63370	Bar, diet, cranberry apple, granola	1 ea	56	220	8	35	1	5	3.5	—	—	5	150
8975	Bar, diet, hi prot & low carbohydrate, peanut butter	1 ea	50	190	22	2	0	5	2.5	—	—	0	0
62875	Bar, diet, hi prot, peanut butter	1 ea	70	250	30	11	2	6	3.5	—	—	0	0
62855	Bar, diet, oatmeal raisin	1 ea	56	220	8	36	2	5	3.5	—	—	3	350
62639	Bar, diet, peanut butter, breakfast & lunch	1 ea	34	150	5	19	2	6	2.5	—	—	5	250
63372	Bar, diet, peanut butter, granola	1 ea	56	220	8	35	1	6	3.5	—	—	5	150

Weight Loss Drinks

Code	Food Name	Unit/ Amt	Wt (g)	Energy (kcal)	Prot (g)	Carb (g)	Fiber (g)	Fat (g)	Sat (g)	Mono (g)	Poly (g)	Chol (mg)	Vit A (RE)
62854	Drink, diet, cappuccino, milk base, rtd can	1 ea	345	220	10	42	5	1	0.5	0.5	0.0	5	350
62648	Drink, diet, choc fudge, milk base, rtd can	1 ea	345	220	10	42	5	3	1.0	1.5	0.5	5	350
63359	Drink, diet, chocolate, soy prot, rtd can	1 ea	345	230	12	39	5	3	1.0	1.5	0.5	0	350

Thia (mg)	Ribo (mg)	Niac (mg NE)	Vit B6 (mg)	Vit B12 (µg)	Fol (µg)	Vit C (mg)	Vit D (IU)	Vit E (mg AT)	Cal (mg)	Iron (mg)	Magn (mg)	Phos (mg)	Pota (mg)	Sodi (mg)	Zinc (mg)	Wat (%)	Alco (g)	Caff (mg)
0.05	0.00	1.19	—	—	—	2.6	—	—	17	0.27	7.8	23	189	245	—	84	0.00	0.00
0.09	0.05	1.17	0.23	0.07	8.4	6.5	6.4	0.0	23	0.28	18.9	48	311	317	0.3	79	0.00	0.00
0.09	0.05	1.12	0.23	0.07	8.4	6.3	8.7	0.1	23	0.27	18.9	47	298	333	0.3	76	0.00	0.00
0.10	0.05	1.23	0.25	0.07	9.4	11.0	6.0	0.4	21	0.27	19.9	50	342	350	0.3	75	0.00	0.00
0.15	0.28	2.43	0.43	0.00	27.0	24.3	—	0.5	292	1.57	49.0	277	970	1061	1.7	74	0.00	0.00
0.15	0.28	2.43	0.43	0.00	27.0	24.3	—	1.3	292	1.57	49.0	277	970	1061	1.7	74	0.00	0.00
0.07	0.01	1.19	—	0.00	—	3.7	—	—	0	0.00	—	—	148	14	—	82	0.00	0.00
0.05	0.03	1.10	0.20	0.00	7.8	11.0	—	0.2	13	1.00	17.5	48	242	32	0.3	80	0.00	0.00
0.07	0.05	0.98	0.20	0.00	7.8	16.2	—	0.1	35	0.46	17.5	48	258	210	0.3	80	0.00	0.00
0.02	0.07	0.80	—	0.00	—	2.4	—	—	40	0.36	16.0	60	265	340	—	75	0.00	0.00
0.09	0.10	3.03	—	0.00	—	21.4	—	—	57	1.02	—	—	601	357	—	—	0.00	0.00
0.05	0.00	0.85	0.18	0.00	5.5	7.8	—	0.0	3	0.20	15.2	30	239	147	0.2	75	0.00	0.00
0.05	0.00	0.85	0.18	0.00	5.5	7.8	—	0.0	3	0.20	15.2	30	239	3	0.2	75	0.00	0.00
0.03	0.02	0.86	0.18	0.00	17.1	5.9	—	0.0	9	0.66	17.1	43	326	149	0.2	75	0.00	0.00
0.10	0.07	2.44	0.54	0.00	48.4	16.6	—	0.1	26	1.87	48.4	121	926	17	0.6	75	0.00	0.00
0.23	0.15	3.70	—	0.00	—	11.0	—	—	27	2.79	—	200	922	8	—	6	0.00	0.00
—	—	—	—	—	—	3.6	—	—	0	0.36	—	—	—	190	—	63	0.00	0.00
—	—	—	—	—	—	9.0	—	—	0	1.08	—	—	—	25	—	59	0.00	0.00
0.07	0.00	1.11	0.15	0.00	7.8	6.4	—	0.1	4	0.62	11.0	42	212	15	0.2	67	0.00	0.00
0.05	0.00	1.03	0.15	0.00	6.0	5.1	0.0	0.1	4	0.62	11.0	41	209	15	0.2	57	0.00	0.00
—	—	—	—	0.00	—	2.4	—	—	0	1.44	—	—	290	35	—	—	0.00	0.00
0.17	0.07	2.25	0.62	0.00	34.1	42.0	0.0	0.0	26	1.65	49.0	121	897	13	0.6	79	0.00	0.00
0.07	—	1.57	—	0.00	—	0.0	—	—	0	0.00	—	—	246	263	—	64	0.00	0.00
—	—	—	—	—	—	7.1	—	—	6	0.58	—	—	355	25	—	73	0.00	0.00
—	—	—	—	0.00	—	0.0	—	—	0	0.00	—	—	120	280	—	—	0.00	0.00
0.11	0.09	2.75	0.37	0.00	46.7	21.8	—	0.1	16	1.21	48.4	125	943	14	0.7	77	0.00	0.00
0.11	0.05	2.34	0.40	0.00	19.2	26.3	0.0	0.1	12	1.26	35.0	77	905	10	0.7	62	0.00	0.00
0.02	0.07	0.80	—	0.00	—	2.4	—	—	40	0.36	16.0	60	245	300	—	75	0.00	0.00
0.07	0.05	1.77	0.36	0.00	12.8	7.8	—	0.0	20	4.07	24.9	59	332	12	0.3	47	0.00	0.00
—	—	—	—	—	—	0.7	—	—	0	0.00	—	—	162	251	—	61	0.00	0.00
0.07	0.07	2.64	0.37	0.00	65.7	21.8	—	0.1	17	1.11	46.7	130	941	12	0.6	75	0.00	0.00
0.09	0.02	1.30	0.30	0.00	—	9.5	—	—	13	0.60	16.2	74	335	42	0.3	68	0.00	0.00
0.07	0.23	2.44	0.60	0.00	28.2	13.3	—	0.7	77	3.40	61.4	133	538	192	0.5	74	0.00	0.00
0.21	0.60	7.00	0.69	2.09	60.0	21.0	140.0	4.8	300	2.70	140.0	400	400	200	2.2	—	0.00	—
0.21	0.60	7.00	0.69	2.09	60.0	21.0	140.0	4.8	300	2.70	140.0	400	400	230	2.2	—	0.00	0.00
—	—	—	—	—	—	0.0	—	—	160	1.00	—	—	—	120	—	—	0.00	—
—	—	—	—	—	—	0.0	—	—	200	1.10	—	—	—	120	—	—	0.00	—
0.21	0.60	7.00	0.69	2.09	60.0	21.0	140.0	4.8	300	2.70	140.0	250	170	100	2.2	—	0.00	0.00
0.37	0.43	5.00	0.40	1.50	40.0	15.0	80.0	3.4	100	4.50	16.0	100	115	65	3.8	—	0.00	—
0.21	0.60	7.00	0.69	2.09	60.0	21.0	140.0	4.8	3000	2.70	140.0	400	400	320	2.2	—	0.00	—
0.51	0.60	7.00	0.69	2.09	120.0	60.0	140.0	13.6	400	2.70	140.0	400	600	220	2.2	—	0.00	—
0.51	0.60	7.00	0.69	2.09	120.0	60.0	140.0	13.6	400	2.70	140.0	400	600	220	2.2	—	0.00	—
0.44	0.50	6.00	0.60	2.09	160.0	30.0	120.0	3.4	400	4.50	100.0	300	700	420	3.8	—	0.00	—

94

PAGE KEY: 2 Beverage and Beverage Mixes   4 Other Beverages   4 Beverages, Alcoholic   6 Candies and Confections, Gum   10 Cereals, Breakfast Type
14 Cheese and Cheese Substitutes   16 Dairy Products and Substitutes   18 Desserts   24 Dessert Toppings   24 Eggs, Substitutes, and Egg Dishes   26 Ethnic Foods
30 Fast Foods/Restaurants   44 Fats, Oils, Margarines, Shortenings, and Substitutes   44 Fish, Seafood, and Shellfish   46 Food Additives
46 Fruit, Vegetable, or Blended Juices   48 Grains, Flours, and Fractions   48 Grain Products, Prepared and Baked Goods

Code	Food Name	Unit/ Amt	Wt (g)	Energy (kcal)	Prot (g)	Carb (g)	Fiber (g)	Fat (g)	Sat (g)	Mono (g)	Poly (g)	Chol (mg)	Vit A (RE)
62650	Drink, diet, milk choc, milk base, rtd can	1 ea	345	220	10	40	5	3	1.0	1.5	0.5	5	350
62646	Drink, diet, orange pineapple, rtd can	1 ea	360	220	7	46	5	1	0.0	0.0	0.0	5	500
62649	Drink, diet, straw cream, milk base, rtd can	1 ea	345	220	10	40	5	2	0.5	1.5	0.5	5	350
63374	Drink, diet, vanilla cream, low carb, rtd can	1 ea	350	190	20	7	5	9	1.5	6.0	1.5	15	350
63024	Shake, weight management, chocolate fudge, rtd	1 ea	250	100	15	5	—	2	0.0	—	—	15	150
63025	Shake, weight management, vanilla, rtd	1 ea	250	90	15	3	1	2	0.0	—	—	15	150
MISCELLANEOUS													
Baking Chips, Chocolates, Coatings, and Cocoas													
23519	Baking Chips, chocolate	31 pce	15	72	1	9	1	4	3.0	—	—	0	1
23012	Baking Chips, chocolate, semi sweet	10 pce	5	23	0	3	0	1	0.8	0.5	0.0	0	0
23200	Baking Chips, chocolate, semi sweet, w/butter	60 pce	28	135	1	18	2	8	5.0	2.8	0.3	5	2
23423	Baking Chips, M & M's, milk chocolate, mini bits	1 Tbs	14	71	1	10	0	3	2.1	1.1	0.1	2	6
23444	Baking Chips, milk chocolate, mini kisses	11 ea	15	80	1	9	0	4	3.0	—	—	5	0
4153	Baking Chips, Nestle Crunch, pieces	1.5 Tbs	15	80	1	10	0	4	2.0	—	—	0	0
23446	Baking Chips, Reese's peanut butter	1 Tbs	15	80	3	7	—	4	4.0	—	—	0	0
28299	Baking Chips, white chocolate, chunks	15 g	15	80	1	9	0	5	3.0	—	—	5	0
23401	Baking Chocolate, bar, semi sweet	0.5 oz	14	70	1	8	1	4	2.5	—	—	0	0
28063	Baking Chocolate, bar, unswtnd	0.5 oz	14	70	2	4	2	7	4.5	—	—	0	0
4355	Baking Chocolate, bar, white, premium	0.5 oz	14	80	1	8	0	4	3.0	—	—	5	0
28208	Baking Chocolate, unswntd, liquid	1 Tbs	15	71	2	5	3	7	3.8	1.4	1.6	0	0
28200	Cocoa Powder, unswntd	1 cup	86	197	17	47	29	12	6.9	3.9	0.4	0	0
Baking Ingredients													
28006	Baking Powder, low sod	1 tsp	5	5	0	2	0	0	0.0	0.0	0.0	0	0
28003	Baking Soda	1 tsp	5	0	0	0	0	0	0.0	0.0	0.0	0	0
51150	Candied Fruit	3.6 oz	100	321	0	83	2	0	0.0	0.0	0.0	0	2
26017	Cream of Tartar	1 tsp	3	8	0	2	0	0	0.0	0.0	0.0	0	0
3977	Pineapple, slices, natural glace	1 pce	63	180	0	46	0	0	0.0	0.0	0.0	0	0
28149	Yeast, active, dry	3.6 oz	100	333	39	43	24	5	1.2	2.6	0.8	0	0
28000	Yeast, baker's, dry active	1 tsp	4	12	2	2	1	0	0.0	0.1	0.0	0	0
Condiments													
9149	Catsup	1 Tbs	15	15	0	4	0	0	0.0	0.0	0.0	0	14
27032	Catsup, low sod	1 Tbs	15	16	0	4	0	0	0.0	0.0	0.0	0	16
90602	Catsup, low sod, pkt	1 ea	6	6	0	2	0	0	0.0	0.0	0.0	0	6
27004	Horseradish, prep	1 tsp	5	2	0	1	0	0	0.0	0.0	0.0	0	0
27000	Ketchup	1 Tbs	15	15	0	4	0	0	0.0	0.0	0.0	0	14
9151	Ketchup, low sod	1 Tbs	15	16	0	4	0	0	0.0	0.0	0.0	0	16
9152	Ketchup, low sod, pkt	1 ea	6	6	0	2	0	0	0.0	0.0	0.0	0	6
90931	Mustard, deli	100 g	100	113	5	10	6	7	0.3	—	—	0	4
27058	Mustard, dijon, Grey Poupon	0.5 cup	125	151	8	13	1	11	0.5	3.9	3.0	0	12
53254	Mustard, honey	1 ea	14	50	0	3	0	4	0.5	—	—	10	2
91801	Mustard, honey, fat free	1.5 Tbs	21	30	0	7	0	0	0.0	0.0	0.0	0	0
27070	Mustard, hot, pkt	1 ea	28	60	1	7	1	4	0.0	—	—	5	4
435	Mustard, yellow, prep	1 tsp	5	3	0	0	0	0	0.0	0.1	0.0	0	1
90211	Mustard, yellow, prep, pkt	1 ea	5	3	0	0	0	0	0.0	0.1	0.0	0	1
7523	Sauce, soy, dark	0.5 tsp	3	0	0	0	0	0	0.0	0.0	0.0	0	0

PAGE KEY: 52 Granola Bars, Cereal Bars, Diet Bars, Scones, and Tarts 52 Meals and Dishes 56 Meats 62 Nuts, Seeds, and Products 64 Poultry 66 Salad Dressings, Dips, and Mayonnaise 66 Salads 68 Sandwiches 70 Sauces and Gravies 70 Snack Foods—Chips, Pretzels, Popcorn 72 Soups, Stews, and Chilis 74 Spices, Flavors, and Seasonings 76 Sports Bars and Drinks 76 Supplemental Foods and Formulas 78 Sweeteners and Sweet Substitutes 78 Vegetables and Legumes 92 Weight Loss Bars and Drinks 94 Miscellaneous

Thia (mg)	Ribo (mg)	Niac (mg NE)	Vit B6 (mg)	Vit B12 (µg)	Fol (µg)	Vit C (mg)	Vit D (IU)	Vit E (mg AT)	Cal (mg)	Iron (mg)	Magn (mg)	Phos (mg)	Pota (mg)	Sodi (mg)	Zinc (mg)	Wat (%)	Alco (g)	Caff (mg)
0.51	0.60	7.00	0.69	2.09	120.0	60.0	140.0	13.6	400	2.70	140.0	400	600	220	2.2	—	0.00	—
0.51	0.60	7.00	0.69	2.09	120.0	60.0	140.0	13.6	350	2.70	140.0	400	500	180	2.2	—	0.00	0.00
0.51	0.60	7.00	0.69	2.09	120.0	60.0	140.0	13.6	400	2.70	140.0	400	600	220	2.2	—	0.00	0.00
0.51	0.60	2.00	0.20	0.60	120.0	60.0	140.0	13.6	400	2.70	140.0	400	400	200	2.2	—	0.00	0.00
0.30	0.34	0.40	—	1.50	120.0	15.0	—	4.1	100	0.00	80.0	150	280	170	3.0	—	0.00	—
0.30	0.34	—	0.40	1.50	120.0	—	—	4.1	100	0.00	80.0	150	170	170	3.0	—	0.00	0.00
—	—	—	—	—	—	0.0	—	—	5	2.00	—	—	—	31	—	4	0.00	—
0.00	0.00	0.01	0.00	0.00	0.1	0.0	—	0.0	2	0.15	5.4	6	17	1	0.1	1	0.00	2.93
0.01	0.02	0.11	0.00	0.00	0.9	0.0	—	0.3	9	0.88	32.6	37	103	3	0.5	1	0.00	17.57
0.00	0.02	0.02	0.00	0.03	0.7	0.1	—	0.1	16	0.17	6.5	24	42	10	0.2	2	0.00	2.50
—	—	—	—	—	—	0.0	—	—	20	0.00	—	—	—	15	—	2	0.00	—
—	—	—	—	—	—	0.0	—	—	0	0.00	—	—	—	25	—	2	0.00	—
—	—	—	—	—	—	0.0	—	—	0	0.00	—	—	—	35	—	—	0.00	0.00
—	—	—	—	—	—	0.0	—	—	20	0.00	—	—	—	15	—	0	0.00	—
—	—	—	—	—	—	0.0	—	—	0	0.72	—	—	—	0	—	3	0.00	—
—	—	—	—	—	—	0.0	—	—	0	1.44	—	—	—	0	—	4	0.00	—
—	—	—	—	—	—	0.0	—	—	20	0.00	—	—	—	15	—	3	0.00	—
0.00	0.03	0.31	0.00	0.00	2.9	0.0	—	0.9	8	0.62	39.8	51	175	2	0.6	1	0.00	7.05
0.07	0.20	1.87	0.10	0.00	27.5	0.0	—	0.1	110	11.92	429.1	631	1311	18	5.9	3	0.00	197.80
0.00	0.00	0.00	0.00	0.00	0.0	0.0	—	0.0	217	0.40	1.5	343	505	4	0.0	6	0.00	0.00
0.00	0.00	0.00	0.00	0.00	0.0	0.0	—	0.0	0	0.00	0.0	0	0	1259	0.0	0	0.00	0.00
0.00	0.00	0.00	0.00	0.00	0.0	0.0	—	0.0	18	0.17	4.0	5	57	98	0.1	17	0.00	0.00
0.00	0.00	0.00	0.00	0.00	0.0	0.0	—	0.0	0	0.10	0.1	0	495	2	0.0	2	0.00	0.00
—	—	—	0.00	—	—	0.0	—	—	0	0.00	—	—	5	40	—	27	0.00	0.00
10.00	5.00	41.00	—	—	—	6.0	—	—	73	6.00	—	898	1361	259	—	8	0.00	0.00
0.09	0.21	1.59	0.05	0.00	93.6	0.0	—	0.0	3	0.66	3.9	52	80	2	0.3	8	0.00	0.00
0.00	0.07	0.23	0.01	0.00	1.5	2.3	—	0.2	3	0.07	2.9	5	57	166	0.0	68	0.00	0.00
0.00	0.00	0.20	0.02	0.00	2.2	2.3	—	0.2	3	0.10	3.3	6	72	3	0.0	67	0.00	0.00
0.00	0.00	0.07	0.00	0.00	0.9	0.9	—	0.1	1	0.03	1.3	2	29	1	0.0	67	0.00	0.00
0.00	0.00	0.01	0.00	0.00	2.9	1.2	—	0.0	3	0.01	1.4	2	12	16	0.0	85	0.00	0.00
0.00	0.07	0.23	0.01	0.00	1.5	2.3	—	0.2	3	0.07	2.9	5	57	166	0.0	68	0.00	0.00
0.00	0.00	0.20	0.02	0.00	2.2	2.3	—	0.2	3	0.10	3.3	6	72	3	0.0	67	0.00	0.00
0.00	0.00	0.07	0.00	0.00	0.9	0.9	—	0.1	1	0.03	1.3	2	29	1	0.0	67	0.00	0.00
—	—	—	—	—	—	0.0	—	—	113	2.09	—	—	—	1553	—	74	0.00	0.00
0.17	0.11	2.55	0.10	0.00	0.0	1.0	—	—	170	3.25	—	273	222	3030	1.9	70	0.00	0.00
0.00	0.00	0.00	0.00	0.02	0.9	0.1	0.0	0.7	3	0.03	0.2	4	6	85	0.0	—	0.00	0.00
—	—	—	—	—	—	0.0	—	—	0	0.00	—	—	—	140	—	—	0.00	0.00
0.00	0.00	0.14	—	—	—	0.0	—	—	7	0.72	—	17	27	240	—	—	0.00	0.00
0.00	0.00	0.01	0.00	0.00	0.4	0.1	—	0.0	4	0.09	1.9	4	8	56	0.0	82	0.00	0.00
0.00	0.00	0.01	0.00	0.00	0.4	0.1	—	0.0	4	0.09	1.9	4	8	56	0.0	82	0.00	0.00
—	—	—	—	—	—	0.0	—	—	0	0.00	—	—	—	150	—	—	0.00	0.00

Code	Food Name	Unit/ Amt	Wt (g)	Energy (kcal)	Prot (g)	Carb (g)	Fiber (g)	Fat (g)	Sat (g)	Mono (g)	Poly (g)	Chol (mg)	Vit A (RE)
53614	Sauce, soy, light	1 Tbs	18	10	1	1	0	0	0.0	0.0	0.0	0	0
53530	Sauce, soy, low sod	1 Tbs	16	8	1	1	0	0	0.0	0.0	0.0	0	0
53471	Sauce, tabasco, rts	1 tsp	5	1	0	0	0	0	0.0	0.0	0.0	0	8
53099	Sauce, worcestershire	1 Tbs	17	11	0	3	0	0	0.0	0.0	0.0	0	2
53457	Vinegar, balsamic	1 Tbs	15	10	0	2	—	0	0.0	0.0	0.0	0	—
27007	Vinegar, cider	1 Tbs	15	2	0	1	0	0	0.0	0.0	0.0	0	0
92153	Vinegar, distilled	1 Tbs	17	2	0	1	0	0	0.0	0.0	0.0	0	0
27204	Vinegar, red wine	1 Tbs	16	0	0	0	0	0	0.0	0.0	0.0	0	0
Salsas													
92617	Salsa, lime & garlic	2 Tbs	32	15	0	3	1	0	0.0	0.0	0.0	0	40
92618	Salsa, rstd peppers & garlic	2 Tbs	32	10	0	2	1	0	0.0	0.0	0.0	0	40
53466	Salsa, rts	2 Tbs	32	9	0	2	1	0	0.0	0.0	0.0	0	10

Thia (mg)	Ribo (mg)	Niac (mg NE)	Vit B6 (mg)	Vit B12 (µg)	Fol (µg)	Vit C (mg)	Vit D (IU)	Vit E (mg AT)	Cal (mg)	Iron (mg)	Magn (mg)	Phos (mg)	Pota (mg)	Sodi (mg)	Zinc (mg)	Wat (%)	Alco (g)	Caff (mg)
—	—	—	—	—	—	0.0	—	—	0	0.00	—	—	—	605	—	—	0.00	0.00
0.00	0.01	0.54	0.02	0.00	2.5	0.0	—	0.0	3	0.31	5.4	18	29	533	0.1	71	0.00	0.00
0.00	0.00	0.00	0.00	0.00	0.0	0.2	—	—	1	0.05	0.6	1	6	30	0.0	95	0.00	0.00
0.00	0.01	0.11	0.00	0.00	1.4	2.2	—	0.0	18	0.89	2.2	10	136	167	0.0	79	0.00	0.00
—	—	—	—	—	—	—	—	—	—	—	—	—	—	5	—	—	—	0.00
0.00	0.00	0.00	0.00	0.00	0.0	0.0	—	0.0	1	0.09	3.3	1	15	0	0.0	94	0.00	0.00
0.00	0.00	0.00	0.00	0.00	0.0	0.0	—	0.0	0	0.00	3.7	0	3	0	0.0	95	0.00	0.00
—	—	—	—	—	—	0.0	—	—	0	0.00	—	—	0	0	—	100	0.00	0.00
—	—	—	—	—	—	1.8	—	—	0	0.00	—	—	—	210	—	89	0.00	0.00
—	—	—	—	—	—	0.0	—	—	0	0.00	—	—	—	230	—	92	0.00	0.00
0.00	0.00	0.01	0.05	0.00	1.3	0.6	—	0.4	9	0.15	4.9	10	96	194	0.1	90	0.00	0.00

Dietary Intake Assessment Forms

Although it may seem overwhelming at first, it is easy to track the foods you eat. One tip is to record foods and beverages consumed as soon as possible after consumption.

1. **Food Record Form.** To estimate the nutrient values of the foods you are eating, consult food labels and the food composition table in this book. If these resources do not have the serving size you need, adjust the value. If you drink ½ cup of orange juice, for example, but a table has values only for 1 cup, halve all values before you record them. Then, consider pooling all the same food to save time; if you drink a cup of 1% milk three times throughout the day, enter your milk consumption only once as 3 cups. As you record your intake for use on the nutrient analysis form that follows, consider the following tips:
   - Measure and record the amounts of foods eaten in portion sizes of cups, teaspoons, tablespoons, ounces, slices, or inches (or convert metric units to these units).
   - Record brand names of all food products, such as "Quick Quaker Oats."
   - Measure and record all those little extras, such as gravies, salad dressings, taco sauces, pickles, jelly, sugar, catsup, and margarine.
   - For beverages
     — List the type of milk, such as whole, fat-free, 1%, evaporated, chocolate, or reconstituted dry.
     — Indicate whether fruit juice is fresh, frozen, or canned.
     — Indicate type for other beverages, such as fruit drink, fruit-flavored drink, Kool-Aid, and hot chocolate made with water or milk.
   - For fruits
     —Indicate whether fresh, frozen, dried, or canned.
     —If whole, record number eaten and size with approximate measurements (such as 1 apple—3 in. in diameter).
     —Indicate whether processed in water, light syrup, or heavy syrup.
   - For vegetables
     — Indicate whether fresh, frozen, dried, or canned.
     — Record as portion of cup, teaspoon, or tablespoon, or as pieces (such as carrot sticks—4 in. long, ½ in. thick).
     — Record preparation method.

- For cereals
  - Record cooked cereals in portions of tablespoon or cup (a level measurement after cooking).
  - Record dry cereal in level portions of tablespoon or cup.
  - If margarine, milk, sugar, fruit, or something else is added, measure and record amount and type.
- For breads
  - Indicate whether whole wheat, rye, white, and so on.
  - Measure and record number and size of portion (biscuit—2 in. across, 1 in. thick; slice of homemade rye bread—3 in. by 4 in., ¼ in. thick).
  - Sandwiches: list all ingredients (lettuce, mayonnaise, tomato, and so on).
- For meat, fish, poultry, and cheese
  - Give size (length, width, thickness) in inches or weight in ounces after cooking for meat, fish, and poultry (such as cooked hamburger patty— 3 in. across, ½ in. thick).
  - Give size (length, width, thickness) in inches or weight in ounces for cheese.
  - Record measurements only for the cooked, edible part—without bone or fat left on the plate.
  - Describe how meat, poultry, or fish was prepared.
- For eggs
  - Record as soft or hard cooked, fried, scrambled, poached, or omelet.
  - If milk, butter, or drippings are used, specify types and amount.
- For desserts
  - List commercial brand or "homemade" or "bakery" under brand.
  - Purchased candies, cookies, and cakes: specify kind and size.
  - Measure and record portion size of cakes, pies, and cookies by specifying thickness, diameter, and width or length, depending on the item.

Food Record Form

Day	Meal	Food Eaten	Amount/Serving Size

II. **Nutrient Analysis Form.** A blank copy of this form is printed for your use.

Name	Quantity	kcal	Protein (g)	Carbohydrates (g)	Fiber (g)	Total fat (g)	Monounsaturated fat (g)	Polyunsaturated fat (g)	Saturated fat (g)	Cholesterol (g)	Calcium (mg)	Iron (mg)
Totals												
RDA or related nutrient standard*												
% of nutrient needs												

*Values from inside cover. The number of kcals is a rough estimate. It is better to base energy needs on actual energy output. †Use RAE values, even though food table is based on RE units. ‡Use DFE values, even though the food table is based on total folate content, irrespective of natural or synthetic source.

Magnesium (mg)	Phosphorous (mg)	Potassium (mg)	Sodium (mg)	Zinc (mg)	Vitamin A (RE)	Vitamin C (mg)	Vitamin E (mg)	Thiamin (mg)	Riboflavin (mg)	Niacin (mg)	Vitamin B-6 (mg)	Folate (µg)	Vitamin B-12 (µg)

III. Dietary Intake Summary

Percentage of kcal from Protein, Fat, Carbohydrate, and Alcohol

Intake			
Protein (P):	____g/day × 4 kcal per gram	=	(P)____ kcal per day
Fat (F):	____g/day × 9 kcal per gram	=	(F)____ kcal per day
Carbohydrate (C):	____g/day × 4 kcal per gram	=	(C)____ kcal per day
Alcohol (A):		=	(A)____ kcal per day*
	Total kcal (T)/day	=	(T)____ kcal per day

Percentage of kcal from protein:

$\frac{(P)}{(T)} \times 100 =$ ____%

Percentage of kcal from fat:

$\frac{(F)}{(T)} \times 100 =$ ____%

Percentage of kcal from carbohydrate:

$\frac{(C)}{(T)} \times 100 =$ ____%

Percentage of kcal from alcohol:

$\frac{(A)}{(T)} \times 100 =$ ____%

Note: The four percentages can total 99, 100, or 101, depending on the way in which figures were rounded off earlier.

*To calculate how many kcal in a beverage are from alcohol, first look up the beverage in Appendix J. Then determine how many kcal are from carbohydrate (multiply carbohydrate grams times 4), fat (fat grams times 9), and protein (protein grams times 4). The remaining kcal are from alcohol.

IV. MyPyramid Diet Analysis.
Record your food intake for one day, placing each food item in the correct category of MyPyramid, with the correct number of servings. A food such as toast with soft margarine contributes to two categories—namely, to the grains group and to the oils group. You can expect that many food choices will contribute to more than one group. Indicate the number of servings from MyPyramid that each food yields.

Indicate the Number of Servings from MyPyramid That Each Food Yields

Food or Beverage	Amount Eaten	Milk	Meat & Beans	Fruits	Vegetables	Grains	Oils
Group totals							
Recommended servings from www.mypyramid.gov							
Overages/Shortages in numbers of servings							

Serving Sizes

MyPyramid provides serving sizes of foods for the various food groups in household units. Pay close attention to the stated serving size for each choice when following MyPyramid. This helps control total calorie intake. See the convenient guide to estimating common serving size measurements.

- **Grains:** 1 slice of bread; 1 cup of ready-to-eat breakfast cereal, or ½ cup cooked rice, pasta, or cereal counts as a 1-ounce equivalent.
- **Vegetables:** 1 cup of raw or cooked vegetables or vegetable juice or 2 cups of raw leafy greens.
- **Fruits:** 1 cup of fruit or 100% fruit juice or ½ cup of dried fruit.
- **Milk:** 1 cup of milk or yogurt, 1.5 ounces of natural cheese, or 2 ounces of processed cheese.
- **Meat & Beans:** 1 ounce of meat, poultry, or fish; 1 egg; 1 tablespoon of peanut butter; ¼ cup cooked dry beans, or ½ ounce of nuts or seeds are all 1-ounce equivalents.
- **Oils:** A teaspoon of any oil from plants or fish that is liquid at room temperature counts as a serving, as do such servings of foods rich in oils (e.g., mayonnaise and soft margarine).

MyPyramid Recommendations for Daily Food Consumption Based on Calorie Needs and Resulting in Twelve Separate Pyramids

Daily Amount of Food From Each Group												
Calorie Level	1000	1200	1400	1600	1800	2000	2200	2400	2600	2800	3000	3200
Fruits	1 cup	1 cup	1.5 cups	1.5 cups	1.5 cups	2 cups	2 cups	2 cups	2 cups	2.5 cups	2.5 cups	2.5 cups
Vegetables[1,2]	1 cup	1.5 cups	1.5 cups	2 cups	2.5 cups	2.5 cups	3 cups	3 cups	3.5 cups	3.5 cups	4 cups	4 cups
Grains[3]	3 oz-eq	4 oz-eq	5 oz-eq	5 oz-eq	6 oz-eq	6 oz-eq	7 oz-eq	8 oz-eq	9 oz-eq	10 oz-eq	10 oz-eq	10 oz-eq
Meat & Beans	2 oz-eq	3 oz-eq	4 oz-eq	5 oz-eq	5 oz-eq	5.5 oz-eq	6 oz-eq	6.5 oz-eq	6.5 oz-eq	7 oz-eq	7 oz-eq	7 oz-eq
Milk[4]	2 cups	2 cups	2 cups	3 cups	3 cups	3 cups	3 cups	3 cups	3 cups	3 cups	3 cups	3 cups
Oils[5]	3 tsp	4 tsp	4 tsp	5 tsp	5 tsp	6 tsp	6 tsp	7 tsp	8 tsp	8 tsp	10 tsp	11 tsp
Discretionary calorie allowance[6]	165	171	171	132	195	267	290	362	410	426	512	648

oz-eq stands for ounce equivalent; tsp stands for teaspoon

[1] Vegetables are divided into five subgroups (dark green, orange, legumes, starchy, and other). Over a week's time, a variety of vegetables should be eaten, especially green and orange vegetables.

[2] Dry beans and peas can be counted *either* as vegetables (dry beans and peas subgroup), *or* in the meat & beans group. Generally, individuals who regularly eat meat, poultry, and fish would count dry beans and peas in the vegetable group. Individuals who seldom eat meat, poultry, or fish (vegetarians) would consume more dry beans and peas and count some of them in the meat & beans group until enough servings from that group are chosen for the day.

[3] At least half of the grain servings should be whole-grain varieties.

[4] Most of the milk servings should be fat-free or low-fat.

[5] Limit solid fats such as butter, stick margarine, shortening, and meat fat, as well as foods that contain these.

[6] Discretionary calories refers to food choices rich in added sugars or solid fat.

Grains	1 yo-yo	=	2 ounces	Bagel or English muffin
Vegetables	1 baseball	=	1 cup	Green beans
Fruits	1 tennis ball	=	½ to ⅔ cup	Medium/small apple
Oils	1 golf ball	=	2 tbsp	Salad dressing, peanut butter, margarine, etc.
Milk	4 dice	=	1 ounce	Cheese
Meat & Beans	1 deck of cards	=	3 ounces	Meat, chicken or fish

Convenient Serving Size Guide. A yo-yo, baseball, tennis ball, golf ball, dice, and deck of cards make convenient guides to judge MyPyramid serving sizes. Additional handy guides include:

Matchbox = 1 oz of meat
Bar of soap = 3 oz of meat
Computer mouse = ½ cup of chopped foods

1 ice cream scoop = ½ cup
Ping-pong ball = 2 tbsp
4 golf balls = 1 cup of dry cereal

Today, nearly all foods sold in stores must be in a package that has a label containing the following information: the product name, name and address of the manufacturer, amount of product in the package, and ingredients listed in descending order by weight. This food and beverage labeling is monitored in North America by government agen-

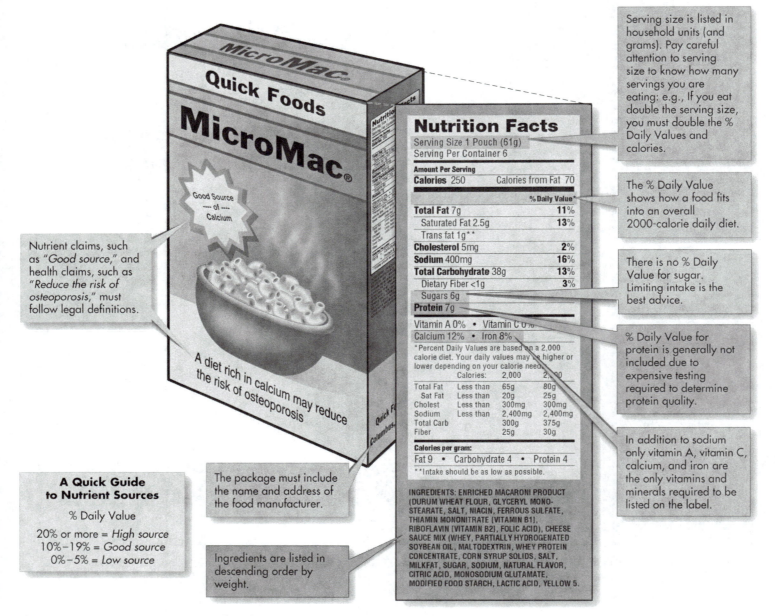

Serving size is listed in household units (and grams). Pay careful attention to serving size to know how many servings you are eating; e.g., If you eat double the serving size, you must double the % Daily Values and calories.

The % Daily Value shows how a food fits into an overall 2000-calorie daily diet.

There is no % Daily Value for sugar. Limiting intake is the best advice.

% Daily Value for protein is generally not included due to expensive testing required to determine protein quality.

In addition to sodium only vitamin A, vitamin C, calcium, and iron are the only vitamins and minerals required to be listed on the label.

Nutrient claims, such as "Good source," and health claims, such as "Reduce the risk of osteoporosis," must follow legal definitions.

The package must include the name and address of the food manufacturer.

Ingredients are listed in descending order by weight.

A Quick Guide to Nutrient Sources

% Daily Value

20% or more = *High source*
10%–19% = *Good source*
0%–5% = *Low source*

Nutrition Facts

Serving Size 1 Pouch (61g)
Serving Per Container 6

Amount Per Serving

Calories 250   Calories from Fat 70

	% Daily Value*
Total Fat 7g	11%
Saturated Fat 2.5g	13%
Trans fat 1g**	
Cholesterol 5mg	2%
Sodium 400mg	16%
Total Carbohydrate 38g	13%
Dietary Fiber <1g	3%
Sugars 6g	
Protein 7g	

Vitamin A 0% • Vitamin C 0%
Calcium 12% • Iron 8%

* Percent Daily Values are based on a 2,000 calorie diet. Your daily values may be higher or lower depending on your calorie needs.

	Calories:	2,000	2,500
Total Fat	Less than	65g	80g
Sat Fat	Less than	20g	25g
Cholest	Less than	300mg	300mg
Sodium	Less than	2,400mg	2,400mg
Total Carb		300g	375g
Fiber		25g	30g

Calories per gram:

Fat 9 • Carbohydrate 4 • Protein 4

**Intake should be as low as possible.

INGREDIENTS: ENRICHED MACARONI PRODUCT (DURUM WHEAT FLOUR, GLYCERYL MONO-STEARATE, SALT, NIACIN, FERROUS SULFATE, THIAMIN MONONITRATE [VITAMIN B1], RIBOFLAVIN [VITAMIN B2], FOLIC ACID), CHEESE SAUCE MIX (WHEY, PARTIALLY HYDROGENATED SOYBEAN OIL, MALTODEXTRIN, WHEY PROTEIN CONCENTRATE, CORN SYRUP SOLIDS, SALT, MILKFAT, SUGAR, SODIUM, NATURAL FLAVOR, CITRIC ACID, MONOSODIUM GLUTAMATE, MODIFIED FOOD STARCH, LACTIC ACID, YELLOW 5.

The Nutrition Facts panel on a current food label. This nutrition information is required on all processed food products. The % Daily Value listed on the label is the percentage of the generally accepted amount of a nutrient needed daily present in 1 serving of the product. You can use the % Daily Values to compare your diet with current nutrition recommendations for certain diet components. Let's consider fiber. Assume that you consume 2000 kcal per day, the energy intake for which the % Daily Values listed on labels have been calculated. If the total % Daily Value for dietary fiber in all the foods you eat in one day adds up to 100%, your diet meets the recommendations for fiber. Food labels also contain the name and address of the food manufacturers. This allows consumers to contact the manufacturer if they desire.

cies such as the Food and Drug Administration (FDA) in the United States. The listing of certain food constituents also is required—specifically, on a Nutrition Facts panel. Use the information in the Nutrition Facts panel to learn more about what you eat. The following components must be listed: total calories (kcal), calories from fat, total fat, saturated fat, *trans* fat, cholesterol, sodium, total carbohydrate, fiber, sugars, protein, vitamin A, vitamin C, calcium, and iron. In addition to these required components, manufacturers can choose to list polyunsaturated and monounsaturated fat, potassium, and others. Listing these components becomes *required* if a claim is made about the health benefits of the specific nutrient or if the food is fortified with that nutrient.

Remember that the Daily Value is a generic standard used on the food label. The percentage of the Daily Value (% Daily Value or % DV) is usually given for each nutrient per serving. These percentages are based on a 2000 kcal diet. In other words, they are not as applicable to people who require considerably more or less than 2000 kcal per day with respect to fat and carbohydrate intake. DVs are mostly set at or close to the highest RDA value or related nutrient standard seen in the various age and gender categories for a specific nutrient.

Serving sizes on the Nutrition Facts panel must be consistent among similar foods. This means that all brands of ice cream, for example, must use the same serving size on their label. (These serving sizes may differ from those of MyPyramid because those of food labels are based on typical serving sizes.) In addition, food claims made on packages must follow legal definitions. For example, if a product claims to be "low sodium," it must have 140 milligrams of sodium or less per serving.

Many manufacturers list the Daily Values set for dietary components such as fat, cholesterol, and carbohydrate on the Nutrition Facts panel. This can be useful as a reference point. As noted, they are based on 2000 kcal; if the label is large enough, amounts based on 2500 kcal are listed as well for total fat, saturated fat, carbohydrate, and other components. As mentioned, DVs allow consumers to compare their intake from a specific food to desirable (or maximum) intakes.

NUTRITION CALCULATIONS

You will use a few mathematical concepts in studying nutrition. Besides performing addition, subtraction, multiplication, and division, you need to know how to calculate percentages and convert English units of measurement to metric units.

PERCENTAGES

The term percent (%) refers to a part of the total when the total represents 100 parts. For example, if you earn 80% on your first nutrition examination, you will have answered the equivalent of 80 out of 100 questions correctly. This equivalent could be 8 correct answers out of 10; 80% also describes 16 of 20 ($16/20 = 0.80$ or 80%). The decimal form of percents is based on 100% being equal to 1.00. It is difficult to succeed in a nutrition course unless you know what a percentage means and how to calculate one. Percentages are used frequently when referring to menus and nutrient composition. The best way to master this concept is to calculate some percentages. Some examples follow:

Question	Answer
What is 6% of 45?	$6\% = 0.06$ or $0.06 \times 45 = 2.7$
What percent of 99 is 3?	$3/99 = 0.03$ or 3% (0.03×100)

Joe ate 15% of the adult Recommended Dietary Allowance (RDA) for iron at lunch. How many milligrams did he eat? (RDA = 8 milligrams)

$$0.15 \times 8 \text{ milligrams} = 1.2 \text{ milligrams}$$

Definitions for Comparative and Absolute Nutrient Claims on Food Labels

Sugar

- **Sugar free:** less than 0.5 grams (g) per serving.

- **No added sugar; without added sugar; no sugar added:**

  - No sugars were added during processing or packing, including ingredients that contain sugars (for example, fruit juices, applesauce, or jam).

  - Processing does not increase the sugar content above the amount naturally present in the ingredients. (A functionally insignificant increase in sugars is acceptable for processes used for purposes other than increasing sugar content.)

  - The food that it resembles and for which it substitutes normally contains added sugars.

  - If the food doesn't meet the requirements for a low- or reduced-calorie food, the product bears a statement that the food is not low calorie or calorie reduced and directs consumers' attention to the Nutrition Facts panel for further information on sugars and calorie content.

- **Reduced sugar:** at least 25% less sugar per serving than reference food

Calories

- **Calorie free:** fewer than 5 kcal per serving

- **Low calorie:** 40 kcal or less per serving and, if the serving is 30 g or less or 2 tablespoons or less, per 50 g of the food

- **Reduced or fewer calories:** at least 25% fewer kcal per serving than reference food

Fiber

- **High fiber:** 5 g or more per serving. (Foods making high-fiber claims must meet the definition for low fat, or the level of total fat must appear next to the high-fiber claim.)

- **Good source of fiber:** 2.5 to 4.9 g per serving

- **More or added fiber:** at least 2.5 g more per serving than reference food

Fat

- **Fat free:** less than 0.5 g of fat per serving

- **Saturated fat free:** less than 0.5 g per serving, and the level of *trans* fatty acids does not exceed 0.5 g per serving

- **Low fat:** 3 g or less per serving and, if the serving is 30 g or less or 2 tablespoons or less, per 50 g of the food. 2% milk can no longer be labeled low fat, as it exceeds 3 g per serving. *Reduced fat* will be the term used instead.

- **Low saturated fat:** 1 g or less per serving and not more than 15% of kcal from saturated fatty acids

- **Reduced or less fat:** at least 25% less per serving than reference food

- **Reduced or less saturated fat:** at least 25% less per serving than reference food

Cholesterol

- **Cholesterol free:** less than 2 milligrams (mg) of cholesterol and 2 g or less of saturated fat per serving

- **Low cholesterol:** 20 mg or less cholesterol and 2 g or less of saturated fat per serving and, if the serving is 30 g or less or 2 tablespoons or less, per 50 g of the food

- **Reduced or less cholesterol:** at least 25% less cholesterol and 2 g or less of saturated fat per serving than reference food

Sodium

- **Sodium free:** less than 5 mg per serving

- **Very low sodium:** 35 mg or less per serving and, if the serving is 30 g or less or 2 tablespoons or less, per 50 g of the food

- **Low sodium:** 140 mg or less per serving and, if the serving is 30 g or less or 2 tablespoons or less, per 50 g of the food

- **Light in sodium:** at least 50% less per serving than reference food

- **Reduced or less sodium:** at least 25% less per serving than reference food

Other Terms

- **Fortified or enriched:** Vitamins and/or minerals have been added to the product in amounts in excess of at least 10% of that normally present in the usual product. Enriched generally refers to replacing nutrients lost in processing, whereas fortified refers to adding nutrients not originally present in the specific food.

- **Healthy:** An individual food that is low fat and low saturated fat and has no more than 360 to 480 mg of sodium or 60 mg of cholesterol per serving can be labeled "healthy" if it provides at least 10% of the Daily Value for vitamin A, vitamin C, protein, calcium, iron, or fiber.

- **Light or lite:** The descriptor *light* or *lite* can mean two things: first, that a nutritionally altered product contains one-third fewer kcal or half the fat of reference food (if the food derives 50% or more of its kcal from fat, the reduction must be 50% of the fat) and, second, that the sodium content of a low-calorie, low-fat food has been reduced by 50%. In addition, "light in sodium" may be used for foods in which the sodium content has been reduced by at least 50%. The term *light* may still be used to describe such properties as texture and color, as long as the label explains the intent—for example, "light brown sugar" and "light and fluffy."

Diet: A food may be labeled with terms such as *diet, dietetic, artificially sweetened,* or *sweetened with nonnutritive sweetener* only if the claim is not false or misleading. The food can also be labeled *low calorie* or *reduced calorie.*

Good source: *Good source* means that a serving of the food contains 10% to 19% of the Daily Value for a particular nutrient. If 5% or less it is a **low source.**

High: *High* means that a serving of the food contains 20% or more of the Daily Value for a particular nutrient.

Organic: Federal standards for organic foods allow claims when much of the ingredients do not use chemical fertilizers or pesticides, genetic engineering, sewage sludge, antibiotics, or irradiation in their production. At least 95% of ingredients (by weight) must meet these guidelines to be labeled "organic" on the front of the package. If the front label instead says "made with organic ingredients," only 70% of the ingredients must be organic. For animal products, the animals must graze outdoors, be fed organic feed, and cannot be exposed to large amounts of antibiotics or growth hormones.

Natural: The food must be free of food colors, synthetic flavors, or any other synthetic substance.

The following terms apply only to meat and poultry products regulated by USDA.

Extra lean: less than 5 g of fat, 2 g of saturated fat, and 95 mg of cholesterol per serving (or 100 g of an individual food)

Lean: less than 10 g of fat, 4.5 g of saturated fat, and 95 mg of cholesterol per serving (or 100 g of an individual food)

Many definitions are from FDA's *Dictionary of Terms,* as established in conjunction with the 1990 Nutrition Education and Labeling Act (NELA).
g = grams; mg = milligrams

THE METRIC SYSTEM

The basic units of the metric system are the meter, which indicates length; the gram, which indicates weight; and the liter, which indicates volume. See next page for conversions from the metric system to the English system (pounds, feet, cups) and vice versa. Here is a brief summary:

> A gram (g) is about 1/30 of an ounce (28 grams to the ounce).
> 5 grams of sugar or salt is about 1 teaspoon.
> A pound (lb) weighs 454 grams.
> A kilogram (kg) is 1000 grams, equivalent to 2.2 pounds.
> To convert your weight to kilograms, divide it by 2.2.
> A 154-pound man weighs 70 kilograms (154/2.2 = 70).
> A gram can be divided into 1000 milligrams (mg) or 1,000,000 micrograms (μg or mcg).
>   10 milligrams of zinc (approximately adult needs) would be a few grains of zinc.
> Liters are divided into 1000 units called milliliters (ml).
> One teaspoon equals about 5 milliliters (ml), 1 cup is about 240 milliliters, and 1 quart
>   (4 cups) equals almost 1 liter (L) (0.946 liter to be exact).

If you plan to work in any scientific field, you will need to learn the metric system. *For now, remember that a kilogram equals 2.2 pounds, an ounce weighs 28 grams, 2.54 centimeters equals 1 inch, and a liter is almost the same as a quart.* In addition, know the fractions that the following prefixes represent: micro (1/1,000,000), milli (1/1000), centi (1/100), and kilo (1000) represent.

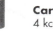

Carbohydrate
4 kcal per gram

Protein
4 kcal per gram

Fat
9 kcal per gram

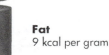

Alcohol
7 kcal per gram

MAKING DECISIONS

Calculating Calories

Use the 4-9-4 estimates for the calorie content of carbohydrate, fat, and protein introduced over the last few pages to determine calorie content of a food. Consider a typical deluxe hamburger sandwich:

Carbohydrate	39 grams × 4 = 156 kcal
Fat	32 grams × 9 = 288 kcal
Protein	30 grams × 4 = 120 kcal
Total	564 kcal

You can also use the 4-9-4 estimates to determine what portion of total calorie intake is contributed by the various calorie-yielding nutrients. Assume that one day you consume 290 grams of carbohydrates, 60 grams of fat, and 70 grams of protein. This consumption yields a total of 1980 kcal ([290 × 4] + [60 × 9] + [70 × 4] 5 = 1980). The percentage of your total calorie intake derived from each nutrient can then be determined:

% of kcal as carbohydrate = (290 × 4) ÷ 1980 = 0.59 (× 100 = 59 %)

% of kcal as fat = (60 × 9) ÷ 1980 = 0.27 (× 100 = 27%)

% of kcal as protein = (70 × 4) ÷ 1980 = 0.14 (× 100 = 14%)

Check your calculations by adding the percentages together. Do they total 100?

Nutrition Calculations

METRIC-ENGLISH CONVERSIONS

Length

English (USA)	Metric
inch (in)	= 2.54 cm, 25.4 mm
foot (ft)	= 0.30 m, 30.48 cm
yard (yd)	= 0.91 m, 91.4 cm
mile (statute) (5280 ft)	= 1.61 km, 1609 m
mile (nautical)	
(6077 ft, 1.15 statute mi)	= 1.85 km, 1850 m

Metric	English (USA)
millimeter (mm)	= 0.039 in (thickness of a dime)
centimeter (cm)	= 0.39 in
meter (m)	= 3.28 ft, 39.37 in
kilometer (km)	= 0.62 mi, 1091 yd, 3273 ft

Weight

English (USA)	Metric
grain	= 64.80 mg
ounce (oz)	= 28.35 g
pound (lb)	= 453.60 g, 0.45 kg
ton (short—2000 lb)	= 0.91 metric ton (907 kg)

Metric	English (USA)
milligram (mg)	= 0.002 grain (0.000035 oz)
gram (g)	= 0.04 oz ($1/_{28}$ of an oz)
kilogram (kg)	= 35.27 oz, 2.20 lb
metric ton (1000 kg)	= 1.10 tons

Volume

English (USA)	Metric
cubic inch	= 16.39 cc
cubic foot	= 0.03 m^3
cubic yard	= 0.765 m^3
teaspoon (tsp)	= 5 ml
tablespoon (tbsp)	= 15 ml
fluid ounce	= 0.03 liter (30 ml)*
cup (c)	= 237 ml
pint (pt)	= 0.47 liter
quart (qt)	= 0.95 liter
gallon (gal)	= 3.79 liters

Metric	English (USA)
milliliter (ml)	= 0.03 oz
liter (L)	= 2.12 pt
liter	= 1.06 qt
liter	= 0.27 gal

1 liter ÷ 1000 = 1 milliliter or 1 cubic centimeter (10^{-3} liter)

1 liter ÷ 1,000,000 = 1 microliter (10^{-6} liter)

*Note: 1 ml = 1 cc

METRIC AND OTHER COMMON UNITS

Unit/Abbreviation	Other Equivalent Measure
milligram/mg	$1/_{1000}$ of a gram
microgram/µg	$1/_{1,000,000}$ of a gram
deciliter/dl	$1/_{10}$ of a liter (about ½ cup)
milliliter/ml	$1/_{1000}$ of a liter (5 ml is about 1 tsp)
International Unit/IU	Crude measure of vitamin activity generally based on growth rate seen in animals

FAHRENHEIT-CELSIUS CONVERSION SCALE

°F	°C		
230	110		
220			
212°F 210	100	100°C	Boiling Point of Water
200	90		
190			
180	80		
170			
160	70		
150			
140	60		
130			
120	50		
110			
98°F 100	40	37°C	Body Temperature
90	30		
80			
70	20		
60			
50	10		
40			
32°F 30	0	0°C	Freezing Point of Water
20			
10	−10		
0			
−10	−20		
−20	−30		
−30			
−40	−40		

To convert temperature scales:

Fahrenheit to Celsius °C = (°F − 32) × 5/9

Celsius to Fahrenheit °F = 9/5 (°C) + 32

HOUSEHOLD UNITS

3 teaspoons	= 1 tablespoon
4 tablespoons	= ¼ cup
5$^1/_3$ tablespoons	= $1/_3$ cup
8 tablespoons	= ½ cup
10$^2/_3$ tablespoons	= $2/_3$ cup
16 tablespoons	= 1 cup
1 tablespoon	= ½ fluid ounce
1 cup	= 8 fluid ounces
1 cup	= ½ pint
2 cups	= 1 pint
4 cups	= 1 quart
2 pints	= 1 quart
4 quarts	= 1 gallon